From Popular Medicine to Medical Populism

From Popular Medicine to Medical Populism

DOCTORS, HEALERS, AND PUBLIC POWER

IN COSTA RICA, 1800–1940

Steven Palmer

DUKE UNIVERSITY PRESS

Durham & London

2003

© 2003 Duke University Press

All rights reserved

Printed in the United States

of America on acid-free paper ∞

Designed by Rebecca Giménez

Typeset in Baskerville by

Keystone Typesetting, Inc.

Library of Congress Cataloging-

in-Publication Data appear on the

last printed page of this book.

To Charles A. Hale and Catherine Legrand

CONTENTS

ILLUSTRATIONS

Maps

Figures

Tables

ACKNOWLEDGMENTS

As I sit down to write this message of thanks, cotton candy clouds float over a graceful suspension bridge glimpsed from my new office window. It is proper that I finish this book just as I take up my first permanent appointment as a historian, for this project was fitfully researched and written during a long period in which I journeyed on the edge of the academic world. Independent scholarship has many rewards. Perhaps they even outweigh the frustrations and anxieties of institutional rootlessness. Still, the condition is precarious, and I am overwhelmed by the sensation of having been indulged by many people who sustained and sheltered me while I compiled the following work. I was not in a position to give them much in return, and so their help was truly selfless and deserves the deepest gratitude.

Preliminary forays into the domain of public health and medicine in 1991–1992 were supported by a generous postdoctoral fellowship from the Social Sciences and Humanities Research Council of Canada. Further research was done while I was a visiting professor in history at the Centro de Investigaciones Históricas de América Central (CIHAC) of the Universidad de Costa Rica in 1995–1996. I would particularly like to thank Victor Hugo Acuña and Yamileth González for making that appointment possible, and the CIHAC for sponsoring a research grant from the Vicerrectoría de Investigación that allowed me to become acquainted with the new Archivo Nacional de Costa Rica.

Since 1995, I have had the intermittent pleasure of working at the wonderful flying saucer of a building that houses Costa Rica's historical memory bank, and while I appreciate the friendly efficiency of the entire staff, I would most like to thank Rocío Vallecillo for gracious support and assistance that allowed me to make the most of often whirl-wind visits. On a number of occasions over the same period, I had the rare luxury of two research assistants, Ana Paulina Malavassi and Soili Buska, who are accomplished historians in their own right. The following pages owe a great deal to their keen eye for relevant material, not to mention their uncommon work ethic and interest in the project. Thanks are also due Gabriela Villalobos and Jorge Quesada for some timely help in the archives. In October 1993, after a red-eye drive through the autumn scents of Vermont, I was able to work at the Rocke-feller Foundation Archives in North Tarrytown, New York, and I thank Tom Rosenbaum for making that brief trip so productive by getting together a mountain of relevant material on short notice.

Catherine Legrand has inspired me from the moment I had the good fortune of taking one of her courses as an undergraduate at the University of British Columbia. She has been a great friend and mentor ever since. While I was in Montreal in 1994–1995, she organized an informal seminar where I was able to discuss early versions of a couple of the following chapters with her, Bob Whitney, and Karen Robert. I thank them for their enthusiasm. Catherine was also kind enough to include me in a wonderful 1995 conference at Yale University, where I presented my findings on hookworm treatment campaigns in Central America — part of which still lives in chapter 7 of this book.

It is my pleasure to acknowledge Herb Klein for asking me to present some ideas about the peculiarities of Costa Rican social policy and public health at Columbia University in January 1996. Over the years, I have profited from Herb's support on a number of occasions that have proved critical to the unfolding of my life. He has pointed me in some fruitful directions, and I have learned a lot from his willingness to encourage work that, although not even within his expansive range of interests, is done with seriousness of purpose.

In November 1999, I was privileged to receive an invitation from Alan Knight to present a paper on medical populism at the Latin American Centre, St. Antony's College, Oxford, some of which appears in chapter 9. I must also express my appreciation to John Crellin for welcoming a rather green historian of medicine into his parlor at Memorial University's medical library, and for offering invaluable advice on how to refine and reframe this study.

A penultimate round of research in Costa Rica was achieved thanks to an invitation to address the Centro de Desarrollo Estratégico e Información en Salud y Seguridad Social and the Academia de Costa Rica. I met many fine students of the country's medical history at that gathering, and am indebted to doctors Edgar Cabezas Solera and José Enrique Sotela for their assistance, and especially Dr. Manuel Aguilar Bonilla for making available to me personal copies of a rare, early Costa Rican medical journal. My gratitude to Ana Cecilia Dwyer and Natalie Niedoba of the Canadian Embassy in San José for making possible that leg of the extended journey of this book. On that occasion, as on so many others over the past thirteen years, I was treated to the warm hospitality of Ana Luisa Cerdas and Julio Jurado, who I must formally thank, finally, for their immense friendship and generosity.

Along the road I renewed contact with Marcos Cueto. I cannot stress how much this happy encounter improved the following study. Marcos is the great animator of the new history of medicine and public health in the Americas. Selfless and self-effacing to a fault, he has deftly brought people together, urging them to go further in their studies, generously providing them with bibliographic and other resources, and of course, leading the way with his own work of understated brilliance and impeccable scholarship. In April 2001, Marcos and Diego Armus kindly asked me to attend what turned out to be a truly illuminating symposium on the new history of medicine in Spain and Latin America at New York University, and I have tried to incorporate into the final manuscript some of the fine exchanges that were had there.

To Charlie Hale goes my deepest gratitude for eleven years of intellectual engagement, advice, and support. He, too, has been a great friend and mentor since the sunny winter afternoon in early 1990 when he welcomed me to Iowa. Needless to say, the following study was improved by his perceptive comments.

Iván Molina Jiménez has sustained and encouraged the research and writing of this book in numerous ways. I cannot even begin to thank him for his generosity in providing resources, data, and administrative help; for his original thoughts on how to improve this work; and most of all, for a friendship filled with the exchange of ideas and laughter that now spans ten years and seven books.

I am grateful to Valerie Millholland at Duke University Press for her patience, enthusiasm, and trust that I would eventually come up with a manuscript that could remain airborne.

Most of all, to my traveling companions, Eylem Rodríguez and our radiant Emil, thanks for waiting — tanto, tanto, tanto.

Windsor, Ontario
August 2001

INTRODUCTION

This book is a history of popular and conventional medical practitioners in Costa Rica, a dynamic periphery of Latin America. It begins in the late colonial era when none of the fifty thousand inhabitants of this southernmost province of the kingdom of Guatemala had access to a titled physician, surgeon, pharmacist, or midwife. In the early 1800s, all Costa Rican medicine was popular medicine. The book closes in the 1940s when the figure of the qualified medical doctor, once extraordinary and alien, was a part of everyday life for a great many Costa Ricans. A people approaching the one million mark were increasingly likely to be treated by licensed doctors and allied health practitioners numbering over a thousand. Almost half the legislators of this relatively prosperous coffee republic were medical doctors, and in 1940 Costa Ricans had elected by an overwhelming majority Dr. Rafael Angel Calderón Guardia, a charismatic physician whose populist program was built on the introduction of medical benefits under Social Security.

The story told here, however, is not the rise and triumph of the modern biomedical doctor. Instead, the book documents the exploits of an ever wider variety of healers over this long period, and maps the interactions among them in a modern medical universe characterized by increasing stratification and heterogeneity. By 1940, schooled and titled practitioners had made an indelible mark on health care in the country, but these included not only doctors in medicine and surgery, not only midwives, pharmacists, and nurses, but also homeopaths, osteopaths, and spiritists. Moreover, the indigenous curer, the empiric midwife, the *curandero* who specialized in herbal medicine or minor surgery, and the home caregiver were still vital figures in the Costa Rican pantheon of practitioners, even if most such healers had modified their repertoire over the preceding century through a growing familiarity with conventional medical practice. Meanwhile, after 1875, Chinese and Afro-Antillean healers arrived in sufficient numbers to introduce powerful new medical traditions to the country. By the mid–twentieth century, this variety of practitioners ministered to a suffering public that tended toward an eclectic approach to illness, capable of comfortably combining an understanding of germ theory, humoral conceptions of common complaints, a belief in the efficacy of homeopathy, and a knowledge of the healing power of saints, spirits, and modern surgical instruments.[1] *From Popular Medicine to Medical Populism* explores the role of practitioners in creating this Latin American world of medical pluralism.

Over the past fifteen years, some excellent work has been done on Latin American medical elites in the century after 1850. Scholars have revealed the emergence of world-class medical scientists and institutions in a variety of settings. They have effectively undermined the notion that Latin American science was "passively derivative" of metropolitan trends, while showing how the politics of medical research on the periphery ultimately limited its global scientific impact and subverted its institutional evolution.[2] A small number of studies have broached the subject of medical professionalism in the region, likewise illustrating that the timing and form of this process depended as much on local political and medical conditions as they did on the adoption of international trends.[3] On the other side of the divide, while curanderos, shamans, and spiritists in Latin America have been intensely studied by anthropologists, properly historical treatment of popular medical practice in the nineteenth and early twentieth centuries has only recently begun.[4] A number of other topics central to the new social history of medicine have been brushed on with promising results: the stature of conventional and popular healers, the role of gender and ethnicity in the formation of practitioner identities, the emergence of a medical marketplace, and the politics of medical regulation.[5]

The following pages combine all these perspectives in an effort to gain a holistic view of medical practitioners in a Latin American society over an extended period of time. The risks of this approach have become obvious to me as this study progressed, but I think they are far

outweighed by the potential rewards that can come from putting together for analysis domains that are usually observed in isolation. It is
no longer controversial to claim that the difference between "irregular" and "regular" medicine is historically constructed rather than reflective of any essential beliefs or practices. The two domains define
their identities in terms of one another, in ways that are mediated by
social and political engagement. As a result, they are highly unstable:
one era's quackery may be another's conventional practice, and vice
versa. Yet conventional and popular medicine in any given period still
tend to be studied separately, and so their dynamic relationship is rarely
reconstructed.[6]

By taking the long view and including as broad a range of practitioners as possible, I hope to show that the rise of a Costa Rican health
system oriented by biomedicine and professionalism was strongly influenced by the dynamic interchange between popular and official medicine. The relationship between the two domains was neither as well-
defined nor conflictive as one might suppose. Conventional medical
practitioners and institutions became more numerous and powerful
over time, sometimes swallowing up or fatally weakening popular rivals
in their wake, or more rarely suppressing them directly. But throughout
this period, strong forms of popular and alternative medicine survived,
renewed themselves, or appeared for the first time in the practices of
unlicensed healers. These, in turn, were often reincorporated into the
sphere of official medicine by governments that persisted in finding
ways to license irregulars and thus recruit them into the expanding web
of state power. The official biomedical array that assumed its modern
form in the 1930s and 1940s still resonated with popular refrains.

The book's nine chapters cover two main phases in Costa Rican
medical practice. The first stretches from the late colonial period to the
end of the nineteenth century. A growing variety of practitioners of
both sexes, many ethnicities and nationalities, and multiple specialties
and approaches emerged in the context of increases in population,
international commerce, and overall social wealth — these latter two
being part and parcel of a booming coffee export economy. Although
by midcentury a small community of titled medical doctors formed,
it was unable to impose norms on the medical universe. The heterogeneity of healing practice was officially enshrined in the young republic's system of medical regulation and unofficially promoted by state

Introduction

tolerance for those practicing medicine without a license. Even as physicians, surgeons, and pharmacists acquired greater professional cohesion and political power starting in the 1870s, the government continued to undermine the medical monopoly they sought by practicing tolerance and selectively appropriating popular medical practitioners into the state's incipient health network.

During the second phase, which extends from the 1890s to the 1940s, physicians and public health experts with growing international connections built an official medical apparatus as an integral part of public power. The drive for professional monopoly was successfully undertaken by an elite of medical doctors who were also members of the Costa Rican oligarchy; this process of professionalization was inseparable from the consolidation of the nation-state, and discourses and images drawn from new medical science were fundamental in solidifying the positivist ideology that shaped and justified the goals of the liberal polity. The institutions of state medicine created during these years promoted the "medicalization" of everyday life. Childbirth was transformed into a clinical procedure that while still largely occurring in the home at the outset of this period, was overseen by titled midwives schooled according to a biomedical model. The population was introduced en masse to the "germ theory" through sustained public health campaigns, and the vast majority of Costa Ricans were subject to a blood and fecal exam by agents of the state, followed by a laboratory-based diagnosis and cure of a disease through targeted pharmacological attack on a specific microorganism, the pernicious hookworm.

Boundaries between conventional and "irregular" medicine were more sharply drawn during this period, as were divisions among a growing number of titled allied health practitioners, with medical doctors more clearly at the apex. Nevertheless, popular as well as new nonstandard medicines thrived, and pharmacists happily acted as general practitioners in managing the common complaints of their clientele (even as they filled prescriptions from physicians and curanderos alike). Though unlicensed practitioners were now subject to persecution by a state formally committed to enforcing professional monopoly, this policing was generally tepid. Indeed, the public power often found ways to license irregular healers in order to extend state medicine into rural areas that were without a physician. And if many popular healers now seemed to imitate physicians more closely, doctors also made concessions to popular health beliefs in order to consolidate their position in the expanding medical marketplace.

Orientations

While a basic division between conventional and unconventional medical practitioners is inevitable and plays a crucial role in defining medicine at any point in time, a consideration of the full spectrum of healers is essential in order to see how that frontier is drawn and redrawn over time. Some healers in Costa Rica clearly practiced on one or the other side of this divide; others are less easy to categorize and displayed an eclecticism that drew from both domains of medicine. With the rise of a more tightly regulated medical profession toward the end of the nineteenth century, these eclectic healers were to be found increasingly on the alternative end of the spectrum. Occasionally they assumed counterhegemonic positions in relation to official practitioners, especially in opposing the monopoly of medical doctors. This book argues, however, that more often than not they served as intermediaries between official and popular medicine. This ultimately meant that a large number of popular healers played significant roles in negotiating the hegemony of biomedicine, translating key notions and ranges of behavior from official medicine into the vernacular while maintaining sites of popular medical practice that promoted pluralistic configurations.

This broad thesis does not easily fit into the literature on conventional and popular medical practice in Latin America. Though the dynamic is only just beginning to be reconstructed in properly historical terms, scholars frequently suggest or assume that the continent's politics of health have been marked by a binary opposition between popular medicine and biomedicine — one that became increasingly rigid as the revolutions in surgery, bacteriology, and medical professionalism gained momentum over the latter third of the nineteenth century. The curandero and shaman are imagined in open combat with the biomedical ideologue.

In 1970, the medical anthropologist Irwin Press noted a "developing stereotype of *the* curandero's style and function," one that was becoming an institution in the Latin Americanist's repertoire; a veritable homage to the peasant milieu which represents Latin America at its 'purist.' "[7] The classic popular practitioner is associated with a healing culture derived from an indigenous or African past as well as the practice of an empirically derived and orally transmitted medicine. The popular medical "system" is characterized by the centrality of magical and religious elements, humoral understandings of illness, herbal remedies, and a close healer-patient relationship in which the healer is of the community and outside the cash nexus.

So, for example, Lynn Marie Morgan's fine recent study of primary care in Costa Rica proposes that "prior to the introduction of biomedicine, indigenous and traditional healers practiced their craft, while a rich herbal pharmacopoeia provided the first line of attack against disease." This Arcadian world entered a period of crisis in the late nineteenth century when a new generation of biomedical physicians, themselves members of the capitalist oligarchy, allied with "two wealthy and powerful United States organizations — the United Fruit Company and the Rockefeller Foundation — . . . gradually [transforming] the health infrastructure and dominant models of medical care along the lines of the germ-theory model of disease etiology, using disease-eradication techniques perfected during the Spanish-American War."[8] Here, typically, the ideal curandero is more sharply defined through juxtaposition with another developing ideal type: the biomedical doctor. The biomedical doctor is defined by his learned, written, and theoretical understanding of disease conceived of in biological, rational, and secular terms; a therapeutic arsenal of pharmaceuticals; official certification by political elites; and an aggressive drive to dominate the medical marketplace. Also crucial to this juxtaposition is that the biomedical doctor represents an alien, neocolonial system of medical control while the popular healer expresses an authentic local culture that is capable of offering resistance to a colonizing biomedicine.[9]

Such a perspective echoes the work on the history of public health done in the 1970s and 1980s in a climate heavy with dependency theory. Its most distinguished exponent, Juan César García, maintained that Latin American states and oligarchies began to promote state medicine in the late nineteenth century in a way that reflected their dependent political economies. That is, their efforts to sanitize port cities and improve the constitution of agricultural laborers directly responded to the needs of imperial powers and the agro-export bourgeoisie as they sought to accelerate capitalist production and the insertion of Latin American economies into the world market.[10] This view meshes with the anticolonial thrust of recent scholarship on medicine and empire — a strand of cultural studies that derived much of its inspiration and rhetorical power from the general coincidence of two broad yet related historical processes during the second half of the nineteenth century. While the medical profession, bacteriology, tropical medicine, and public health were consolidated in the West, the countries in which this matrix was most successfully articulated were the same ones that created a new imperial order in Africa, the Asian subcontinent, Southeast Asia, and the Caribbean.[11]

The Latin American case was left out of important studies on imperial medicine, perhaps due to the lack of a clear and discrete moment of biomedical intrusion. Because of the early and hybrid colonial experience of Latin America, "Western" medicine was "indigenous" to the region long before its biomedical guise was fully donned.[12] Moreover, as a number of recent studies of the Rockefeller Foundation in Latin America have shown, it is not always possible to portray the arrival of U.S. public health institutions in the region in such a straightforwardly imperial fashion. Without losing sight of the general backdrop of unequal geopolitical relations between the United States and host countries, scholars have given center stage to questions of how foundation missions were transformed through their engagement with concrete local conditions.[13] As this study reveals, even in peripheries like Costa Rica, established groups of medical and public health practitioners were there to greet the agents of imperial public health with their own agenda. Costa Rican physicians had discovered that hookworm disease was endemic to the country in 1895, some years before researchers made the equivalent finding in the United States, and the Costa Rican state authorized a local treatment campaign for hookworm disease in 1906, even before Rockefeller philanthropy decided to make hookworm the focus of its foray into public health work in the U.S. South. When agents of the Rockefeller Foundation arrived in Costa Rica in 1914, the organizational model and solidity of funding that accompanied them were novel, but they brought little that was new in epistemological or scientific terms.

Nevertheless, the dependency and neocolonialism perspectives remain compelling for Latin America, where popular medicine so often overlapped with subordinate ethnicity, and where after 1850 the medical elite were frequently members of both the agro-export oligarchies and positivist governments. The liberal modernizing states of Latin America, in finally establishing political control over disparate indigenous, black, and mixed-race population groups in the urban barrios and rural areas, displayed real similarities to the contemporary European colonizing regimes of Africa and Southeast Asia. These "civilizing" programs generally involved the imposition of authoritarian public health measures that met popular resistance. One classic episode of such biomedical intrusion in Latin America was the 1904 mandatory smallpox vaccination campaign in Rio de Janeiro that provoked serious riots and general resistance to yellow fever control measures. A fine recent study by Sidney Chalhoub has made a strong case that the "vaccinophobia" motivating some of the rioters was partly based in Afro-Brazilian medical beliefs.[14]

Studies like Chalhoub's, as well as David Sowell's pioneering history of the popular Andean healer Miguel Perdomo Neira and the tumultuous 1870 confrontation between his followers and the medical elites of Bogotá, offer detailed historical confirmation of the powerful rebellious and counterhegemonic strains in the region's popular medicine. It may well be that the characteristics associated with the ideal type curandero are also those most likely to motivate such episodes of resistance. The focus on these dissident dimensions of popular healing is also a response to the traditional historiography of Latin American medicine — much of it written by physicians — that typically derided the alleged superstition and ineffective, when not actually dangerous, therapeutics of popular practitioners.[15] Contemporary scholars have tried to understand popular medicines on their own terms, while turning a more critical and skeptical gaze on the supposed virtues of biomedicine.[16]

This trend has obscured a significant part of the spectrum of Latin American healers. In his study of the Argentine medical profession in the second half of the nineteenth century, Ricardo González Leandri notes that physicians of the era concentrated their attacks on precisely those rural curanderos who closely corresponded to the ideal type I have outlined. They "converted this sector, which represented only a fraction of irregulars, into the stereotype of the activity." By making "curanderismo" synonymous with superstition and miracle cures — with "el médico de la bolita" (the doctor of the crystal ball) — physicians could more easily exalt their own allegedly special attributes.[17] Modern scholars have inverted this perspective to good effect, revaluing important dimensions of popular medicine. In doing so, however, they may also adopt a restricted, bipolar field of vision.[18]

Concentrating too heavily on the ideal type curandero, according to Irwin Press, risked "a rather monolithic and limiting approach to curers and curer-related phenomena" in which more mundane illness is relegated to a minor position and "a wide range of practitioners is ignored or assigned to some residual category such as 'marginal' or 'limited.' "[19] Though Press was referring to a wide range of *popular* practitioners, I think it can equally be said that by focusing on the biomedical zealot, a diverse array of conventional, certified practitioners is also excluded from view. The historian of popular and professional medicine in France, Matthew Ramsey suggests that the concept of a modern "official medicine" is not nearly as self-evident as one might like to think. "We can perhaps agree in recognizing it as a domain in which the activities of certified expert practitioners of medicine intersect with the activities of certified experts in the production of scientific knowledge. But this is very abstract, and the key question of how, historically, such a domain was constituted in different social and political contexts has not received the sort of attention that scholars have devoted to . . . the development of the modern medical profession and the construction of scientific authority."[20]

In this spirit, the following study tries to move beyond the binary framework that currently governs the view of medical practice in Latin America. It proposes that popular medicine was not synonymous with oral tradition, unlettered empiricism, and religious and magical belief, nor was conventional medicine practiced by a homogeneous group of highly trained biomedical ideologues applying alien techniques and medicines. It calls into question the dichotomous representation of popular practitioners as authentic expressions of the local community versus biomedical doctors as agents of neocolonial intrusion. I will also challenge the idea that official medicine engaged in a consistent campaign to suppress and eradicate popular medicine. Though such a fantasy existed in the minds of many an official medical zealot, and was often on the formal government agenda, it never came anywhere near fruition. The relationship between popular and conventional practitioners was characterized by coexistence, complementarity, and dialogue more than outright rivalry and ideological warfare.

Perhaps more important, the state never consistently displayed an interest in suppressing irregular medical practice. Indeed, one of the most intriguing and paradoxical findings of this study is that although the professionalization of medicine was an essential part of the formation of the Costa Rican liberal state, that same public power persistently subverted professional monopoly by finding ways tacitly and explicitly to certify untitled healers to practice medicine. Moreover, police and judicial agents were generally soft on unlicensed medical practitioners — so much so that one can speak of an informal, but widely accepted state policy of tolerance in this domain. It was through such "everyday forms" of negotiation among agents of the state, medical professionals, and popular practitioners that the contours of modern medical hegemony were established.[21] On the one hand, the empirics tolerated and licensed by the state were generally those who practiced conventional styles of medicine. The state, in this sense, did not call into question the legitimacy of conventional medicine as defined by the professional community of doctors, but it did throw into doubt the legitimacy of professional monopoly. On the other hand, though a majority of popular practitioners appear increasingly to have emulated key elements of conventional medical practice, precisely because they were not subject to professional strictures they maintained autonomous sites of popular medicine that might — and often did — exceed medical orthodoxy without necessarily threatening its dominion.

Comparative Relevance of the Costa Rican Case

Among the laudable qualities of the specialized historians of medicine whose work appeared in the wake of Aristides A. Moll's monumental 1944 compendium *Aesculapius in Latin America* was their transcontinental scope.[22] The insistence on a comparative perspective has been revived to excellent effect in the recent work of Marcos Cueto and Nancy Leys Stepan. Inspired by these efforts, I have made a concerted attempt to situate the Costa Rican case through comparative references in order to make this book as much as possible an "embedded" case study of medical practitioners in Latin America.

I propose that the history of medical practitioners in Costa Rica might be taken as representative of an important Latin American "midrange." This proposition will surprise readers who best know Costa Rica for its alleged "exceptionalism." The label is accurate to the degree that

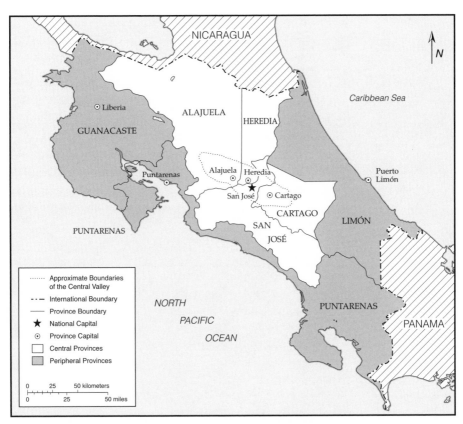

Map 1. Costa Rica. Courtesy of Fabrice Lehoucq and Iván Molina.

a highly literate populace, long periods of unbroken electoral democracy, infrequent military intervention in politics, and a state that has consistently displayed mild reformist tendencies are all, sadly, exceptional in Latin America. On the other hand, one does not have to search too carefully in the country's past to find essential ingredients of the Latin American polity. The country's colonial period was marked by a conflictive Spanish and Native American cultural encounter with the admixture of an African slave population. The development boom of the nineteenth century was based on the cultivation and export of a single crop: coffee. This was subsequently "complemented" by the rapid implantation of a banana enclave on the Caribbean coast, crucible of the United Fruit Company that made Costa Rica the original banana republic. The development between 1880 and 1914 of Limón province, attracted a large Afro-Caribbean population. Beginning in

Introduction

Table 1. Costa Rican epidemics and related phenomena, 1805–1927

1805	Threat of smallpox: first vaccination campaign
1814	Malaria and hepatitis in Cartago province
1816	Smallpox in Nicaragua: first quarantine of ship in Puntarenas
1823–1826	Official concern over leprosy leads to building of Lazareto (completed 1835)
1831	Smallpox (worst epidemic of century)
1832	Cholera in Mexico: creation of Juntas Generales de Sanidad
1836–1837	Cholera in Nicaragua: creation of cordon sanitaire on border
1839	Fevers in Cartago and Heredia
1845	Infant cholera (summer diarrhea) throughout country
	Smallpox in Guanacaste
	Fever among coffee carters journeying from Central Valley to Puntarenas
c. 1850	Typhoid (remains endemic thereafter)
1852	Smallpox in Cartago and subsequent localized outbreaks throughout country
1853	Yellow fever in Puntarenas
1856–1857	Cholera claims 8 to 10 percent of populace
1860	Yellow fever in Puntarenas
1861	Whooping cough
1862–1863	Smallpox in Puntarenas and Guanacaste
1863	Whooping cough and measles (simultaneous)
	Typhoid (virulent upsurge)
1865–1866	Scarlet fever in San José, Alajuela, and Cartago
1867–1868	Smallpox in isolated areas
1869	Yellow fever in Puntarenas
1875	Smallpox in Limón
1881–1882	Yellow fever in Puntarenas
1884	Smallpox in isolated areas
	Cholera in Europe: preparation of quarantine islands on each coast
1888	Dysentery in Heredia
1891	Smallpox in isolated areas
	Whooping cough and influenza (simultaneous)
1892–1893	Whooping cough: 8,000 child deaths attributed to disease
1895	Infant cholera, measles, and mumps (simultaneous)
1895–1896	Yellow fever in Puntarenas
1898–1899	Whooping cough in San José and Cartago

Table 1. (*continued*)

1899–1900	Yellow fever in Puntarenas, spreads to Alajuela; quarantine of Alajuela
1902	Smallpox outbreak in isolated area
1919–1920	Influenza pandemic reaches Costa Rica: 2,300 deaths attributed to disease

Sources: Lachner Sandoval, "Apuntes de higiene," 190–200; República de Costa Rica, *Memoria de Gobernación y Policía, año 1920* (San José: Imprenta Nacional, 1921), xxii; and República de Costa Rica, *Memoria de Salubridad Pública y Protección Social correspondiente al año 1927* (San José: Imprenta Nacional, 1928), vii–viii.

the 1870s, an oligarchic liberal state was constructed according to positivist principles, and though the political balance of forces promoted the evolution of a functional electoral democracy, the system was fragile and succumbed to military dictatorship between 1917–1919, and later to civil war in 1948. In these terms, as much revisionist historiography has shown recently, Costa Rica is as exemplary a Latin American country as it is an exception.[23]

Costa Rica's population, typical of Latin America as a whole, grew significantly in the second half of the eighteenth century and continued to increase at an average rate of 1.5 percent per year throughout the nineteenth century, growing sixfold to reach 300,000 in 1900.[24] The country's coffee boom, beginning in the 1840s, integrated Costa Rica more closely into the global network of maritime commerce dominated by English capital. The trend was intensified after 1880. With the building of a railroad that linked the Central Valley to the Caribbean coast, and the rise of banana cultivation in Limón province, Costa Rican society was drawn into the Caribbean and North American web of shipping and human migration spun by the dynamic banana companies.

Costa Rica's nineteenth-century disease ecology closely resembled the classic patterns of other Latin American countries in the throes of export booms and foreign market integration. During the period of this study, smallpox, malaria, yellow fever, typhoid, and cholera posed the greatest epidemic threats to the country on a schedule that would not have seemed unusual to its continental neighbors. Dysentery, malarial fevers, and syphilis were endemic, and they accounted for the largest share of adult deaths. Diarrhea, malnutrition, and a tight cycle of whooping cough epidemics decimated an infant population that was also jolted periodically by infant cholera (summer diarrhea), scarlet fever, diphtheria, mumps, and measles.[25]

Obviously, Costa Rica's historically Hispanic and mestizo cultural ballast separates it from countries in the continent that have strong African and indigenous social bases like Peru, Mexico, Guatemala, and Brazil (though it resembles mixed-race cultural spaces within these same countries). The dynamic of Costa Rican medical practices is, in many respects, drastically different from that found in such countries. Also, the very development of a cultural and political order in Costa Rica based on consensus rather than conflict has undoubtedly promoted a similar muting of confrontation in the medical realm. Nevertheless, even in these terms I think the study of Costa Rica might offer a significant alternative perspective. Studies in countries with strong indigenous and African medical traditions have led to the equation of Latin American popular medicine with the figures of the shaman and herbalist, subordinate ethnicity, and counterhegemonic cultures. Studying Costa Rican popular medicine provides a picture of that other, perhaps less spectacular but no less important domain of common Latin American healing — one that more often than not complemented and emulated the realm of official medicine, even while contesting its pretensions to monopoly and final truth.

As for conventional medicine, the Costa Rican story is, in crucial respects, more representative of the Latin American experience than that of the places that have received the lion's share of attention from scholars: Mexico City, Rio de Janeiro, and Buenos Aires. Such metropolitan centers, with their deeply sedimented and variegated communities of titled practitioners, as well as their institutional network of hospitals, schools, and regulatory agencies reaching back into the colonial past, make them exceptional indeed in the continental scheme of things. The Costa Rican case thus allows one to perceive the evolution of medical practice in a secondary, Hispanicized zone of Latin America with residual and peripheral indigenous and African influences. At the same time, it allows an appreciation of the evolution of medical politics in a Latin American nation-state. If there is any country suitable for a study of medical practice at the national level over the long haul it is Costa Rica, since its relatively small size makes the evidence potentially manageable—though whether or not I have succeeded in managing it is a question I will leave for the reader to decide.

A Note on Terminology

The quest to provide a definitive terminology for differentiating between the two basic domains of the medical universe has not led to any consensus. There has been a move away from using such terms as "irregular," "folk," and "traditional" medicine due to the mildly pejorative or antiquarian overtones they carry. Terms such as "alternative" and "non-standard" still nonetheless suggest that mainstream, standard medical practice is the yardstick (while generally begging the question of exactly what constituted standard medicine in any period).[26] In fact, as the following pages reveal, the only accurate labels are "licensed" versus "unlicensed" practitioners, and this distinction generally, but not always, corresponded to that between the medicine whose authority came from the people (which I refer to as popular medicine) versus the medicine whose authority came from state, professional, and academic officialdom.

I use the terms "empiric" and "curandero" throughout this study when referring to practitioners of popular medicine. No pejorative overtones are attached to either term, though in Western medical history, empiric in particular is often used as a synonym for charlatan, and Costa Rican medical elites sometimes used both terms in a derogatory way to signify quackery. Even in official medical discourse, however, the terms were also used neutrally. For example, from the 1840s through the 1880s, the state granted licenses to a variety of healers authorizing them to practice as "empirics in medicine" (*empíricos en medicina*) in any part of the country that was without a titled physician or surgeon, the designation of empiric simply being a recognition that they had demonstrated knowledge and competence in the art of medicine. There was no hard-and-fast distinction between the kind of healer who might be called an empiric and the one that might be labeled a curandero. Empiric tended to suggest someone who had acquired some formal knowledge of healing through study and apprenticeship with more conventional types of medical practice, while curandero tended to connote a more rustic healer who practiced in their locale (a distinction that I tend to employ here). Nevertheless, even in the 1860s, the country's

Introduction

leading medical regulator, referring to the authorization of empirics, stated that "the law permits authorizing *curanderos,* and the selling of certain classes of medicines, in the areas where there are no *pro-fesores.*"[27] Here, curandero is interchangeable with empiric.

The use of profesores is particularly curious in Costa Rica, where there was essentially no medical school throughout my period of study. In the Iberian tradition, all doctors in medicine were *facultativos*—that is, members of the official medical body that would also serve as the faculty of the university should one exist. This terminology was simply adopted by the emergent community of official practitioners in Costa Rica, regardless of whether they were bachelors, licentiates, or doctors of medicine or surgery. At the nineteenth century's end, it was incorporated into the name of the country's first true professional body: the Facultad de Medicina. Of course, the idea was always there that eventually its members would serve as the staff of a medical school, though one was not functional until the 1960s.

Finally, from the 1840s onward, Costa Ricans employed the term "*farmacéutico*" to describe a schooled and titled preparer and dispenser of medicines. I have translated this throughout as "pharmacist," while translating the generic term "*boticario*"—which referred to an untitled preparer of medicine, though often one who was knowledgeable and experienced due to a conventional apprenticeship—as "apothecary." Other clarifications are made as necessary in the text.

1

Healers before Doctors

When Costa Rica gained its independence from Spain in 1821, there was not a single physician or surgeon in the province of fifty thousand people. This was typical of most places in Latin America at the time: outside of Lima, Mexico City, Buenos Aires, and Rio de Janeiro, practitioners with full academic training were scarce. There were less than twenty titled medical doctors in all of Central America with its population of one million, despite medical faculties at the University of San Carlos in Guatemala and the University of León in Nicaragua. Even important Mexican centers like Querétaro, with a populace of thirty-five thousand, had only two physicians in 1787; Bogotá had only two for twenty-five thousand in 1800. As far as the governor of Puerto Rico could tell, there was not a single licensed practitioner of surgery or medicine on the island in 1812.[1]

Shocked by the scarcity of schooled and titled medical practitioners in Spain's American colonies, John Tate Lanning concluded that "the whole history of colonial medicine, as it really was, is the story of the all-too-natural filling of this awesome gap in doctors."[2] A growing literature on "medicine without doctors" has undermined the idea that popular medicine is a lack—an "awesome gap in doctors." I will instead follow the recent generation of social historians in conceiving of popular medicine as an expansive domain characterized by the interaction of common sufferers with their families, and with a wide variety of practitioners, many of whom had neither orthodox training nor official certification.[3] In doing so, I will avoid any presumptions about the motives, skills, or efficacy of unlicensed practitioners.

Titled physicians, surgeons, pharmacists, and midwives remained relatively few in number throughout Costa Rica's nineteenth century—indeed, outside the principal cities and towns, they remained scarce right up until the end of my period of study. One must try to form an idea of the way that the large majority of people addressed their health during the first half of the nineteenth century, and with limited evidence, develop a portrait of the popular healers who were all but unrivaled by certified doctors at this time. This will provide a basis for understanding the medical culture that physicians, surgeons, and pharmacists encountered when they began to arrive in small, but significant numbers during the 1840s and 1850s. It is significant that Costa Rica's first curers were not authorized by anyone but the community of sufferers, yet it is equally essential to note that official and learned medical knowledge and technique were incorporated by many sufferers and lay practitioners even prior to the arrival of licensed healers.

Domestic Medicine

Healing begins in the home. The essential value of domestic medicine in the nineteenth century was similar to what it is today: the constant, focused care available and affordable only within a household economy. This was touchingly expressed in 1867 by the poor of Puntarenas, Costa Rica's main Pacific port, in the course of petitioning the president to license an empiric who could provide attention in the home for reasonable fees. The "*parte proletaria*" could not afford to pay for visits by the local district physician, who would only treat the poor without charge on the dreaded condition that "the patients resign themselves to moving to the hospital, depriving themselves in the process of the affectionate and concerned care of their family."[4]

Characterizations of popular medicine in the Latin American past invariably emphasize the role of herbs, magic, and faith. These certainly loomed large in Costa Rica's common culture of healing. From at least the second half of the eighteenth century, most Costa Rican homes had a small garden planted in herbs known for their medicinal properties. Common knowledge of herbal medicine was used to prepare remedies that might alleviate dysentery, respiratory problems, stomach ailments, nervous conditions, muscle and joint stiffness, and a host of other more or less minor illnesses. Typically used as the basis for emetics, purgatives, febrifuges, and tonics, herbs were also employed as contraceptives and abortifacients.[5]

In every village, region, or country of Latin America, people also turned to constellations of healing deities in which icons of local renown combined with universal figures to provide divine coverage for the entire spectrum of health problems. Appealed to in prayers or sayings; represented in statues, paintings, prints, medallions, and necklace figurines; hidden beneath the clothing of patients — these were the mystical physics called on to attend the vast majority of sufferers over the course of the nineteenth century. Though the particular Costa Rican pantheon has not been researched, Lydia Cabrera has re-created a marvelous litany of such saintly intercessors in nineteenth-century Havana: San Antonio for inflammations, San Quintín and San Fermín for dropsy, San Hilario for gout, San Caralampio for plagues and miasmas, Santa Elena for catarrhs and epilepsy, and so on.[6] Often, of course, these were syncretic expressions of deities that had once been indigenous or African, as in the syncretism of African *orixás* and Catholic saints common to Bahian medical culture in the nineteenth century.[7] Belief in the healing powers of these religious figures might span an entire faith, as in the case of San Lázaro, the Catholic patron saint of lepers. In other instances, the saintly figure was of local significance (frequently derived from a particular vision of the Virgin Mary), although its healing powers might be general. The most important Costa Rican example is the cult of the Virgin of Los Angeles, which revolves around an icon found at the wellspring where the Virgin appeared to an Indian girl in the seventeenth century. Both the icon and waters were (and still are) believed to have miraculous healing powers.[8]

The herbal and spiritual dimensions of popular healing are attractive because they conjure up an aura of transcendental purity — the good life in the garden. Often overlooked is the fact that much popular medical practice was mundane, pragmatic, and mechanical. For example, Wilhelm Marr, a German immigrant to Costa Rica in the 1850s, fell ill from chiggers, tropical burrowing fleas that caused sores and swelling on the entire surface of his body. A wealthy compatriot sent over each morning "his big-nosed Indian, Casimiro, who removed the *niguas* with marvelous skill using a needle."[9] Such mundane popular medical skills, then, could bring profound relief from suffering. Yet, although they might be enhanced by local knowledge and experience, they could hardly be categorized as part of a distinct medical "system" standing in opposition to conventional medical practice.

Given the tendency to romanticize "herbal medicine" as inherently organic and outside the cash nexus, it is also worth noting that common medicinal herbs were not necessarily available to be plucked freely from the garden or forest. The culture of herbal healing in Latin America as elsewhere had been part of a highly developed international commerce since the sixteenth century. In large Latin American centers such as Mexico City, medicinal substances were imported from other parts of the Americas, the Levant (via Bayonne), and Manila. Sufferers and healers on a periphery like Costa Rica probably did not have access to such variety. Nevertheless, the country was historically part of the large-scale overseas commerce in herbal medicinals. In the early eighteenth century, for instance, a local expert spotter was sending hundreds of boxes of *copalchi* (probably copal, an astringent resin) and *chirraca* (Peruvian balsam) to a buyer in Panama who subsequently shipped them to Europe.[10]

Nor was knowledge of herbal remedies necessarily part of local, oral lore. Written compilations of herbal recipes have been circulating in many cultures for centuries, serving as textual references for domestic medicine. In Latin American outposts like Costa Rica where specialized medical help was rare, such *recetarios* were especially important in the eighteenth and nineteenth centuries.[11] In 1833, Costa Rica's official news sheet adopted the tradition of the recetario, publishing a number of home remedies for those suffering from smallpox. The fact that the remedies were differentiated by the price of ingredients underlines the fact that not all herbs were affordable to the common sufferer. Some of the ingredients listed also show that a range of imported medicines was available, including chemical ones like mercurous chloride, which had long been in use in Latin America. Other prescriptions published in the official paper in 1833 required imported items like laudanum and Epsom salts (sometimes called "English" salts).[12]

It is possible that even prior to independence and the liberalization of trade, the active contraband of the late colonial period on Costa Rica's Caribbean shores gave the wealthier residents of the Central Valley access to the British patent medicines that already made up a large part of the North American market by 1750. Patent medicines certainly were known in Mexico by this time, and some prominent Mexican pharmacists were producing their own.[13] In 1833, at the outset of the experiment in coffee cultivation for export by the leading agriculturalists of San José, a French merchant, Adolphe Carit, established Costa Rica's first *botica*, or drugstore, in the capital (the store also specialized in the sale of wines and spirits).[14] The market for prepared medicines grew and diversified in step with Costa Rica's insertion into the world economy. By 1859, a pharmacy in the bustling port of Puntarenas, the principal point of export-import exchange, alerted newspaper readers that the establishment was "well-stocked with medicines, chemical products and perfumes, all imported recently and available on reasonable terms."[15]

Even distant peripheries like Costa Rica participated in the popularization of learned medicine that had characterized the eighteenth century. In 1815, the estate of one prosperous San José farmer contained a Spanish edition of William Buchan's *Domestic Medicine*. A classic expression of Enlightenment populism, Buchan's text saw three Spanish translations after its publication in 1769, and was the most popular of such layperson's guides in Latin America.[16] The Costa Rican market for these home guides to medical theory and practice was significant enough that one of the first editions printed in the country after the arrival of the printing press in 1830 was a pirated version of Thomas John Graham's *Modern Domestic Medicine*. The Costa Rican edition, a weighty tome of 750 pages, was certainly not cheap to buy.[17]

As was the case in Anglo-America, unauthorized translations of Buchan printed in Brazil, like those of Manuel Joaquim Henriques de Paiva (which saw four editions between 1788 and 1841), came with annotations concerning local variations in climate and suggestions on how the reader might adapt Buchan's advice to local conditions.[18] There is no extant copy of the Costa Rican edition of Graham's work, so it is not known if the work was so adapted. Still, the popularity of such manuals indicates a secular, pragmatic, and rationalist vector in popular medical culture. As Charles Rosenberg notes, Buchan's manual provided prudent rules for maintaining good health while attacking the false promises of quacks as well as criticizing the "sometimes superstitious and always uncritical therapeutics of folk medicine." Though the book took issue with the wild theorizing and "mystical jargon" of the medical profession and implicitly legitimized some lay practice, *Domestic Medicine* counseled nothing that was not in accordance with the conventional medicine of the time, and promoted a sensible adherence to expert surgical and medical care.[19]

On a more popular scale, in 1846 in Heredia, one of Costa Rica's four main towns, the estate of a priest who had been known for his interest in the art of healing contained sixty copies of *The Discourse on Medicine*, which he was presumably selling to the public. The notary valued the books at fifteen pesos for the lot; even if the priest had been selling the books for one peso each, the manual was easily within the reach of a comfortable peasant family.[20] So, though much domestic medicine might have included traditional home remedies and the invocation of divine assistance, it was not necessarily devoid of knowledge derived from written reference texts, technical pragmatism, and secular understandings of illness. Moreover, home remedies were not always herbal and entirely outside the market, nor were the herbs used always local in origin.

Main Systems of Medicine

Common sufferers shared some basic notions of illness and health with popular healers. At the beginning of the nineteenth century, humoral principles governed the medical cultures of Latin America (they continue to play a large role in the continent's popular medicine today). Anthropologists have recently debated whether the humoral principles found in Native American and African American medicine are parts of distinct ethno-medical systems or were the result of the more or less forced adoption of European humoral principles following the cultural devastation of the conquest and slavery.[21] What is at stake in this debate is whether indigenous and African ethno-medical systems survived in the Americas or can be treated together with popular Hispanic medicine as variants developed on the basis of the same essential principles. The debate has reached something of a stalemate, but since it is impossible to propose a competing indigenous medical system that survived the conquest and subsequently informed Costa Rican mestizo popular medicine, I will describe the basic principles of humoralism according to the European tradition.

With a genealogy stretching as far back as Greek medicine in the sixth century B.C.E., humoralism understands illness as the result of an upset of the body's (or parts of the body's) natural balance of fluids. As this system was absorbed into Western medicine via the medieval revival of ancient texts, the four humors established in the Galenic current of Greek medicine became the norm: phlegm, blood, black bile, and yellow bile. These were actual bodily fluids to which were ascribed, through hypothesis and symbolic association, different vital functions. The humors also corresponded with the four basic corporal states — hot, cold, wet, and dry, which were environmental states as well — the four elements, four seasons, four stages of life, and four cardinal points in the universe. These complementary symmetries and oppositions gave the theory of humors a great, commonsensical weight along with broad interpretative possibilities.

Each individual had different circumstances, and the same disease varied in its character with every individual precisely because it was inseparable from that person's particular mode of humoral imbalance. Diet, medicines, mood, and the bodily issues associated with ill health were invested with humoral qualities, and regimes of treatment or prophylaxis logically worked out according to the particular circumstances of each individual — the end result of all medical intervention being to maintain or reestablish humoral equipoise. Although the range of therapies was great, they often involved purging and bleeding, because these were considered the quickest and most effective ways of evacuating corrupt and excess fluids from the body.[22]

Nevertheless, the mental aspect of health was integrated with the physical. In humoral medicine as in most forms of world medicine, there was no "disease without suffering" (as one author puts it in discussing the characteristics of biomedicine).[23] Neither sufferers nor practitioners dissociated disease from the individual, or from his or her spiritual, social, and environmental state. Because humoral medicine had so much hermeneutic flexibility, typically including considerations such as the age of the patient, astrology, faith, diet, and so on, the ideal practitioner was one who had great interpretative skill, long-term knowledge of the individual, and the ability to offer an explanation of curative or preventive treatment that would ring true within the worldview of the patient.

The principal opposition in Latin American popular medicine was, and is, between hot and cold. This was common to both popular and conventional medical theory. Thus, for example, because cholera spread more rapidly in warm climates or seasons, it was a "hot" disease, something confirmed by the symptoms. In 1833, when the century's second cholera pandemic reached Mexico, the official Costa Rican newspaper explained that the disease was "produced by the effect of a hot atmosphere, whose air produces an excessive increase in bile by irritating the liver." The balance of bodily humors was tipped toward a state of excessive, acrid bile that caused vomiting and diarrhea. The recommended treatment focused on "softening or liquefying the bile" with doses of barley water, corn gruel, and warm water in order to avoid damaging or overheating the alimentary canal. If the evacuations became excessive and overly irritating, the application of laudanum was suggested to stop them and reduce the swelling.[24]

The stress on an atmospheric source was not the only explanatory model at this time, but it was a common, conventional one for cholera transmission in the United States, Mexico, and Guatemala during the pandemic's 1832–1833 passage through the Americas.[25] Until the end of the nineteenth century, environmental understandings of disease causation were common to popular and conventional medicine, and honed in on miasmas as well as fetid waters and their corruption of neighboring air, which created locations propitious for disease. Though there was never any precise theoretical conception of how diseases were transmitted via miasmas, there was a sensible association of corruption with disease along with an empirical apprehension of a link between fetid sites and illness.[26] One manifestation of this in Costa Rica was that, from 1840 to the end of the century, miasmism informed conflicts between communities and local coffee processing facilities over the safety of drinking water since the detritus of the fruit and husk separated off by water from the bean collected in mass quantities in the rivers and streams, generating a foul odor as it rotted.[27]

The spontaneous generation of disease by miasmas was often combined with a notion of "predisposition" among those who came in contact with the corrupt air. As a learned priest from Heredia, José Emigdio Umaña, observed in the official paper in 1833, "The cause of the illness called smallpox is the same as all the others with which living beings can be smitten; that is, a degeneration in the mass of the humors, in proportion to the contagion, and poor state of disposition of the same humors in the individual when they are attacked."[28] This formulation is unusually simple in that few medical thinkers believed all diseases to be contagious — that is, transmissible from person to person. It is also typically complex, however, to posit a humoral imbalance in the environment that has created a proportionate contagion that will produce sickness when encountered by an individual whose humoral imbalance predisposes them to such an illness.

David Sowell has made explicit a historical presumption found in much scholarship, proposing that a basic tension arose between popular and certified medicine in Latin America across the nineteenth century. A "highly social, Catholic influenced set of beliefs that drew upon humoral principles" was juxtaposed with "an emerging, secular, scientific system that envisioned the body to be a knowable machine whose maladies could be corrected."[29] According to anthropologist Arthur Kleinman, such "biomedicine" is unique to Western conventional medicine, with its "extreme insistence on materialism as the grounds of knowledge"; its search for single, causal chains to explain the course of disease and provide a rationale for effective therapy; and its commitment to understanding nature in purely physical terms, as a "thing" that can be "laid bare in morbid pathology."[30]

As we will see, the juxtaposition of biomedicine with spiritual beliefs about healing and humoral medical systems did animate a number of key disputes between popular and conventional practitioners in Costa Rica, especially as a powerful professional community of doctors organized itself in the latter part of the nineteenth century. But it is important to avoid a presumptive association of neatly categorized medical systems with specific groups of healers. Notions of spiritual healing, humoralism, miasmatism, and the teachings of clinico-pathological and bacteriologic schools were to some degree common currency available to all practitioners, and were frequently capable of coexisting — often within a single practitioner or network of practitioners. Some popular healers incorporated clinical approaches to the body and ideas of infection derived from bacteriology as the nineteenth century progressed. And while some physicians were undoubtedly biomedical positivists, many remained Catholic, and skeptical of radical materialism and scientism (as was Louis Pasteur himself); into the early twentieth century, most physicians continued to use in their daily practice deeply embedded notions drawn from both humoral medicine and the environmentalist suppositions of miasmatism.[31]

If family care was the foundation of the medical edifice in Latin America, the base was a huge variety of unlicensed practitioners. Among them were healers with magical powers: indigenous *brujos,* mestiza sorceresses, and Afro-American practitioners of Santería, Condomblé, and Obeah, to name a few. Specialists in spiritual healing included the *benzedor* or *rezador,* men or women who cured with prayers, and the thaumaturge, a miracle healer often relying on the laying on of hands or application of saliva.[32] There were also a great number of curanderos and curanderas who specialized in treating illness with a largely herbal therapeutic arsenal (though the fact that animal and mineral ingredients were used as well in medicines is often overlooked). For Brazil, Lycurgo de Castro Santos Filho notes that a further distinction was sometimes made between *raizeiros,* specialists in medicinal roots, and *herbanários,* experts in remedies made from leaves, flowers, fruits, and resins. There was also a variety of specialists of manual skills that closely corresponded to the list compiled by Guenter Risse from sixteenth-century Valencia: the *algebrista* or bonesetter, *hernista* who reduced and managed hernias, phlebotomist, bladder stone remover, cataract coucher, tooth puller, and midwife. The list should probably be extended to include spider, fly, and snakebite healers along with the *comadrón* (or male midwife).[33] Nor would the taxonomy of popular practitioners be complete without mentioning the eclectic assortment of usually foreign healers who began to circulate in Latin America toward the end of the colonial period, equivalent to the "old-style mountebank and other charlatans" who, according to Matthew Ramsey, experienced a golden age during the period of mercantile capitalism in northern Europe.[34] Such healers became especially visible in Costa Rica in the second half of the nineteenth century, no doubt motivated to add the country to their itinerary due to a growing population and the commercial prosperity of the coffee boom.

But such a variety of healers was rarely to be found in any one place at the same time, and particularly not in a peripheral province with a small populace. Take the case of Alajuela in the 1840s, still without a licensed physician, surgeon, or apothecary even though the town was prospering in the orbit of San José's coffee trade, and serving as a service center on the route of peasant migration toward the agricultural frontier in the north and west of the Central Valley. According to a list compiled in 1845 by the municipality, 10 curanderos—6 men, of whom one was a priest, and 4 women—provided medical services to approximately 7,000 people (if one includes the outlying barrios). The following year the flamboyant foreigner, Count Adolfo Salisch, began to offer his medical services. The town thus supported 11 curanderos, or roughly 1 for every 640 people (for reasons I will go into below, this figures does not include midwives, five of whom were listed in Alajuela in the first census of 1864).[35] What kind of healers were they?

As in other parts of Latin America, the most common male healer in Costa Rica during the first two-thirds of the nineteenth century was the practitioner who combined barbering, phlebotomy, and minor surgery with medicinal prescription and preparation.[36] They might be likened to the "surgeon apothecary" that characterized English country practice in the eighteenth and early nineteenth centuries, and the diversity of practitioners that might be included in the general category was equally large.[37] They were often called *sangradores* (bleeders), reflecting one of their most common procedures: bleeding through venesection or the application of leeches, which was believed to both cure illness by ridding the patient of excessive or unhealthy humors and maintain health by ensuring that humors retained their proper balance.[38] The practice was also common in conventional therapeutics, of course (although it was becoming controversial by the late eighteenth century), and in Mexico City and Lima, the colonial Protomedicato bestowed titles and licenses on the most educated in the art. Though none were so recognized in Costa Rica, in 1820 the town council of San José, already experiencing some prosperity from commercial agriculture, contracted a licensed doctor from outside the province. Only two practitioners were singled out for suppression in the wake of his arrival. Both were unlicensed sangradores who operated in the center of the town.[39] While there are no details about their establishments, they were likely similar to the little shops of the sangradores that dotted the main thoroughfares of the principal cities of Brazil and Mexico at this time, and served as social gathering spots.[40] As late as 1852, the popularity of bleeding was sufficient for an itinerant "barbero y sangrador," don Jacinto Guzmán, to set up shop in the Costa Rican capital offering to "perform cupping, extract teeth, and apply gold fillings."[41]

Others who might be placed in this category seem to have developed an identity more as apothecaries. A portrait of one such Costa Rican healer can be sketched from the 1850 inventory of the estate of Nicolás Brenes, who lived in the city of Cartago. A father of six, separated from his wife for the last twelve years of his life, Brenes's tools included four pairs of scissors, combs, hand mirrors, three razors in their case, thirteen razor blades, six whetstones, and shaving soap. He also possessed tweezers, four lancets (including a large one "for pricking animals," suggesting he also did veterinary work), three small syringes, and a package of forty-five needles.[42] If his surgeon's armamentarium seems rather restricted, it roughly corresponds to the classic kit described by Santos Filho for Brazil in the early nineteenth century, where the scarcity of more specialized tools was a constant complaint of practitioners. Like his Brazilian counterparts, Brenes probably devoted much of his surgical attention to lancing abscesses and removing skin growths, extracting teeth and bleeding. He may also have reduced fractures, cauterized wounds, and performed amputations.[43]

The notaries recorded "two stones for grinding remedies [*remedios*]" and the remnants of a scale as well. Brenes's medicinal ingredients were all essentially herbal except for a small quantity of monkey fat in a bottle and twelve ounces of verdigris. The medicines were stored in a large assortment of glass bottles and jars, many chipped and without lids. They included melon, known for its cooling properties in cases of fever; linseed, used in poultices, decoctions, and infusions to soothe chest pains, coughs, and hoarseness; ipecac, commonly used as an emetic; two jars of the classic laxative rhubarb (perhaps different varieties); and a large quantity of astringent copalchi resin. Whatever training Brenes may have had was checked against "a treatise on medicine by Juan Calixto Geore." An old horse carried Brenes about when need be.[44]

He was not successful in financial terms, his house and simple possessions placing him if not on the lowest rung, among the lower strata of Cartago society. More than three-quarters of his wealth was made up of a promissory note (perhaps from a patient) and a title to some distant land. The net fortune after the funeral and inventory costs was a paltry ten pesos, to be divided between seven heirs.[45] Perhaps because his trade was not a lucrative one, he followed other common healers of the era in offering nonmedical services. The presence of a small and large vihuela among his possessions suggests that he also practiced another trade: that of musician (a typical combination for barber-surgeons; in

Rio during the first half of the nineteenth century, they often also played the violin or clarinet for their customers).[46]

In a land where university-trained physicians were rare, the populace frequently turned to a priest for healing help. As John Tate Lanning puts it, "They knew he could read medical works, and because he was often obliged to try his hand at prescriptions and cures, he gained both a knowledge and a reputation he could not escape."[47] Indeed, a number of priests and friars left their mark as healers during this period in Costa Rica. In 1787, a few years before he established and administered the province's first, short-lived hospital, Friar Pablo Bancos of Cartago was denied the agreed-on payment of one hundred pesos by the widow of a man he had treated for a cerebral hemorrhage by prescribing a mercurous ointment, which indicated to the respectable patient that he was being treated for syphilis (a diagnosis he considered erroneous as well as logically impossible). Father Rafael Arnesto of Bagaces carried out Costa Rica's first vaccinations on the Pacific lowlands in 1805, and Father C. Benavides of Esparza acquired fame in the 1830s for curing snakebites with an antitoxin made from powdered rattlesnake and viper bile. I have already mentioned the Heredian priest, José Emigdio Umaña, who sold popular medical books and published medical advice in the official newspaper. And at the top of a list of curanderos banned from practicing medicine in Alajuela in 1845 was the parish priest, José Antonio Benavides, who had a large house in the center of town and an estate worth almost eleven thousand pesos when he died three years later.[48] Their learning, charitable vocation (although they sometimes charged handsomely for their medicines), and special knowledge of the connection between body and soul all made them attractive to sufferers. The strong and semiofficial correspondence between religious and healing offices was underscored in 1856 by Anselmo Llorente y Lafuente, the first bishop of Costa Rica, when he ordered all priests to treat the sick during the fearful cholera epidemic of that year.[49]

A good example of the culture of the healer priest comes from Cartago in 1864. A new cleric from Guatemala, Father Juan Corredor, immediately developed a following as a healer among popular and elite families. He was denounced by four local doctors, who alleged that he had charged for his medical services. Corredor defended himself by claiming ignorance of the country's laws (in his country of origin, he maintained, practicing medicine was not so closely policed) and insisting that he had simply recouped the cost of his medicines rather than charging for a consultation. The testimony of one of his patients, a woman with a fever, suggests that he employed conventional humoral therapy and confined his remedies to herbs: some unidentified drops to dilute in a cold water enema, liquid to make a poultice to apply to her belly, and a regimen of cold water baths with crushed ginger (used as a diaphoretic for colds and fevers). In criticizing the physicians, Corredor contended that he had been "naturally inclined to the study of medicine" and had "learned this science from the same books as the doctors with titles."[50]

If evidence on male healers is hard to come by, women practitioners are even more elusive. During the first half of the nineteenth century, women curers accounted for about half of the healers notable enough to be singled out by Costa Rican authorities. In Cartago in 1839, three of seven curanderos prohibited from practicing medicine during an epidemic were women, and four of the ten mentioned by name in an edict in Alajuela in 1845 were curanderas.[51] Women healers were sometimes labeled in a way that implies a slightly higher stature than the generic popular term curandera. During an epidemic of fever in 1853, in the face of a prohibition against unlicensed practitioners, the middling barrios ("*el pueblo mediano*") of Cartago presented a petition to the municipality "soliciting that the empiric [*la empírica*] María Echavarría be allowed to continue exercising the occupation of doctress [*el oficio de médica*]."[52] She was probably the same "María de Jesús Chavarría" named in the ban fourteen years earlier, suggesting a long specialization and notoriety as a healer.

Because the evidence from Costa Rica is slight, it is worth mentioning some clearer cases from other parts of Latin America. In 1830, the Peruvian Protomedicato charged Dorotea Salguero with acting as a "doctora," visiting the sick and running a hospital in her home where she "acted as a physician and surgeon." She claimed that she treated only simple diseases — particularly venereal complaints and wounds — referred patients with serious problems to physicians, and used only herbal medicines rather than "drugstore medicines." Her testimony, however, was contradicted by patients (after a lengthy legal battle, she was fully exonerated in 1837).[53] In early nineteenth-century Toluca, Mexico, the Spanish-born Tiburcia Reynantes ("María la Gachupina") ran a practice quite similar to Salguero's, though incorporating indige-

nous medicine and shamanism that she had learned through apprenticeship as a servant in the household of an indigenous medical practitioner.[54]

In neither case did midwifery figure in their practices. I will look
more closely at the role of midwives in a later chapter. For now, suffice it
to say that midwives were certainly curanderas to the degree that they
commonly treated problems relating to pregnancy, postpartum recovery, the inducing of abortions, and vaginal conditions, including venereal disease.[55] Yet women healers should not be conflated with midwives
—that is, a curandera was not necessarily the same as a *partera* or
comadre.[56]

Healing and Ethnicity

Indigenous and African healers were important in many parts of the
Americas, although the history of their ministrations inside their communities in the nineteenth century, if it can be written at all, is separate
from their participation in the general medical marketplace, and there
is virtually no information that would allow one to try to write the
former.[57] Part of the popularity of indigenous and African medicine
with people of other ethnicities stemmed from the magical promise of
shamanism and the "secret" knowledge of the herbalist. These were
fetishized, particularly by mestizos and Creoles, who would appeal to
them "outside" their own medical culture. So throughout the nineteenth century indigenous Kallawaya herbalists, natives of the Andes,
made annual mercantile circuits into coastal areas and neighboring
countries to trade on the mystique and renowned effectiveness of their
skills as well as therapeutic arsenal. Likewise, the mestizo Andean surgeon Miguel Perdomo Neira, who made a controversial entry into
Bogotá in 1872, claimed to have acquired special knowledge and secret
medicines through apprenticeship with an indigenous group in Ca-
quetá, thereby allowing him to perform surgery without the patient
feeling pain.[58] This cross-cultural engagement transformed indigenous
or African medicine into something quite distinct, complicating any
attempt to identify "authentic" forms.

One recorded interaction from late colonial Costa Rica between a
Hispanic resident and native healer indicates both that the standard
distinction between herbal and shamanic indigenous healers is often

overdrawn, and that such healers could perform the role that Hispanics expected of them while practicing more conventional medicine.[59] Manuel de Cruz Méndez was described as a brujo from the town of Tres Ríos, situated on the road between Cartago and San José. The town had been founded in the 1740s as a *reducción* of newly conquered indigenous people from the Talamanca region of southern Costa Rica. Cruz Méndez, then, may have been what one visitor to the remaining Talamanca Bribri in the 1870s called an "*awa*" — a doctor or sorcerer who cured diseases and controlled the rain.[60]

Charges were brought against Cruz Méndez in 1775 by a dissatisfied patient from Cartago who had sought out the Indian healer believing himself bewitched by two women. In justifying himself before the court, Cruz Méndez surprised the judge by explaining that even though he did not contradict the man's belief that he had been bewitched, his treatment had begun with an examination of the man's urine. After considering other symptoms, which included sores, Cruz Méndez diagnosed the patient as suffering from "the gallic disease." He prescribed a drink made of *bejuquillo* (possibly liana), and applied to the sores powders made from salt and "*cáscara de candelilla*" (probably willow bark, a common febrifuge but also sometimes used as an antaphrodisiac to suppress sexual desire).[61] Cruz Méndez's diagnostic approach, which included urinoscopy, may have been learned from the missionary priests who had ministered to the sick after the establishment of the reducción. It is a reminder that indigenous healers were exposed to European medical culture from the time of the conquest onward, and this exposure continued into the nineteenth century: in 1805–1806, for instance, indigenous healers in Costa Rica were trained in vaccination by a number of university-educated men such as the surgeon Manuel del Sol, a member of the Guatemalan Protomedicato.[62] It is likely that most native healers who did participate in the medical marketplace combined elements of indigenous medicine with the techniques, pharmacopoeia, and idiom of European medicine, either for better therapeutic effect, purposes of translation, or reasons of demand.

The same was true for black practitioners who often mixed rituals and cures deriving from African- and European-based systems.[63] Whether or not they continued to incorporate dimensions of African medicine into their practice, free blacks and mulattoes dominated the ranks of healers — and not just in their "folk" variety — in many parts of colonial Latin America, particularly Brazil and the tropical lowland areas of the Spanish colonies. In Brazil, the professions of barber and midwife, certified by municipal examining committees, were "both virtually monopolized by persons of African descent," according to A. J. R. Russell-Wood.[64] This was also the case in places like Peru and Venezuela. Simón de Ayanque, a late colonial voyeur of the market in Lima's central plaza, satirically remarked, "Que la pública salud / Está en manos de los negros, / De los chinos, los mulatos / Y otros varios de este pelo ("The public health is in the hands of blacks and zambos, mulattoes, and others of that ilk).[65] In discussing Venezuela on the eve of independence, Ricardo Archila writes matter-of-factly and unequivocally that "medicine was practiced by whites, and surgery, obstetrics and pharmacy by *pardos.*"[66] As John Tate Lanning has established, even in regions such as Chile, where African slavery was not fundamental in demographic or economic terms, a racist equation between healing and impure caste was one reason that young Creole men of good family had no interest in pursuing even academic medicine.[67]

With independence, emancipation, and a general tendency toward assimilation, the question of black and mulatto preponderance in the healing trades becomes occluded in Spanish American republics like Costa Rica where Africans had made up a relatively small proportion of the total populace. Perhaps 10 percent of Costa Ricans at the time of independence were mulatto or black, and by the mid–nineteenth century most Costa Ricans with African ancestry, at least in the Central Valley, were doing their best to be fully assimilated.[68] Still, future research may well find that they played a significant role as healers, and this strain in Latin American medical culture would be quickly revived in Costa Rica after 1880 with the arrival of large numbers of Afro-Antillean migrants to the Caribbean region of Limón.

Foreigners

During the late colonial period in Spanish America, according to Lanning, sufferers with some education and money who did not have access to a physician preferred "the foreign intruder."[69] The "foreign doctor" was actually a European, and in the nineteenth century also a North American, who claimed to be a qualified physician, but had inevitably "lost his title" on the Atlantic passage. English, Scottish, and French practitioners were especially common in the Spanish Empire, followed closely by Italian and Portuguese, and they were tolerated by the authorities — and occasionally even accredited — as long as they played their social cards right and did not undercut the business of any licensed peninsular or criollo physician in the area.[70]

The case of "Doctor" Esteban Courtí provides an idea of why such foreign practitioners seemed so desirable. Courtí was an eccentric Milanese empiric and the son of a physician. After a series of adventures in Spain, he gained entry to the colonies by posing as a Catalan physician and insinuating himself into the entourage of the newly appointed governor of Costa Rica as the latter was about to sail from the peninsula. Courtí spent two years in the province in the late 1780s astonishing the populace with his cures, vast knowledge of medical botany, and new discourses on physics, mineralogy, and medicine. He was the first practitioner to compose a report in legal medicine. Courtí also engaged in bizarre episodes of blasphemy, fell under suspicion of being a philanderer, and was denounced by a widow of Cartago who claimed he had pressured her for sexual favors during a consultation. Finally accused of witchcraft and spreading heretical "Voltairean" ideas, he was arrested and taken to Mexico to be tried by the Inquisition. There Courtí acquired huge fame as a healer while imprisoned for his trial and continued to exercise the trade even after his conviction (he subsequently escaped from Havana while awaiting transportation and died some thirty years later in Philadelphia, then the leading center of medicine in the United States).[71]

More foreign healers came in his wake, and the allure of the marvelous foreign physic, no matter how dubious he might have been, remained a strong element of local medical culture and a large problem for Costa Rica's small community of licensed practitioners. Count Adolfo Salisch, who claimed to be a Silesian aristocrat with special curing powers, caused a stir when he set up practice in Alajuela in 1846, and a large number of patients from all social classes quickly began to arrive at his door. Even though the town still had no titled or licensed practitioner of medicine, Salisch was forced to flee after being investigated by the authorities and fined.[72] In 1857, among the chief reasons given for establishing a Costa Rican Protomedicato was to protect against "the many foreigners who under the name of doctors visit our towns, settling there in some cases, or in others passing through like birds of ill omen."[73]

Popular medicine in late colonial and early republican Costa Rica was not an Arcadia of organic knowledge, local herbs, and community-based or ethnically "pure" healers. Though the evidence is slight, it suggests a number of trends that run counter to standard portraits. Healers were part of an incipient medical marketplace whose reduced size led to general practice versus specialization and promoted transience among the foreign healers who were attracted to the area. The country was connected to an international commerce in medicinals, and sufferers were already being encouraged by the public power and merchants to become consumers of medicines, including patented ones. Some popular healers engaged medical texts that espoused conventional, secular conceptions of illness and therapy. Indeed, the overall impression is not one of a deep-seated traditionalism but rather a popular medical culture open to new influences and eager to discover the most effective means to treat illness.

The U.S. adventurer and diplomat John Lloyd Stephens discovered this firsthand during his voyages through Central America in 1839 and 1840. Everywhere he went, Stephens was beset by people expecting him to supply special medical assistance, and his trip through Costa Rica was no exception. At a ranch halfway between Puntarenas and San José, the mistress ushered him into a darkened and sealed room to see her daughter, ailing with intermittent fever (probably malaria). The distressed mother begged him for *remedios,* allowed him to examine the young woman, and heeded his insistence that air and light be allowed into the room and that her daughter be bathed ("according to the obstinate prejudice of the country, her face had not been washed for more than two months").[74] It is an arresting image of the anguished and isolated family caregiver side by side with the learned traveler, one desperately seeking the trick, the secret, the commodity, the knowledge that the other might have acquired along the way.

There were also historical reasons for this pronounced "allure of the foreign" in the medical marketplace of Costa Rica, from the new knowledge brought from Spain by colonial officials, to the novel remedies brought back to their land of origin by traveling merchants, to the visits of marvelous medical men like Courtí.[75] The allure did not fade, in large measure because, as we are about to see, the first wave of qualified physicians, surgeons, and pharmacists was made up predominantly of foreigners, a majority of these professional practitioners were immigrants throughout the nineteenth century, and even the few titled practitioners of Costa Rican origin had left the country to acquire their learning.

2

First Doctors, Licensed Empirics,

and the New Politics of Practice

Between independence in 1821 and 1870, the government gave about fifty medical men full license to practice anywhere in the country. Almost all of them arrived after 1840 as immigrants, although a handful were Costa Ricans returning home following medical studies in foreign lands.[1] With few exceptions, this first wave settled in the four main towns, and the majority of those in San José. They were a heterogeneous group in terms of nationality, medical training, and extramedical commercial ventures, and did not forge an active scientific community as occurred in some Latin American countries at this time, most notably Mexico and Brazil.

When in 1857 the government of Costa Rica passed legislation creating a Protomedicato of the republic, it enshrined an institution that went back to the beginning of Spanish colonialism. This had ramifications for the status of titled and untitled practitioners. Neither the young and fragile state nor the tiny and loosely knit community of physicians were usually in a position to suppress popular medicine, and they faced public protest and appeal when they tried. The model of the Protomedicato was flexible enough to incorporate a heterogeneous array of healers. The Protomedicato gave the immature state a mechanism to institutionalize its authority through irregular medical practitioners, granting some of them license to practice and a series of official rights and duties that effectively extended public power, especially in secondary or isolated parts of the country. While some types of popular healers were officially banned, they were tacitly accepted and even selectively mobilized by the state during epidemics.

This first wave of physicians and surgeons did not, then, effect a systematic displacement or suppression of the array of healers that I recreated in the first chapter. Rather, they completed it, installing themselves at the apex of the healing pyramid—a superior space that had been held in reserve for them by government officials and members of eminent society since the late eighteenth century. The resultant official medical model involved a selective incorporation of all but the lowest echelons of healers into an official public health apparatus and a tolerance, born of necessity, for even those lowest ranks who were excluded.

Early Birds and Postcolonial Patricians

Titled medical practitioners were eminences rarely seen in colonial Costa Rica, but they were not entirely unknown. As in many peripheral parts of Spanish America, the province spent long stretches without certified doctors or surgeons, punctuated with the occasional arrival of an immigrant who had, or claimed to have, a title recognized by colonial authorities. As early as 1608 there is reference to a "surgeon," Manuel Farfán, who prudently demanded that a fee be contractually agreed on prior to treating a man whose wound the surgeon correctly guessed was fatal. In the first half of the eighteenth century, the "physician and surgeon" Francisco Lafons brought to the province an immigrant's knowledge from Bayonne in the Basque region of France, and his commercial peregrinations likely continued to serve as a conduit for new medical practices (he died during a voyage to Acapulco). In 1750, the priest of Villa Vieja (the original name of Heredia), Father Dr. Juan de Pomar y Burgos, had unspecified credentials recognized by the viceroyalty of New Spain and the Protomedicato of Panama. And in 1806, a member of the Protomedicato of Guatemala, the Licenciado in Surgery Manuel del Sol, spent two years on an official mission to propagate the smallpox vaccine in Costa Rica, during which time he also ministered to the local notables.[2]

In the late years of the colony, such occasional visits convinced the elites that a permanent group of learned practitioners was indispensable for civilization and progress. In 1820, the town council of San José, "considering that public health is one of the first necessities that must be provided to the body and enduring a rigorous necessity in this town of a licensed practitioner," adopted an old colonial practice by raising a subscription among the leading residents to contract Licenciado José Benigno Castro to serve them, but he did not stay long.[3] Three or four others like him made brief appearances in the new polity between 1825 and 1835, and were charged with propagating the smallpox vaccine or planning a leprosarium, but none stayed on.[4] Apparently only a single native son ventured to an imperial center to study medicine prior to the independence era, Friar Antonio de Liendo y Goecoechea (born 1735), who became a key figure in the brief flourishing of medical instruction at the University of San Carlos in the late eighteenth century (the so-called "Guatemalan medical Enlightenment"). If there were others, they either failed to graduate or, like Goecoechea, never returned home.[5]

Costa Rican independence was achieved with almost no bloodshed, as a corollary of the Mexican and Guatemalan break with Spain. Skirmishing subsequently broke out among the four major municipalities, all situated within twenty miles of one another in the Central Valley. Already the center of a buoyant commercial agriculture based on sugar and tobacco, San José emerged triumphant and replaced Cartago as the capital of Costa Rica.[6] San José and its hinterland experienced an early export boom in coffee whose effects on social wealth were manifest by the 1840s, and this was registered in the distribution of the country's first wave of medical doctors, surgeons, and pharmacists.

It was not until the 1840s, twenty years after Costa Rica achieved its independence, that the first native-born physicians and surgeons returned home from their studies. Even so, they accounted for only eleven of the fifty-five fully licensed practitioners in the five decades following independence. Almost all of these Costa Ricans were products of a pilgrimage whose colonial overtones are striking: born to the patrician families of the colonial capital, Cartago, they traveled to the University of San Carlos in Guatemala to study medicine before returning home. Of the eight Costa Ricans who acquired a license to practice prior to the founding of the Protomedicato in 1858, six fit this pattern; of the other two, both from eminent San José families, one had also studied at San Carlos.

The vestigial colonial aura of these first Costa Rican physicians was captured in 1860 by Alexander von Frantzius, a German doctor and naturalist resident in Costa Rica. During an expedition to the thermal waters in the valley of Orosi, west of Cartago, he stopped in on Lucas Alvarado at his estate adjacent to a monastery. "Don Lucas, the hacienda's proprietor, is a physician in Cartago, but he has been living here with his large family for the past two months. . . . He is considered a grand protector of the Indians, who also from time to time give testimonies of their gratitude through gifts and other reciprocal services."[7] That Alvarado still enjoyed the condition of a virtual *encomendero* should not be too surprising. The last names of the Cartago physicians — Alvarado, Bonilla, Sáenz, and Jiménez — are a litany of Costa Rica's colonial criollo elite.

The postindependence "hajj" of the old provincial elite to the former colonial capital of the Audiencia to study medicine in an antiquated institution, more than simply a morbid echo, was a first attempt to re-center and internalize ideal forms of political rule that had never been fully realized. Prominent families sought for their sons a title that in the recent past, would have consolidated their preeminence. It certainly did them no harm in the new republican polity, but the ornament of academic title had lost some of its value in an emerging political economy driven by a capitalist agro-export sector based in the new capital, San José. This is illustrated in counterfactual terms by the trajectory of José María Montealegre, one of only two licensed practitioners in this first wave who was a native of San José. The son of an influential colonial official (his father held the powerful post of factor de tabaco, or comptroller of the tobacco monopoly), he was sent to England as a boy and later moved to Scotland, graduating from Edinburgh's Royal College of Surgeons in 1838. But by the time Montealegre returned to San José the following year, his parents had large interests in the budding coffee economy, and according to a Scottish traveler who met him in 1844, Montealegre was too busy amassing coffee wealth to bother exercising a profession that paid so poorly. Montealegre did later practice medicine in various public advisory and charity roles, but he does not seem to have engaged in private practice (although he may have ministered to laborers on his coffee properties, and he effectively cured the Scot's severe gastric attack).[8]

Immigrant Merchants

During these early years of the coffee boom, sons of the Costa Rican elite tended to devote themselves to commercial agriculture rather than study and professional office. As a result, intellectuals from other parts of Central America, many displaced by the incessant civil wars and intolerant politics in their home territories in the three decades following independence, were attracted by the young country's relative peace and prosperity as well as its shortage of educated men.[9] One such émigré, the Guatemalan Nazario Toledo, became the country's preeminent medical practitioner during the middle third of the nineteenth century. When this licenciado in surgery from the University of San Carlos took up residence in San José in 1835, there was only one other recognized "doctor" in the country (the Englishman Richard Brealey, who resided in Cartago). Toledo was already known in Costa Rica for the twelve-page pamphlet he had published in Guatemala in 1833 outlining methods for preventing and combating cholera—reprinted by the federal government in 1837 when the disease appeared again in Belize and worked its way south to Nicaragua. In 1839, Toledo was charged with creating "a complete course in medicine" at San José's general school, the Colegio de Santo Tomás. Although the program did not prosper, Toledo was named official doctor of prisons and the leprosarium, and won appointment as the rector of Santo Tomás when its status was upgraded to a university in 1844. The appointment registered a rise in the stature of medical practitioners since during the colonial era, a physician (let alone a licentiate in surgery) was ineligible for the position of university rector. Toledo went on to occupy a seat in the legislative assembly in 1846–1847, serve as director of the state press and editor of the official newspaper in 1849, head up the government commission that evaluated the credentials presented by physicians, surgeons, and empirics, become the country's first protomédico and head of the Medical Association in 1858, and act as a senior government minister in the same year.[10]

Four of the fully licensed medical practitioners prior to 1870 were from neighboring Nicaragua and Colombia, two were natives of Spain and graduates of peninsular universities, and thirteen others, whose nationalities cannot be determined, had Hispanic names and were probably from Spain and Spanish America in roughly the same proportions (see figure 1).[11] Two of the three Englishmen had been drawn to Costa Rica via the imperial Caribbean trade. Brealey was a ship's doctor who frequently docked in Costa Rica and decided to try his luck there in 1830. Charles Salmon, who set himself up in Costa Rica as a farmer in 1856, arrived just in time to earn the distinction of treating sufferers of

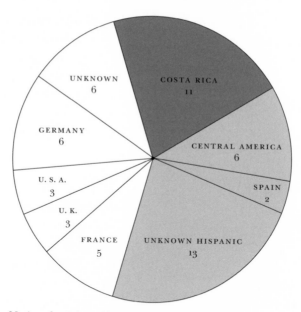

Fig. 1. National origins of licensed medical practitioners in Costa Rica, 1830–1870.

cholera during three separate epidemics (he had treated victims in Panama in 1832 and had control of a hospital in Jamaica during the epidemic of 1850). Five doctors were from France. The United States contributed three practitioners of dubious academic pedigree who nonetheless managed slowly to earn themselves a place in the medical establishment.[12]

As in other Latin American peripheries like Venezuela, it was the Germans who made the strongest impact of any single nationality, accounting for at least six of the physicians and pharmacists of the period.[13] This group included Juan Braun, Francisco Ellendorf, and Guillermo Joos, who arrived hard on the heels of the failed 1848 revolution, perhaps as political refugees. They were followed five years later by Frantzius, a graduate of the University of Heidelberg, and Karl Hoffman, a doctor in natural science, medicine, and surgery from the University of Berlin. The two were able to present themselves to President Juan Rafael Mora with a letter of introduction from Baron Alexander von Humboldt.[14]

These immigrants benefited from the fact that most of the native Costa Rican practitioners were from Cartago and reestablished them-

selves there rather than in San José on their return. Heredia and Alajuela, demographically and economically dynamic towns to the west of
San José, did not see the return of a titled native son practitioner until
the last third of the nineteenth century. So foreign surgeons and pharmacists were able to set themselves up in these three centers without the
obstacle of an entrenched native establishment. In 1845, after the return of two native son physicians, Brealey moved from Cartago to Heredia. The Germans Braun, Ellendorf, Joos, and Hoffman established
surgeries and pharmacies in San José between 1848 and 1854, along
with the Catalan José Ventura Espinach in 1858. Frantzius, meanwhile,
set himself up in Alajuela for four years before moving to the booming
market of San José in 1859. In the latter year there were nine pharmacies in San José (population eight thousand), each apparently functioning in tandem with a doctor's surgery; of the seven pharmacies
whose proprietors are known, five were run by European immigrants.[15]

Costa Rica's large proportion of immigrant physicians in the postindependence era was typical of many places in Latin America. In Chile,
three of five members of the first republican Protomedicato, reconstituted in 1830, were foreigners (an Irishman, a Welshman, and a
Spaniard), four professors of the first medical school faculty, established in 1833, were from Britain or France, and until the 1840s almost
all the physicians in the country were foreign-born. Brazil also began
the century in this condition, although medical instruction was instituted soon after the transfer of the Portuguese court in 1808, and
medical schools were formally created in 1832 in Bahia and Rio. Even
here though, as Nancy Leys Stepan points out, foreign physicians accounted for four of the eight founding members of the Medical Society
in 1829, and as Julyan Peard has shown, foreign doctors (albeit with
deep roots in the country) continued to play the vanguard role in medical science until the 1870s. In the late 1820s, of the first fifteen members of the Buenos Aires Academy of Medicine, seven were foreigners.[16]

Costa Rica did not have a medical school, but even those countries
that did have a functioning university medical program did not necessarily produce many graduates given the relatively low esteem of the
profession and the erratic nature of university instruction in most countries. In Chile, the medical school did not graduate any of the first class
of 18 until 1842 — almost a decade after their enrollment — and even
then, only 4 managed to make it through. In the decade between 1833

First Doctors

43

and 1843, of the 2,000 students enrolled in Rio's medical school (presumably the great majority native Brazilians), only 100 became licensed physicians. In Lima, only 10 of 143 students enrolled at the University of San Marcos in 1854 were studying medicine — theology and law remaining the primary attractions. Prior to 1858, according to Bradford Burns, most of Nicaragua's patrician sons likewise considered the study of medicine at the university in León "a poor third choice," and even the chairs in medicine were often vacant.[17] In Havana, only about 30 students were enrolled in the courses of San Ambrosio in 1825. The numbers did not rise rapidly after that, and Ross Danielson underlines that "increasing medical immigration was especially significant for Cuba."[18] Indeed — and this is worth stressing — Mexico was unique in having a strong preponderance of schooled and certified native-born practitioners of medicine and surgery during the first fifty years of independence. As Luz María Hernández Sáenz has established, this had already been the case in the late colonial era, with foreigners making up a mere 11 percent of the titled physicians and surgeons between 1740 and 1826.[19]

By the first two decades of the nineteenth century, the top half of these physicians in Mexico City, if not yet among the highest ranks of society, were wealthy and enjoyed significant stature. Though their riches may also have derived from inherited earnings and other mercantile activities, the medical profession was integral to their preeminence, and its fees essential to their fortune.[20] In Costa Rica, this was not yet the case even by midcentury. No Costa Rican physician was dedicated exclusively to medical practice. Medicine was instead often combined with operation of a pharmacy, which in turn was part of broader mercantile activities. Many of the physicians and surgeons of the capital were associated with particular pharmacies, as sole owners or in partnership with a titled pharmacist or merchant specializing in medicines. Many of the Germans participated in a failed capitalist venture to promote immigrant agricultural colonies, and the immigrant, Henrique Roches de la Tour tried to build a spa near the thermal springs east of Cartago.[21]

Many physicians shared the Costa Rican dream of the dance of the millions, and tried to become *cafetaleros* (coffee barons). Richard Brealey was involved with the development of mining concessions, and achieved some prosperity in the early 1840s as a grower and exporter of coffee. Reproducing an old peninsular mercantile strategy, the Catalan physician José Ventura Espinach emigrated to Costa Rica at the behest of his uncle, Buenaventura, who had done well with a mining concession in the 1830s and married into the well-to-do Giralt family of Cartago. Espinach and Giralt had a joint import-export venture in the 1840s that placed them among the earliest coffee barons. With his uncle, Espinach was able to mount a pharmacy in San José in the 1850s, showing that medicine and pharmacy could be conjoined with coffee as significant components of a merchant family strategy.[22] Native Costa Rican doctors also sought coffee riches, some like José María Montealegre with notable success. At least one of the physicians of Cartago, Lucas Alvarado, shed the colonial skin and embarked down the road to agroexport capitalism. When Frantzius visited him at his hacienda in 1860, Alvarado was in the early stages of converting the property to coffee groves, and the intense managerial focus required kept him from practicing medicine during most of the growing season.[23]

Practice

After arriving in San José in 1859 and securing a license from the Protomedicato "with the idea of staying some time in this Republic," Epaminondas Uribe, a doctor in medicine and surgery, advertised his services in the *Crónica de Costa Rica*. He assured readers that he would be available at any hour and no matter where the call might come from. Also, "in his room on the lower floor of the Hotel Costa Rica he will hold free consultations every day from ten until noon, and make his small selection of medicines available free to the needy."[24] Although Uribe was just getting started in practice, offering his services at the most comfortable rates possible in order to establish a clientele, his advertisement is a small window into some of the characteristics and limitations of a physician's practice at midcentury.

Doctors commonly set aside one or two mornings each week for free consultations for the poor as part of their charitable vocation (this may also have been a way of ensuring that their decent clientele did not have to rub elbows with the poor and destitute). Unlike Uribe, most doctors saw patients in their home or, at this point in San José, the pharmacy that might also have been the storefront of the practitioner's house.[25] It is not clear how much of a physician's or surgeon's earnings would come from actual consultation fees. The cost of medical services was fixed by the government.[26] Doctors might charge a global fee for the comprehensive treatment of an illness, like the sum of sixty pesos one physician exacted for treating a San José patrician's venereal disease in 1821 (at the time, the monthly salary of a day laborer was three to five pesos).[27] If treatment required surgery, the fee was larger. More involved surgery, like "common amputations," could be charged in Costa Rica at one hundred pesos for the rich and twenty-five pesos for common folk. For more delicate operations, like the removal of gallstones, "if they save the life of the patient, and that patient is rich, one can demand up to 1,000 pesos; if they are not [rich], up to a quarter part of that sum."[28] Fees might differ, then, according to the wealth of the patient and the outcome of the treatment.[29] This responded in part to the fact that medicine was still not fully detached from a government-regulated moral economy. It might also have reflected the notion that the intervention of an educated and qualified practitioner was considered more of a necessity the higher one rose on the social scale; the plebeian, more inclined to be satisfied with a curandero, might have been better wooed with a fee that was just in range, given a serious enough condition. That the physician's free consultations for the poor usually did not include medicine is suggested in Uribe's advertisement, since he underlines that his medicine chest would be made available free of charge to the destitute. The price of medicines could be substantial, although the average profit margins are unknown. After performing their official duties during Costa Rica's time of cholera in 1856, physicians, surgeons, and pharmacists submitted large claims for the medicines they had dispensed; the San José surgeon, Bruno Carranza requested that the government reimburse him over one thousand pesos, a large sum at the time.[30]

The potential earnings of Costa Rican physicians were limited by the lack of public health or medical institutions. In 1839, the central government agreed to pay Nazario Toledo four hundred pesos annually to establish a teaching program at the Colegio de Santo Tomás, and to be the official doctor of the leprosarium and prison.[31] This was the only public medical post in the country at the time, and things would not change a great deal before the 1870s. In the great urban centers of the Americas, charity hospitals for lepers, slaves, and indigenes had a long history. Hospitals provided salaries and prestigious positions to physicians, surgeons, pharmacists, phlebotomists, and midwives, and continued to do so even after independence when many went through difficult financial times. In Costa Rica, there would be no functional hospital until the 1870s.[32]

The only public institution of this period that could help sustain a physician's livelihood was the office of Médico del pueblo, or town doctor. Appearing in its first form in 1845 as the *propagador de la vacuna*— propagator of smallpox vaccine—the town doctor designation was formally created by the central government in 1847 to answer a variety of official needs for medical services. The office eventually evolved into one of public relief and public health oversight, while ensuring that a physician would be available for consultation to all residents in secondary towns, even if they had to pay for the services. In normal times, the town doctor was expected to visit the prisons and barracks of his respective town, and provide medical certificates to those who could not work due to debilitating illness, allowing them to beg for charity without fearing that they would be transported to a penal colony for vagrancy.[33]

The post was to be paid for by the municipalities, with the doctor given the added incentive of exclusive privileges over billable matters of legal medicine. A lengthy process of redefinition began almost immediately, with impoverished municipal councils unable to offer enough to attract candidates, and tugs-of-war between the central government and town councils over who should foot the bill.[34] When salaries were paid by the municipality in the early 1850s, they were in the range of ten to twenty pesos monthly, though the physician could also bill for medicines dispensed.[35] As a result, unless the posts seemed likely to provide a newcomer an entrée into a prosperous community like Alajuela or Heredia, they were unattractive and often left unfilled.

The marginal nature of a town doctor's practice is revealed by the case of Juan Echeverría, who contracted with the government in October 1858 to perform for free the duties of town doctor in the port of Puntarenas in return for a monopoly right to sell medicine in the town and surrounds. By December, he lodged a formal complaint with the president, saying that many stores continued to retail in medicines and demanding the authorities intervene to make the monopoly effective. The provincial governor's secretary claimed ignorance regarding any sales of medicine in contravention of Echeverría's patent. By the end of January 1859, the disappointed physician published the following notice in the country's newspaper, the *Crónica de Costa Rica:*

> Because the professional practice of medicine in Puntarenas is not very lucrative I have resolved that I will only practice in future when I have the time and interest in doing so. My decision takes effect one month from the publication of this notice, so that the residents of the area can provide themselves with a new physician should they so desire, and not say later that being the only medical practitioner in the town, I stopped prescribing medicine without prior warning.[36]

During the cholera epidemic of 1856, all available doctors were mobilized and paid by the central government at the rate of two hundred pesos per month. Initially an exception for extraordinary circumstances, the central government would eventually return to this sum in the 1860s when it begrudgingly assumed responsibility for town doctors' salaries.[37] This improved the profile of the post, but even so, in the smaller and more traditional markets of the periphery, for the office of town doctor to be profitable the official subsidy had to be combined with the political clout to rein in rival unlicensed healers.

Medical Science

In the United States at this time, physicians embarked to Europe, and especially Paris, for lengthy clinical apprenticeships in new medical specialties that would give them a niche in the crowded marketplace of the Northeast on their return and the chance for a hospital appointment.[38] Costa Rican practitioners were all generalists, and even the rough distinctions between physicians, surgeons, dentists, and pharmacists were becoming intentionally blurred. To what degree did these medical practitioners cultivate a scientific identity? The community was too small to produce any professional journal, there was only the most sporadic and rudimentary medical instruction at the University of Santo Tomás, and its library's impoverished and outmoded thirty-six-volume collection of works on medicine, anatomy, and pharmacy was no source for research, or for keeping up with developments in the field. On the other hand, the fact that all of the country's physicians had studied outside of Costa Rica, some of them in leading centers of medical instruction like the University of Berlin, and maintained mercantile links abroad meant that they shared a certain cosmopolitanism, probably maintained relatively up-to-date personal libraries, and were in a position to pool knowledge learned in a wide variety of settings.[39]

A Costa Rican Medical Association was mandated by government in 1858 as the twin of the Protomedicato, in recognition that a certain critical mass of practitioners had been reached and as an acknowledgment of trends in other countries.[40] The association originally included thirty-six members, twelve of them pharmacists. While it was supposed to serve as a forum for professional debate and the circulation of knowledge, there is no evidence that it ever functioned in this manner — or indeed in any way at all. This is not to say that there was no public medical culture. In May 1854, when yellow fever first appeared in Puntarenas and threatened the coffee trade, eight San José practitioners of different nationalities came together to answer a government request for current knowledge on the cause and nature of the disease. Their report demonstrated that they were aware of the emergence of yellow fever in coastal areas of the American tropics, conversant with the contagionist versus anticontagonist debates of the day, and inclined to see the disease as a result of local conditions (the miasmas of nearby swamps sweeping into the port during the hottest months of the year) and individual predisposition.[41] Many of these same physicians and surgeons volunteered for the country's great patriotic war against William Walker in 1856–1857, and served heroically on the battlefields of Santa Rosa and Rivas (the German Karl Hoffman was even credited with engaging the enemy during one particularly harrowing struggle). They also rallied to treat those ill with cholera during the horrendous return to Costa Rica following the victorious campaign of 1856.[42]

Basic notions of humoralism and miasmatism still directed the therapeutic and prophylactic strategies of the everyday physician, but in this Costa Rican practitioners were little different from their educated brethren throughout the West. Toledo's 1837 pamphlet promising a "curative method for Asiatic cholera" placed a heavy emphasis on diet to avoid the onset of the disease or minimize its effect.[43] Twenty years later, Hoffman was asked to prepare the official instructions for treatment and prophylaxis during the epidemic that decimated Costa Rica. The recent graduate of Berlin — almost certainly a veteran of the 1848 cholera epidemic in Germany — retained the stresses on constitution, diet, and temperament that were at the heart of humoral medicine. People were instructed to avoid emotional turmoil, especially "fits of rage," and dedicate themselves to pleasurable social activities while avoiding fruits and alcoholic beverages. For those suffering from the disease, Hoffman proposed treatment with the usual assortment of Dover's Pills (whose opium was intended to stanch the flow of diarrhea), laudanum enemas, and calomel rubs (whose mercury caused the suppurating gums that were considered a sign of recovery).[44]

Though these did not effectively combat the cholera, and many of their results were detrimental to the health of the sufferer, they were common in the medical therapeutics of the day, according to Charles Rosenberg's classic study of the response to cholera in the United States at the time (similar therapies were employed in Brazil during the epidemic of 1855–1856).[45] Hoffman's fellow naturalist physician Frantzius perhaps demonstrated a more flexible incorporation of the local folk pharmacopoeia in his preparations for cholera sufferers. As well as the standard camphor, laudanum, Dover powder, and "choleric drops" (probably opium based), he included yucca starch alongside more traditional herbals like mint, ipecac, and chamomile.[46]

In any case, Costa Rican practitioners displayed no great tendency toward the dogmatism or wild theorizing associated with scholastic medicine. If anything, a secular, Enlightenment spirit of observation and experience — more the province of the new clinical medicine — was the rule of thumb. In the preface to his cholera pamphlet, Toledo recognized that popular and professional opinions were contradictory as well as capricious, and that "while we are ignorant of the real nature of the disease, we shall closely observe the symptoms the better to combat them most actively."[47] His major effort was to provide a reasoned tone to offset the terror, panic, and extraordinary theories that the disease caused in the populace at its onset. In 1856, the Englishman Charles Salmon was more eloquent and, for the time, accurate. Although he supplied the government with a treatment regime based on humoral principles, he concluded his report by saying that he had twenty-five years of experience with cholera, and "as such I think I have cause to know the disease in all its stages as well as caprices and can confidently assert there is no specific mode of treatment."[48]

What medical and surgical instruction there was in Costa Rica weakly echoed the promotion of surgery and clinical medicine in other areas of Latin America at the end of the eighteenth and beginning of the nineteenth centuries. Autopsies were performed as part of legal medical procedures from the 1840s onward, and the veterans of the 1856–1857 war were probably more experienced in surgical techniques than they had ever hoped to be. Although Costa Rica's physician-historians of medicine contend that anesthesia was not introduced to the country until the 1870s, this seems unlikely since ether and chloroform were in use in many parts of Latin America (including Guatemala, where all native Costa Rican physicians had studied) within a year of being employed in the United States and Europe in 1846.[49]

Vaccination was a well-known procedure. After a recurrence of smallpox in 1852, increasing efforts were made to maintain an indigenous source of vaccine from local cattle herds, and the district physicians were more systematic in their prophylactic efforts. In 1853 Bruno Carranza, the acting town doctor for San José, reported to the minister of the interior that he was engaged in "extensive inoculation with the vaccine that arrived from Germany, which was in excellent shape," and had "begun the system of vaccinating in the barrios at the same time that I have another central vaccination established for the city, which seems to me a better way to ensure the conservation of the serum."[50] The report suggests that a spirit of technical innovation and improvement was alive among Costa Rican practitioners.

Still, with such a small community of practitioners, there was no renaissance in medical research of the kind that distinguished the Tropicalista School in Bahia and, according to the recent work of Julyan Peard, founded a Brazilian medical identity. Had they had the inclination to engage international currents of medical science, Costa Rican physicians lacked clinical facilities, subjects, and research instruments. Even in an important center like Bahia, the nucleus of foreign-born medical scholars along with inquisitive and rebellious young Brazilian physicians was just barely large and influential enough to constitute a scientific circle, and much of their clinical success was made possible by their ability to work out of a second-rank hospital. Costa Rica had no hospital. And while Bahian physicians could refer to a significant Brazilian medical bibliography, written by local and foreign scientists, Costa Ricans could not count on a single published work in local medicine. Nor does the 1854 report on the causes of yellow fever in Puntarenas provide any indication that Costa Rican physicians might have been developing a sense of a particular, local "medical distinctiveness" of the kind that John Harley Warner has proposed in the U.S. South.[51]

The only scientific pursuit shared by many of Costa Rica's practitioners was natural history. Following in the footsteps of eighteenth-century physician travelers to the Caribbean as well as the new world colonies of Spain and Portugal, Hoffman not only arrived with a blessing from Humboldt but carried out a number of expeditions to collect plant specimens for the Berlin Herbarium, and published at least one major work in Germany on the flora and fauna of Costa Rica.[52] Frantzius had a broader range of interests still, spanning natural history and anthropology. He not only published a sequence of prickly articles in the German scientific press disputing the findings of previous vulcanologists, cartographers, and nature biologists but he also penned the first ethnographic studies of indigenous groups who lived in the frontier regions of Costa Rica. He left his practice and pharmacy in San José in 1869 to work at the Smithsonian Institution for five years prior to returning to Germany. The naturalist vocation was also shared by at least one Costa Rican physician, Lucas Alvarado, who Frantzius noted was "a great friend of the natural sciences and possesses some collections." The two joined forces during at least an 1860 expedition to Orosí, and Alvarado served as an intermediary in arranging for Indians to hunt and harvest specimens for his European colleague.[53]

The Republican Protomedicato

The large majority of the first postindependence wave of doctors may have been immigrants, but over half were shaped by a Hispanic medical culture (thirty-two out of fifty-five). The five men appointed to the Protomedicato on its creation in 1858 were Nazario Toledo, Lucas Alvarado, Andres Sáenz, Manuel María Esquivel, and Bruno Carranza — the first a Guatemalan, and three of the remaining four natives of the former colonial capital, Cartago. All five were criollo graduates of Guatemala's University of San Carlos, a scholastic academy whose medical program had fallen into pronounced decay following a brief period of scientific florescence in the late eighteenth century. Given this lineage, it is not surprising that the new administrative edifice of republican medicine and public health was based on colonial blueprints.[54]

The need for some kind of formal council of medical and public health oversight was underlined in dramatic fashion by the nightmarish epidemic that accompanied the great patriotic war of 1856–1857 against William Walker's filibusters in Nicaragua. In the preamble to the legislative proposal to create a Protomedicato, Toledo wrote of "the time when cholera invaded and many converted themselves into frantic merchants, poisoning people with their drugs in the midst of desolation and death." The council also responded to the need for a "professional authority" to establish a fee schedule for medical practitioners, and to normalize the naming of juntas of health as well as the appointment of physicians to a growing number of public duties.[55] Of course, none of these issues needed to be addressed through the specific form of the Protomedicato.

The institution of the Protomedicato, of peninsular origin, was transferred to New Spain soon after the conquest and subsequently extended throughout the empire, proliferating especially with the rise of the regional bureaucracies that characterized the Bourbon reformism of the 1770s. At the helm of this council of distinguished doctors was the protomédico, the leading physician or first professor, his position inherently attached to an academic chair. The Protomedicato established the pharmacopoeia, and inspected the quality of medicines sold by pharmacists and apothecaries; investigated and suppressed dangerous medical practices; and examined and licensed a range of practitioners, including physicians, pharmacists, surgeons, midwives, barber-surgeons, and surgeon-algebraists.[56]

In Mexico and Peru, the Protomedicato enacted the Bourbon state's Enlightenment reformism by elevating the status of surgery, creating a Royal School of Surgery in Mexico in the 1760s and promoting the development of anatomy in Lima.[57] In a similar vein, during the second half of the eighteenth century the Protomedicatos developed a public health advisory role in the context of a general upsurge of imperial and cabildo concern for hygiene. These ripples were felt in the secondary areas of the empire, and Costa Rica was no exception.[58] Between 1770 and 1810, in conjunction with the Guatemalan Protomedicato that had jurisdiction over colonial Costa Rica, local governors promoted public health measures typical of the era such as the cleaning of garbage and filth from the streets along with the removal of lepers from the towns. Costa Rica also participated in the 1805 smallpox vaccination campaign initiated by the Guatemalan Protomedicato even prior to the arrival of the famous Balmis expedition (whose officers often found that local efforts had rendered their mission somewhat redundant). Vaccine and instructions were sent from Guatemala, and Governor Tomás de Acosta created Costa Rica's first Junta of Health to oversee the campaign.[59]

As functioning institutions the Protomedicatos had a rather intermittent and nebulous existence outside of Mexico City and Lima. For reasons relating to the relative scarcity of fully qualified practitioners, the conciliar positions were often left unfilled and the council was inactive. Nevertheless, the institution was not so much a dead letter as it was an elaborately codified medical and public health "ideal" — one that could be invoked in each jurisdiction in the Spanish Empire regardless of the actual presence of licensed medical experts. After independence, while Costa Rica participated in the Central American federation (1823–1838), the province remained under the sway of the republican incarnation of the Guatemalan Protomedicato (where the institution was maintained without interruption). The Costa Rican government enacted health decrees in accordance with those emanating from the federal capital. Starting with the threat of cholera in 1833 and continuing in times of epidemic through the 1850s, Juntas of Health, modeled on the 1805 experience with smallpox, were convoked in each of the four main towns.

Costa Rica's republican Protomedicato, then, was revived from a direct line. Still, its formal reconstitution in the mid nineteenth century was a classic reprise: a self-conscious republican attempt to effectively realize, through re-centering, a colonial model that had long been part of the ideal type of government. The creation of such a neocolonial form of medical oversight was not unusual for Latin America. Some countries abolished the Protomedicato for good: for instance, in Gran Colombia in 1827, where liberals implemented complete laissez-faire in medical practice as had been done in the United States; and Mexico in 1831, after which jurisdiction over public health regulation devolved to the municipalities and federal states (which in itself suggests the reclaiming of a different colonial tradition of municipal sovereignty over questions of health).[60] But many countries retained it (Peru until 1848, and Guatemala until 1870) or like Costa Rica created it anew (Bolivia in 1830 and lasting through 1892; El Salvador in 1849 in conjunction with the founding of a university that included a medical faculty; and Honduras as late as 1869). Chile disbanded its Protomedicato at independence, then revived it in 1830 and maintained the institution through the 1880s.[61]

While it is still unclear how the Protomedicatos worked in these other countries, in Costa Rica its redeployment allowed for the combination of hierarchical and informal mechanisms characteristic of an older style of corporatist oversight, with the monopolistic licensing restrictions and policing techniques demanded by the emerging medical profession. The elaborate hierarchy of expertise and license that had been codified in the colonial Protomedicato was dissolved in the draft legislation of 1857. Gone entirely were the barber-surgeon, phlebotomist, and surgeon-algebraist.[62] The classic distinction between physicians and surgeons was upheld, but only for the purpose of establishing fee structures for different lists of practices. Physicians were not explicitly restricted from practicing surgery, and vice versa. Moreover, "specialists be they oculists, obstetricians, [or] surgeons of the urinary tract, the ears, or the mouth" were recognized under the category of surgeon, and so were technically invested with the same stature as both surgeons and physicians. The distinction between medical practitioners and pharmacists was implicitly recognized (but not codified) in the regulations, and the latter were invested with elite medical stature. Though both groups wished to acquire the right to trespass on the other's professional jurisdiction (and did in fact do so anyway), neither group was willing to cede legal ground to the other, and the foundations of a testy relationship were laid.[63] Perhaps most important, however, a homogeneous "fully qualified medical practitioner" category had appeared: *el médico*. This despite the fact that along with their disparate origins and schooling, the credentials of those who called themselves médicos were not equivalent. In the 1864 census, seven practitioners identified themselves as "doctors in medicine," five as "licenciados in medicine," and twenty-six simply as "médicos." Notably, "surgeon" does not appear as a separate census label.[64]

So although a colonial artifact, Costa Rica's republican Protomedicato also contained in embryo the modern division of labor in the health professions, and reflected major developments in Western medicine such as the professional conflation of medicine and surgery. Of course, as Ross Danielson points out in his study of Cuba, even during the colonial era "the jealously disputed working boundaries of the early professions were legally unclear and often circumstantially irrelevant."[65] Nevertheless, by conflating different types, the republican incarnation of the Protomedicato sanctioned the formation of an incipient, elite professional body of "medical practitioners" who were also invited to join the medical association that was mandated alongside the Protomedicato: a "literary body composed of all the doctors and licenciados in medicine and surgery, pharmacists, obstetrical surgeons, and dentists who now reside in the country."[66] In one sense, this was a move in the direction of medical monopoly by schooled and titled practitioners. Yet the Protomedicato also recognized a medical heterogeneity in a manner held over from its colonial predecessor — one that would prove alien to the maximalist professional line of modern medical regulation.

Training, Licensing, and Co-opting Empirics

The Protomedicato regulations also formally recognized a category of healer called "empírico," whose fees were established at "a fourth part of the rights that correspond to the *licenciados* [in medicine and surgery]."[67] At least a dozen of those listed as médicos in the Costa Rican census of 1864 were not in fact fully qualified graduates of medical or surgical training but empíricos.[68] They were practitioners who could demonstrate some measure of experience or schooling in conventional medicine or surgery and who might be given official permission to practice as empirics in areas of the country that were without a titled physician or surgeon. Who were they?

It must be recalled that medical education in the West was not yet standardized between or even within countries. Apprenticeship retained great currency. Although surgeons were tending to reach a par with physicians in professional status, they still often earned their doctor's stripes through apprenticeship, particularly as military surgeons on the countless battlefields of Latin America's bloody nineteenth century.[69] The wars transformed many a barber-surgeon into a fully licensed medical practitioner. As Ricardo Archila puts it in discussing the independence era in Gran Colombia, "A very interesting phenomenon, produced by the wars, is that from that time onwards social barriers were erased at the same time that careers or ascent were made easier for doctors and surgeons without titles."[70] Meanwhile, Latin American medical faculties generated many alumni who did not complete their studies but had knowledge of and association with academic medicine.[71]

The incipient public power had an interest in incorporating such men and women rather than persecuting and excluding them. Costa Rica's agricultural frontier continued to expand while the small number of physicians and surgeons remained clustered in the main urban settlements. Already in the late 1830s the political elite was expressing a worry about the lack of healthy, laboring bodies for the agricultural economy, and by the 1840s the central government was moving to extend its tenuous authority outward by providing charity and legal medical services in new parishes (and old ones still unable to sustain a physician). In April 1839, the government established a "complete course in medicine" at San José's general school under the tutelage of the Guatemalan surgeon Nazario Toledo. Each of the four main municipalities was ordered to select and send to San José two literate "children" (*niños*) who would be supported by a state subvention for the four-year duration of the program. Nevertheless, undoubtedly on the assumption that the youths might not make it through the full course, the first two years were to be dedicated to "the principal branches of Surgery." Rather than graduate doctors or licenciados in medicine, the Costa Rican government hoped to create a contingent of educated *bachiller* empirics of basic medical and surgical techniques to replace "curanderos who, perhaps without even knowing how to read and write, assume power over men's lives, sacrificing a portion of them with impunity when, had [these patients] been in the hands of *inteligentes,* their lives might have been preserved."[72] This might be likened to the famous Chinese effort to train "barefoot doctors" to bring basic medical skills to the countryside in the 1950s and 1960s. The creation of the school offers an interesting example of how the Enlightenment and Bourbon moves toward the integration of medicine and surgery, and the elevation of the stature of practical, anatomic, and clinical knowledge, were manifest in the peripheral areas of Latin America.

The school was dissolved after six months under mysterious circumstances when one student was denounced as a leper, fearful parents withdrew their children, and municipalities withdrew their support. The Colegio (and after 1844, University) of Santo Tomás periodically provided courses in medicine and appointed doctors as professors in the "faculty" of medicine. Though records of students and courses are not available, a library inventory of 1858 listed multiple copies of medical and pharmaceutical textbooks, suggesting that classes in both subjects were given intermittently.[73] Even in this shoestring institutional environment, then, formal instruction in medicine did likely produce a number of empirics or provide some training to curanderos.

Between 1840 and 1889 the state commonly granted empiric's licenses to those who could demonstrate a measure of medical learning and clinical experience. A good example comes from December 1853 when José María Cardona applied for permission to "exercise [his] profession in the republic." Originally from Guatemala, Cardona presented documents showing that he had taken courses in medicine, practiced surgery in "the Hospitals of Guatemala," and been "named" to an unspecified medical position in El Salvador. His petition was passed on to Nazario Toledo, head of the Commission on Public Instruction that decided medical licensing matters prior to the creation of the Protomedicato. Toledo determined that Cardona's credentials were "worthy of consideration" and recommended that he be allowed to practice surgery in "exceptional cases." Based on this report, the government, much less cautious, decided that "in consideration of the knowledge in Medicine and surgery" possessed by Cardona, he should be granted "permission to exercise both professions with the status of empiric [*en calidad de empírico*] in those areas of the republic where there are no professors invested with the legal formalities."[74] Empirics might be hired by the state for specialized purposes, too. This was so in the case of Rafael Jarret, paid twenty-five pesos a month in 1853 to serve as "vaccinator general" in the province of Guanacaste in the wake of a bad outbreak of smallpox. It is probable that he practiced more than vaccination.[75]

Costa Rica's medical landscape was not so frequently traversed by the war surgeon during the first half of the nineteenth century, likely because of the country's felicitous escape from intense independence battles and postemancipation civil strife. This changed after 1856–1857 when the country endured its surrogate war for independence, for two years combating William Walker's attempt to gain control over Central America from his base in Nicaragua. The clearest instance of the ascent of the war surgeon-empiric as a result of this conflict is Francisco Bastos, originally from Nicaragua. After serving the Costa Rican army in this capacity during the war against Walker, he emigrated south with the returning troops. Denied full recognition as a licenciado in medicine and surgery when he failed to present the title he claimed to have from the Protomedicato of Nicaragua and refused to subject himself to exams, Bastos nonetheless tried his luck in San José, Cartago, and Alajuela. According to Bruno Carranza, who reviewed his case for the Protomedicato, "In every place he acquired a reputation as a very bad doctor."

Gradually relegated to the periphery, Bastos was appointed official town doctor for the northwestern town of Liberia in 1865 (perhaps he hoped eventually to jump the border back home and make his reputation there on the basis of having achieved official standing as a practitioner in Costa Rica). While serving in this office, he was accused by the Protomedicato of giving a substandard legal medical report and having caused through faulty treatment the death of the wounded man in the case. Carranza concluded that Bastos possessed "no knowledge of Medical Science and Surgery beyond a fleeting grasp of a few basic theories [*ligeras teorías a su modo*] and a collection of technical terms that he still does not know how to apply."[76]

Others were more fortunate. Henry Guier also entered the country in the aftermath of the so-called National Campaign of 1856–1857, probably as one of the many former soldiers of Walker's defeated army who were incorporated into Costa Rican society. Though he had no medical title, he secured an appointment as the town doctor for Santa Cruz, a small center on the distant periphery of Guanacaste. The subject of complaints by the residents for his alleged assiduous persecution of local curandero competitors, he later moved to Cartago with his brother, who was also without title, and they successfully set themselves up as a physician-pharmacist team. By 1864, Guier felt confident enough of his status as a legitimate practitioner to band together with local physicians to press charges against a rival curandero for the unlicensed practice of medicine.[77]

So the legitimate empiric sanctioned in the laws of the Protomedicato was not an empty category. A large number of men with proof of medical schooling and experience, and influential enough referees, acquired restricted title to practice in medical markets of no interest to fully qualified physicians and surgeons. This general category of restricted legitimacy encompassed the range that had formerly been occupied by romancistas, phlebotomists, midwives, and so on. The restriction, however, was now usually defined in terms of geography rather than specialty. A geographically restricted but licensed "general practitioner" had been created, the Costa Rican equivalent of the nineteenth-century French *officiers de santé* who were given license to practice in areas without qualified professionals.[78]

How did unlicensed empirics—common curanderos—fare in this new politics of healing? In normal circumstances, any unlicensed empiricism was officially illegal yet widely tolerated. Cases from throughout Latin America reveal that up to the mid–nineteenth century, the limits of tolerance were defined by the type of malady treated and nature of the medicines prescribed. A healer's use of simple herbs to alleviate mundane complaints were not grounds for prosecution but, according to the charges brought against Dorotea Salguero in Lima in the 1830s, the treatment of patients with "serious ills" (*graves malos*) using "drug-store medicines" (*remedios de botica*) was a criminal transgression.[79] Thus, the threshold of tolerance was defined by the vague border between serious and common illness, and between simple and complex medicines.

In Costa Rica this same logic was applied in time of epidemics, but here the official government policy was revealing. Initially, all curanderos would be actively suppressed to the extent possible. Subsequently, however, male curanderos would be selectively mobilized to provide care under the command of a licensed doctor. This strategy of creating an integrated, hierarchical circuitry of titled practitioners, officially sanctioned empirics, and provisionally legitimate unlicensed healers dated back at least to the 1805s vaccination campaign—in Costa Rica and throughout Central America. The governor, Tomás de Acosta, unable to appeal to any physicians, passed on the technical instructions and lymph to a learned resident, Licenciado Manuel Lacayo, who formed a network of religious and indigenous curanderos to propagate the vaccine. Acosta was not convinced by the results, displaying the official preference for sanctioned medicine when he secured the visit of a member of the Guatemalan Protomedicato, Manuel del Sol. Still, Sol probably mobilized a similar or identical network of curanderos, which had been the official strategy throughout the isthmus.[80]

The 1839 edict issued by Cartago's Junta of Health during a fever epidemic banned curanderos from "curing in any fashion and in all types of illness *until they receive the corresponding pass from the doctors who are knowledgeable on the subject.*"[81] An 1851 law passed by the central government stipulated that "in the towns without professors of medicine, the judge will call two empirics or *peritos* to declare" in questions of legal medicine.[82] Again and again, the postcolonial state sought to enlist popular healers by giving them conditional authority over health emergencies following some rapid and rudimentary training in conventional medicine.[83] The practice was still employed during the cholera epidemic of 1856. The government instructed physicians to prepare a treatment strategy and store of medicines to be passed on free of charge to the afflicted (they would be reimbursed later). At the same time, as Dr. José Fermín Meza of Heredia described it, "I was told to give the necessary medicines to the curanderos of the barrios [the popular neighborhoods and adjacent villages]."[84] Government records show that not only were twelve curanderos provided with medicines and instructed in official treatment, they were also commissioned at a salary one-third that of the town doctors to treat the sick.[85]

Notably, though, all those listed were men. The fragmentary evidence indicates that slightly less than half of irregular healers were women (see chapter 1). So the way in which curanderos were mobilized during epidemics shows that female practitioners occupied the lowest echelons of the official healing hierarchy, and were excluded entirely from the medical "system" overseen by the Protomedicato (this corresponded to an old taxonomy indeed: the Spanish chronicler of the conquest, Fray Bernardino de Sahagún had divided Aztec physicians into "good, poor, and female").[86] As we have seen, the exclusion contrasted with the support one woman healer enjoyed among the middling and lower orders of Cartago when her practice was suppressed during an 1853 epidemic. One might hypothesize that beneath the Protomedicato's provisionally legitimate, third category (the unlicensed male healer), there was an illegitimate, fourth one (the unlicensed female healer). This category also included empiric midwives, who were constantly criticized yet for reasons of necessity never suppressed, and it should be stressed that even doctresses were tolerated unless an epidemic was afoot.

Hierarchies and Rivalries

The Protomedicato system reflected the dual domains of medical culture: a heterogeneous one that existed everywhere outside the four main towns; and a more homogeneous one, initially peculiar to the capital city, but gradually applying also to Cartago, Alajuela, and Heredia where the medical marketplace became more complex during the

1850s and 1860s. To take the case of Alajuela, the city acquired its first licensed physician and pharmacist, the German immigrant Alexander von Frantzius, in 1854. Though the elite almost certainly began consulting him by preference, the numbers of practicing healers continued to increase, as evidenced by the network of twelve barrio curanderos identified during the 1856 cholera epidemic by the town doctor of Heredia, a place of comparable size, yet keeping in mind that this did not include women healers.[87] Even using a conservative estimate, there were a dozen popular healers in the mid-1850s for a town of this size.

Ten years later, in the census data of 1864, the province of Alajuela registered one doctor of medicine, one dentist, two pharmacists, three general practitioners of medicine, and five midwives (one curandero also had the audacity to list this as his occupation). Some of these were certainly located in the new parish centers on the agricultural frontier, but it is safe to say that at least the doctor, dentist, one of the pharmacists, and two of the midwives practiced in the town of Alajuela. Even assuming that the number of barrio curanderos had remained equal (it had probably increased), the town had seventeen regular and popular practitioners for a populace of 11,521, or 1 for every 670 residents (in the previous chapter, I calculated a ratio of 1 to 640 in 1845). The ratio of practitioners to populace had remained roughly the same over the twenty-year period, but the range of types was broader.[88] In essence, Alajuela had completed the kind of mature colonial market configuration of a significant secondary center like Querétaro, in Mexico which in 1787, according to John Tate Lanning, had two licensed physicians, two friar empirics, two "foreign doctors" with dubious titles, and two other tolerated empirics for a population of 35,000. Taking into account that these figures leave out pharmacists, barrio curanderos, and midwives, Querétaro in 1787 and Alajuela in 1864 were probably roughly similar marketplaces.[89]

The story in San José was more complex. In the 1850s, the city quickly outpaced the gradual evolution of a colonial-style medical marketplace in the rest of the country and became something qualitatively distinct, approaching a market in professional medical services and pharmaceuticals. By the census of 1864, on the other side of the great coffee divide, the city's 8,500 residents (21,000 if the surrounding villages are included) could avail themselves of the services of 17 of the 38 men in the country who registered themselves as doctors, and 9 of the

18 who called themselves pharmacists. There was a licensed practitioner for every 800 inhabitants (recall that the 1 to 670 ratio calculated for Alajuela was for all practitioners, both licensed and unlicensed).[90]

This sanctioned heterogeneity did not mean that Costa Rican licensing categories were loose. Quite the reverse, they were the site of some intense struggle and were apparently enforced more stringently than in many other Latin American countries. In applying for a license to practice as an empiric in Puntarenas in 1863, Manuel de la Guardia of New Granada (Colombia) wrote that to practice medicine "in our country it is not necessary to have any titles beyond those of public confidence in accordance with our laws, [while] in this nation they demand titles I do not have."[91] A year later, Father Juan Corredor, recently arrived from either El Salvador or Guatemala (both origins were attributed to him) and denounced by the doctors of Cartago for practicing medicine without a license, explained to the governor that "I came from a Republic where there are no restrictions on curing."[92] If these might be dismissed as the hollow protestations of foreigners caught committing crimes in their new land, the memoirs of the German traveler and fortune hunter Wilhelm Marr offer more certain confirmation of the tight medical policing in the capital. Arriving in San José in 1853, even before the formal creation of a Protomedicato, he briefly thought about continuing to make his way by posing as a physician, only to realize that "the practice of medicine did not turn out to be so easy in Costa Rica as it had been in Nicaragua."[93] Feeling himself under the sharp scrutiny of doctors Bruno Carranza and Nazario Toledo, Marr decided instead to sell his camera equipment to survive.[94]

In San José, a rivalry developed among those who did have full license to practice medicine and pharmacy, and perhaps led to some commercial specialization. In an intriguing article on the diversification of consumption patterns in San José in the 1850s, Patricia Vega Jiménez has shown that European physician-pharmacist pairings had connections with continental suppliers and continued to expand the offerings of patent medicines. In 1860, the German pharmacist Juan Braun, who operated with the physician Francisco Ellendorf, offered to the public "a complete selection of new drugs and medicines, in addition to syringes, trusses, nursing bottles, mortars, pillboxes, a genuine remedy to kill rats and flies, and corrosive sublimate for anthills. New pills for intestinal worms, a new powder guaranteed to combat colic in infants."[95]

Adolphe Carit and Son, advertising themselves in 1858 as a "drugstore and wine shop," offered at retail and wholesale prices "a selection of drugs from Germany and France" along with "good wines of every kind, and pure wines especially selected for the use of invalids."[96]

Bruno Carranza, meanwhile, established himself as the exclusive representative of the English makers of Holloway's Pills, whose international popularity was echoed in San José. The Guatemalan Nazario Toledo specialized in "Central American products and spices," guaranteeing their "freshness" by offering only samples in his shop, which would then be ordered from suppliers on the basis of customer needs.[97] Dr. Salvador Riera, likely a dental surgeon, offered an "anacardine balm" manufactured locally to cure "toothache and pain in the ears and face in ten minutes."[98] The German merchant specialized in chemical-based pharmaceuticals and pesticides, the French in spirits, the Guatemalan in medicinal herbs and spices, and the only Costa Rican, Carranza, whose family's coffee connections were almost certainly with an English firm, established a specialty in an English line of natural patent medicines.

It is worth noting that as was the case throughout Latin American urban markets of the time, the protagonists in this rapid diversification of goods and services were Europeans with specialized skills and commercial connections.[99] The pharmaceutical explosion of the 1850s provided a greater variety of medicinal and technical alternatives for sufferers. That nine shops could maintain themselves in San José suggests a positive response from the populace (though a notable emphasis on natural ingredients in many of the advertisements for patent medicines perhaps indicates a backlash against the heroic treatments that were used so widely during the cholera epidemic of the mid-decade).

Commercial competition both motivated and frustrated demarcation between legitimate and illegitimate practice. For example, the proliferation of pharmacies in midcentury San José led to some fierce competition over professional legitimacy. In 1866 Dr. Bruno Carranza, then head of the Protomedicato as well as the owner of a pharmacy, ordered one of his competitors, "Carit and Son," to stop dispensing medicine or suffer fine and closure on the grounds that neither father nor son possessed recognized credentials. Alphonse Carit, in turn, criticized Carranza and other physicians for simply being medical fronts, allowing untrained clerks and even servants to dispense medicine while they pursued other business. Carranza questioned the Carits' contention that they provided excellent, experienced, and sober service, charging that "the pharmacy foments the charlatanism of curanderos [by] selling pomades, unguents, medicinal wines, and other substances under absurd and capricious names that they invent, like Lion and Elephant butter [and] Unicorn powder . . . [and] that they exploit the credulity of the people, diagnosing and prescribing for anyone who arrives to consult them about illnesses."[100]

Carranza argued on the basis of titular legitimacy and medico-pharmaceutical standards. Yet this was the same professor of medicine who made the panacean claim in an 1858 newspaper advertisement that the Holloway's Pills he had for sale in his pharmacy were "totally inoffensive in their operation and effect, while they seek out and remove illnesses of any type, of any severity, no matter how old or established they are."[101] Moreover, Carranza himself, though protomédico, was a licenciado rather than a full doctor of medicine, and likely only occupied the senior position due to his status as a rare titled national living in the capital. Carit countered by urging the state to judge the legitimacy of his practice on informal and commercial criteria: "the seniority [*antiguedad*] of our establishment, the good it has done for the people, the considerable quantity of our merchandise, and the losses that would befall us if the protomédico's order were executed." Still, in 1866, this argument won the day; the minister responsible ordered the police to ascertain the age of the business and determine that the empiric owners did indeed oversee it.[102] The Carits remained pillars of the pharmaceutical community and the San José elite, major charitable donors to the country's most important medical institutions, and in 1903, founders of the first maternity hospital, which bears their name to this day.

By the 1860s Costa Rica's physicians, surgeons, and pharmacists were characterized by a cultural split with political overtones, and another geographic division with a marked commercial and professional expression. Costa Ricans, Central Americans, and immigrant practitioners from other Hispanic countries occupied the political heights of the profession, but those among them who should have inherited the leadership mantle — native-born Costa Ricans — lived in the former colonial capital, Cartago. Meanwhile, medical and pharmaceutical practice in San José, the booming economic and political capital of the republic, was dominated by European immigrants. An antique institutional model of the Protomedicato, leprosarium, and charity hospital, hobbled together by local men forged in the embers of the colonial bonfire, contrasted with an emerging modern medical marketplace.

The threat that this contradiction posed to the institutional and political edifice of Costa Rican medicine was quite evident to Dr. Andres Sáenz. Sáenz was yet another Carthaginian who had studied medicine at Guatemala's San Carlos. As a representative to Congress in 1867, he pointed out the difficulty of maintaining the law requiring that the members of the Protomedicato be Costa Rican citizens. "There are scarcely seven or eight doctors who qualify . . . and the greatest share of them do not live in the capital." The situation caused a good deal of difficulty every year in electing a new tribunal and was "so great an anomaly that it has almost nullified the existence of the Protomedicato."[103] But the lack of native physicians in this dynamic medical marketplace was a vacuum that could not last, and even as Sáenz spoke, a new generation of young men from San José's preeminent families was abroad preparing to fill the void. Within thirty years Costa Rican-born physicians, most trained in Europe and the United States, would have a steady grip on a revamped network of medical institutions in the capital and take over practices throughout the republic.

3

The Formation of a Biomedical Vanguard

Between 1870 and 1900, the postcolonial Protomedicato system that had incorporated and regulated a heterogeneous range of practitioners was gradually displaced by a model of professional monopoly and biomedical reformism. A new generation of native-born physicians and surgeons, most from patrician San José families, was primarily responsible for this transformation. Over the last third of the century, the medical profession was nationalized and its stature dramatically elevated. Elite physicians acquired great political and ideological influence in the republican polity, and not only because they were members of the powerful merchant families of the oligarchy. The dramatic advances in surgery and the revolution in bacteriology that reshaped the scientific identity of medical doctors throughout the world during this period gave the Costa Rican profession a central symbolic role in the liberal polity, for in essential ways the promise of the new scientific medicine and its public health applications was a metaphor for the promise of the positivist project as a whole. The rise of this vanguard and the professionalization of medicine was integral to the building of a modern Costa Rican state apparatus.

The Costa Rican experience was a reproduction in miniature of a process occurring throughout Latin America in the last decades of the nineteenth century. Due to the small size of the professional community and the meager sums of public money available for institution building, the consolidation of a biomedical vanguard was in some ways less complete in Costa Rica than it was in large metropolitan centers like Mexico City and Buenos Aires. Yet in other ways, young, reform-minded Costa Rican physicians were able to make rapid and bold strides due to the relatively unencumbered spaces that they could occupy when they returned from their medical studies abroad. By the turn of the twentieth century, a small nucleus of medical scientists and public health reformers occupied the heights of society, politics, and the profession in the capital city, and had successfully embarked on some ambitious projects of medical modernization.

Medicine, Positivism, and Liberal Reform

Physicians played a central role in the rise of positivism as a governing ideology in Latin America, becoming key members of what Charles Hale calls "the liberal establishment." Though its basic principles were influential in political reform throughout the West, in Latin America positivism became a kind of official, secular religion, justifying and organizing the so-called liberal states that took shape after 1870. Politicians and intellectuals everywhere on the continent espoused a new faith in social engineering, often with notoriously tragic results. In an effort to accelerate the spread of capitalist production and secular modernity, existing carceral institutions, civil and penal codes, education systems, public bureaucracies, and militaries were analyzed, declared to be rife with antiquated Luso or Hispanic traditions (which could be read in Latin America as "colonial"), and systematically reconstructed with reference to models found in the United States and Europe. At the same time, civilizing campaigns were waged — sometimes with arms — against embodiments of ethnic or spiritual difference who were deemed a threat to the health of the national organism. All too often the result was genocide.[1]

The link between positivism and medicine was strong as well as unique. To begin with, Auguste Comte's founding texts of positivist philosophy explained society as a physiological organism. In both the *Cours de philosophie positive* (1830–1842) and *Système de politique positive* (1851–1854), biology was accorded a paradigmatic status in the hierarchical classification of the sciences, just below, and directly informing, "social physics." Appropriately, it was a young Mexican student of medicine, Gabino Barreda, who first introduced Comte's philosophical system to the Americas after attending his 1850 lecture series in Paris, and the earliest and among the strongest advocates of Mexican positivism was the Asociación Metodófila Gabino Barreda, a philosophical society of physician-disciples of Barreda.[2]

The basic positivist metaphor of society as an organism was made more compelling by the Pasteurian revolution of the 1870s and 1880s, plus the 1890s' "boom" in microbiology. As bacteriology won a series of spectacular triumphs, apparently promising humanity protection from some of its oldest threats, the metaphor became more convincing still, and proponents of positivist politics received greater acceptance. The new breed of medical doctors benefited from a reciprocal aggrandizement, and the physician became the very figure of the scientific savant capable of regulating the condition of the body politic, through prophylaxis or drastic intervention, in order to preserve its health.[3]

Latin American physicians achieved tangible political power due to their prior position in the local oligarchies and the vital status of their professional discourse within positivist ideology.[4] As Mauricio Tenorio-Trillo has noted, "Physicians were the most important receptors and disseminators of idealist, positivist, hygienist, and to a large extent, liberal ideas in nineteenth-century Mexico." The coterie of hygienist physicians led by men such as Eduardo Liceaga, Porfirio Parra, and Domingo Orvañanos transformed their posts at the medical school, in scientific institutes, and in various levels of government sanitation councils into the spaces and sources of power that made them part of the group of *científicos* who provided the compass to Porfirian public policy.[5] Ricardo Cruz-Coke has shown how in Chile, the new generation of physicians were members by birth or marriage of the positivist political class, and played a crucial role in the parliaments and cabinets of the period 1890–1925.[6] Indeed, a strong representation of physicians in national government is one of the unique aspects of Latin American medicine.[7]

In a cabinet, physicians might find themselves at the helm of any portfolio, but the one that most corresponded to their mission was Ministerio de Gobernación — the Ministry of the Interior — responsible for matters of public health (the physicians Guillermo Rawson and Eduardo Wilde of Argentina, for example, effected legendary urban sanitation reforms in this capacity as part of liberal governments).[8] Indeed, most historical work on the medical dimensions of Latin America's liberal-positivist regimes has focused on *higienismo* — the discourse and practice of the expanding municipal and national public health bureaucracies. Particularly in Argentina and Brazil, the strong hygienist bent to medical reform arose in conjunction with the rapid urbanization of metropolises like Buenos Aires, Rio de Janeiro, and São Paulo, and secondary centers like Rosario.[9]

Because San José's urban growth rate remained relatively benign (the city had only slightly over twenty thousand residents in 1900), Costa Rica's body of physicians did not throw up a specialized corps of activist hygiene reformers until the twentieth century was well underway. There was no one like Wilde or Emilio Coni, the titans of municipal hygiene in Buenos Aires in the 1880s; no Oswaldo Cruz, the anointed vaccinator of the new Rio, rebuilt by the Rodrigues Alves government according to the precepts of modern sanitation; no activist scientists with international profiles like the Cuban, Carlos Finlay, who first proposed the mosquito theory of yellow fever transmission in 1881, or Domingos José Freire, whose hunt for a yellow fever vaccine won acclaim in Brazil and abroad in the 1880s and 1890s.[10] Due to the small size of their professional community, and the limited dimensions of the urban polities on which they relied for their livelihood, Costa Rican physicians had no incentive for such specialized, full-time activism. Instead, their leading lights maintained an eclectic interest in a variety of domains, and pursued a general goal of progressive reform of medicine and public health. Nevertheless, their power was in many ways more immediate and palpable than that of their counterparts in other Latin American countries. Between 1890 and 1916, physicians accounted for 21 percent of the members of the Costa Rican Congress, while others occupied crucial cabinet posts and, in one instance, the presidency.[11]

Generational and Social Transformation

If the first influx of medical doctors after 1840 was characterized by eclecticism in terms of nationality, education, and commercial and professional ambition, the new medical vanguard was much more homogeneous in these terms, and self-consciously sought to reinforce the tendency toward standardization of professional practice, credentials, and identity. Beginning in the 1860s, as the coffee economy centered in San José achieved a mature prosperity, a steady stream of young men from wealthy families left the country to study medicine. This time the majority of them were from the new capital, and rather than study in Guatemala, they tended to journey further afield to Western Europe and the

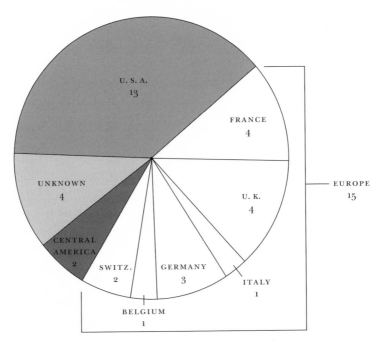

Fig. 2. Country of study of native Costa Rican physicians, 1870–1910.

United States. The country's body of medical practitioners began a dramatic metamorphosis. Between 1870 and 1910, one hundred and ninety-five physicians and surgeons had their credentials recognized and began to practice in the country (four times more than in the previous forty years). Of the fifty-four whose nationality can be determined, thirty-four (63 percent) were natives of Costa Rica, and almost half of these were from San José. The remaining twenty were an eclectic assortment of Latin Americans, North Americans, and Europeans.[12]

There was also a marked change in the places that the young nationals studied (see figure 2). Of those thirty-four who are known to have been Costa Rican by birth, just under half journeyed to Europe for medical studies, most of them to France, Germany, and the U.K. Almost the same portion received their training in the United States. Most significantly, the University of San Carlos lost its hegemonic role in Costa Rican medical education almost overnight; based on existing evidence, only two Costa Ricans had Guatemalan degrees. Many now attended institutions closer to the mainstream of modern medical studies like Guy's Hospital (three), the University of Pennsylvania (two), New York University, and the Universities of Strasbourg, Geneva, and Paris.[13] For the fifty years following independence, Guatemalan-trained physicians had been among the elite practitioners; during this second phase, the native or immigrant physician with a Latin American degree would tend to occupy the lower rather than upper ranks of the professional ladder.[14]

The San José municipal census of 1904 presents a striking picture of the rapid nationalization of the profession and the greater vitality of the new community of native doctors. Of the twenty-nine medical doctors resident when the census takers arrived, twenty were Costa Rican by birth; of those twenty, fourteen were originally from San José. The other nine doctors registered in the census were assorted foreigners.[15] Moreover, the immigrant physicians had an average age of 51, compared to an average age of 38.5 for the practitioners of Costa Rican origin. Ten of the Costa Ricans had graduated in Europe, ten in the United States, and only one in Guatemala — the seventy-eight-year-old Andres Sáenz, originally of Cartago.[16]

Many of these Costa Rican nationals were members of the oligarchy, as a brief description of their background and households suggests. Dr. Mauro Fernández was the son of the like-named grand liberal reformer of education (Costa Rica's Sarmiento); in the year of the census, he lived at home with his widowed mother, six siblings, and six servants. Jorge Lara Iraeta was the son of a wealthy planter, and his patrimonial household boasted a family of fifteen spread over three generations and attended by five servants. Fernando Iglesias Tinoco, the offspring of a marital union of two of the country's most politically powerful families, lived with an aunt and two sisters, and enjoyed the comforts of five servants. José María Soto Alfaro, from an influential and prosperous Alajuela clan and brother to Bernardo Soto, the former president of the republic, indulged his single lifestyle with two servants and the ostentation of a "colored" (Jamaican) coachman to ferry him about the streets of the capital city. Dr. Carlos Durán, who both personified and propelled the transformation of elite medical practice in Costa Rica during the last thirty years of the century, was the son of a prosperous merchant and had inherited small yet valuable coffee fincas on the immediate outskirts of the capital; in 1904 he, his wife, and his five children were maintained by eight servants.[17]

Carlos Durán traveled to Paris in 1869 to study medicine, but after the outbreak of the Franco-Prussian War, switched to the medical school of Guy's Hospital in London — still preeminent among the city's medical colleges. Durán trained in a charged and polemical atmosphere of reform. Joseph Lister's experiments in, and arguments in favor of, antiseptic surgery and wound management had shaken the discipline, although they were greeted with skepticism by many English surgeons because Lister's assumptions rested on Pasteur's still controversial germ theory. Durán apprenticed with Henry Howse, not only the newly appointed assistant surgeon at Guy's but also recently returned from a journey to Edinburgh to make a careful study of Lister's antiseptic system. During Durán's years at Guy's, the institution underwent a precocious conversion to Listerism (carbolic spray producers were in general use in the wards there by 1873).[18] His London training also coincided with a great debate over hospital design and the related sweeping reform of nursing spearheaded by Florence Nightingale. After receiving his title from the Royal College of Surgeons, Durán embarked on the Latin American junior reforming oligarch's grand tour, visiting the hospitals of Brussels, Paris, Milan, and Vienna before returning home.[19] According to a later disciple, on the young Dr. Durán's first visit to the Hospital San Juan de Diós, with operations still performed in the dirt-floored corridor, he witnessed Dr. Bruno Carranza amputate the leg of a man without using anesthetic and surrounded by patients who, "some in amazement, others faint of heart and fearful, witnessed the extraordinary spectacle."[20]

Durán was appointed the first hospital surgeon in the late 1870s, then named to San José's Junta of Charity and invested as protomédico in 1881, enabling him to initiate a series of hospital reforms. He designed and had built modern surgical facilities and new hospital pavilions, reorganized the nursing staff, and installed basic laboratory facilities. An interesting comparison could be made between Durán's reform of the Hospital San Juan de Dios and the contemporary proposal for the state-of-the-art Johns Hopkins Hospital, which was influenced by an 1876 tour of European facilities by designer John S. Billings that closely shadowed that of Durán's (Billings visited hospitals in London, Leipzig, Berlin, Vienna, and Paris). Billings was especially concerned with breaking down the block hospital into smaller, separate buildings to prevent institutional hospitalism. Though there was still no consensus on the best means for overcoming the endemic infection, the modern hospital world was embracing antiseptics as well as a new stress on improved ventilation that reflected persistent miasmatic theories of infection. Of course, Durán's Hospital San Juan de Dios was a poor man's Hopkins, but by 1900 the entire original block had been broken down into separate pavilions, and the new operating room was described by a physician just returned from studies in Germany as "built according to the most modern rules for best service and disinfection."[21]

Durán was at the center of a collegial group of young physicians and surgeons who pioneered a number of operations, like ovariotomies, that were paradigmatic of the new surgery, made possible by the combination of antiseptic (and increasingly, aseptic) practices, the use of anesthetics, and the development of new invasive techniques. Durán also began to combine clinical findings with basic bacteriology and parasitology, which led him to make the Costa Rican discovery of hookworm disease (a subject I will return to below).[22] If one put together a Latin American pantheon of reformist titans of the "heroic age" of modern medicine, Durán would be the Costa Rican representative.[23]

In 1885, President Bernardo Soto appointed Durán secretary of the interior (responsible for matters of public health). He thus became the medical intellectual of the "*Olimpo*" — the Olympians, Costa Rica's generation of brilliant young positivist intellectuals who coalesced in the radical reformist cabinets of the 1880s. In 1889, the Church successfully led a popular rebellion against the anticlerical Olympian coterie (who were attempting to perpetrate a fraud to keep the Church-backed candidate from winning the presidency). As part of the brokered ceasefire, Durán, who was third designate to the presidency, had broad enough respect to serve a transitional six-month period as head of state (an office he was never able to recapture, though he was a candidate for the presidency on a number of occasions, served as a congressional deputy for eight terms, and occupied ministerial portfolios in various governments).[24]

With certain key variations, Durán's career was shadowed by Juan Ulloa Giralt, who was an even more criollo personification of the change in Costa Rican medicine. Ulloa's father was the government minister responsible for granting a charter to the Brotherhood of Charity in

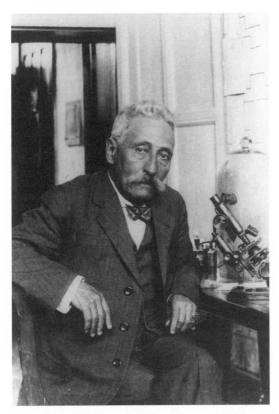

Fig. 3. Carlos Durán, patriarch of Costa Rican biomedicine, c. 1910. Courtesy of Carmela Velázquez.

1864, an oligarchic council that finally ensured the Hospital San Juan
de Dios would reopen on firm financial ground; his mother was a member of the original group of señoras who served on the "committee of
ladies" that supported the brotherhood. In 1877, Ulloa was one of
three students who received the title of bachelor of medicine from the
University of Santo Tomás after the institution experienced a minor
renaissance in medical instruction based on the clinical experience that
was finally available in the hospital (the presence of Durán was probably
principally responsible for this). The young medical apprentice then
embarked for New York University, receiving his doctorate in medicine
in 1879 before returning to Costa Rica.[25]

Ulloa was simultaneously named protomédico and rector of the University of Santo Tomás in 1888. While serving in both capacities, he

made an unsuccessful effort to build a permanent medical program at the university. Appointed minister of the interior in 1894, he presided over a series of important reforms in medicine and public health.[26] Never a pioneer of medical or surgical procedures, nor interested in laboratory research, Ulloa became a key figure in the early internationalization of public health in the Americas. Like most Central American politicians of the era, he was allied to the U.S. drive for hegemony in the game of "Pan-Americanism." He was Costa Rica's first representative at the Pan-American Medical Congress in Washington, D.C., in 1892 and a member of the board of the International Sanitary Bureau of the Union of the American Republics from its inception in 1902 through to the holding of the bureau's fourth congress in San José in 1909. In 1900, while on a diplomatic mission to the United States, Ulloa was immediately able to translate and forward a report on the breakthrough in the U.S. military's yellow fever trials in Cuba (of major interest in Costa Rica, which had suffered a serious outbreak of the disease in Alajuela the previous year).[27]

The best-known liberal reforms in Latin America are those in the areas of public education, civil and penal law, and church-state relations. The Costa Rican state recapitulated the classic continental patterns of reform in each of these areas between 1880 and 1888. It is also valid, however, to speak of a "liberal medical reform" in Costa Rica beginning in the 1880s and culminating in the mid-1890s. Part of this echoed the hygienist heyday of Latin American metropoles. For example, starting in the late 1890s the leaders of the medical community promoted the rebuilding of San José's waterworks, the development of systems to purify water discharges from coffee-processing facilities, the construction of hygienic houses, and the training of mothers in hygienic child-rearing practices — the latter three concerns subjects of prizewinning essays in a competition sponsored by the new professional organization.[28] In 1894, the state and medical profession also embraced the standard Latin American *higienista* obsession with the registry, examination, and treatment of prostitutes, codified in the new Law on Venereal Prophylaxis.[29]

Atypically for Latin America, the boldest and most sustained efforts in Costa Rican state medicine were undertaken in the rural sector. Much of this was organized around the treatment of hookworm disease after 1906 (a subject I will deal with in a separate chapter). But this orientation was already manifest in the 1893 legal redefinition of the office of town doctor and the rapid expansion in the number of posts. The district physicians were invested with much more explicit jurisdiction over questions of public health in their regions and charged with a more systematic provision of statistical data in quarterly reports to the Ministry of the Interior. Their numbers were expanded from eight to as many as forty, corresponding to the new cantonal administrative units. The medical community was now conceived of as an integral component of the state infrastructure and technically the network of official medical knowledge was now coextensive with all areas of significant population in the country.[30] The hospital reforms of the 1880s and 1890s might also be situated as part of this positivist reform since the makeover of the Hospital San Juan de Dios was part of a project to create a modern architecture of the state in the capital city. Finally, and perhaps most important, the liberal medical reform was capped in 1895 with the creation of a new professional association — the Faculty of Medicine, Surgery, and Pharmacy — to replace the Protomedicato. Again, Durán and Ulloa were at the heart of this process.

Professional Association

A Medical Association had been decreed in 1858, and it was common during the country's first era of medical professionalism for eminent practitioners to come together at the request of the government to prepare an official response in times of public health emergency. No doubt doctors exchanged opinions on medical matters in social settings, during activities relating to natural science, or while collaborating professionally. But if the Medical Association itself ever had a moment of effective existence, it was certainly moribund when Ulloa returned from his studies in the United States in 1879. He soon teamed up with Durán to found the Costa Rican Medical Society. In the first issue of the *Medical Gazette*, which was to serve as the official organ of the new society, Durán explained that "for some time now the physicians of the republic have felt the need for a society where we could meet to discuss issues related to the profession, and thereby foment union and brotherhood between the members, and make possible the establishing of rules of medical ethics that would regulate the professional relations of doctors." For its part, the journal was aimed at contributing, "even if only in a small way, to the progress of medicine in our country" by making the latest medical knowledge "available to all those who wish to have it."[31]

Although an initiative of the young Costa Rican nationals, twenty-three of the country's thirty-five doctors joined the society, including some of the resident German and French physicians. Members would gather each month in San José to present clinical and epidemiological findings. Only twelve of the twenty-three members were from the capital, and doctors from other towns, including Puntarenas, made rather arduous journeys to attend the meetings.[32] Three or four clinical cases were presented for discussion, members compared notes on epidemic diseases such as yellow fever, and new surgical techniques were outlined. There was an exchange of the latest medical news culled from the members' combined journal subscriptions (usually from countries where they had studied). Summaries of the talks were to be printed in the *Medical Gazette,* and significant reports from the foreign medical press were reproduced. For example, Durán translated one of Lister's articles on microorganisms as pathogens from the *British Medical Journal,* which Spanish-speaking physicians in Costa Rica could peruse in their own language within seven months of its appearance in England.[33]

This first Costa Rican professional journal was tardy for Latin America, where medical publications were closing a second cycle by the 1880s. The initial, short-lived batch had appeared where one might expect to find them: the *Anales de la Academia Nacional de Medicina* in 1823 in Argentina (the academy had been founded the year before), *Propagador das ciencias médicas* and *Semanaria de Saude Pública* in Brazil on the heels of the founding of the Royal Medical and Surgical Society in 1829, and in Mexico, *Higia* in 1833, coinciding with the founding of the new medical faculty and school. Durán and Ulloa's journal was inspired by similar energies: to organize the voice of a community of scientifically oriented practitioners rather than serve as a mere institutional expression. The Costa Rican Medical Society and its journal dissolved in 1881, victims of the limited size of the community of physicians and the overwhelming time commitment required of the two main sparkplugs to keep the project going. The effort resembled many other premature Latin American attempts to give upstart medical faculties a forum for discussion during the 1840s and 1850s, most of them similarly short-lived.[34]

Rather than burning out, however, the energies of Durán and Ulloa were redirected into reforming the Hospital San Juan de Dios, which during the 1880s started to become a focus for the clinical, surgical, and research interests of a de facto medical society. At the same time, the Protomedicato entered into a period of crisis, with a series of conflicts over the norms of medical licensing and policing culminating in 1889 with the resignation of the entire board. But in the first congressional session of 1890, following Durán's transitional presidency, the physicians in the legislature introduced a proposal on behalf of their professional colleagues to reform the Protomedicato and replace it with a Faculty of Medicine. The bill was particularly concerned with eliminating the fee schedules established in 1872, now considered outmoded due to inflation; doctors called for a free market in fees, with the rates to be posted in their offices. The legislation did not pass during the tumultuous Rodríguez government (1890–1894), which closed Congress and imposed a state of emergency for much of its mandate. The reform project was revived and immediately approved, though, under the subsequent government of Rafael Iglesias, whose minister of the interior was Ulloa.[35]

The Protomedicato was formally dissolved in April 1895, and the venerable Andres Sáenz brought to order the first session of the Faculty of Medicine, Surgery, and Pharmacy, the direct ancestor of Costa Rica's current College of Physicians. The faculty consolidated the professional tendencies that had been expressed only weakly in the Protomedicato and Medical Association. It gave complete authority to the association of physicians to elect their own leadership, define their own professional strictures, and set medical and public health norms throughout the country. This organization acquired exceptional clout when Ulloa was elected as the faculty's second president in 1896 while still serving as the minister of the interior. Once Ulloa's dual tenure ended in 1900 and he took up a diplomatic post in the United States, some members complained that the new organization had less influence over public policy than the Protomedicato because its leaders had no formal position within the state and so government officials did not have to obey their wishes. This obviously reflected a deeply held conviction on the part of physicians, perhaps born of frustration over the unwillingness of government to police irregular medicine more strictly and enforce the de jure monopoly of physicians. Nevertheless, during the twenty-seven-year period stretching from the founding of the faculty until the creation of a Subsecretariat of Hygiene in 1922, this technically private association of professionals enjoyed almost complete jurisdiction over questions of medicine and public health — an extraordinary power that physicians had never had until that time, and one they would never experience again after they were unceremoniously pushed aside in favor of a ministerial model in 1922.[36]

But if the creation of a Faculty of Medicine in 1895 did not immediately translate into the effective policing of the association's professional monopoly, it was crucial in articulating a more coherent and homogeneous set of licensing standards as well as medical ethics for practitioners, alerting practitioners to scientific and professional news, and fomenting a collegiality and professional identity that was inseparable from a sense of national and scientific mission. The faculty also gave institutionalized expression to a national medical elite who set standards and goals for the profession, and defined hierarchies for practitioners throughout the country.

The election of Ulloa in 1895 inaugurated a veritable golden age in Costa Rican medical professionalism. Ulloa dominated the faculty board for the first five years, was succeeded by another young patrician, Rafael Calderón Muñoz, for the next five, and then Durán reemerged as the guiding light of the profession for the five years beginning in 1905. The mainstays of the faculty during these fifteen years were the medical elite of San José. Virtually all were nationals, although foreign physicians were still welcome to play an important role, particularly if they were *gente* like the Ecuadoran César Borja (in temporary political exile, and who would return directly to his country to take up a senior cabinet post in 1903) and Spanish oculist Juan Arrea y Cosp. Although there were sometimes distinguished physicians from outside of San José on the board (usually from Heredia, the closest of the major towns to the capital), and physicians from all the major towns including Limón and Puntarenas infrequently attended sessions and corresponded, the board of the Faculty of Medicine, Surgery, and Pharmacy was dominated by the doctors of the capital city.

The board met each week for an evening session that lasted two to four hours. An average meeting considered petitions from newcomers for incorporation into the faculty, and if necessary, set dates and committees for qualifying exams; if these had already taken place and the candidate was successful, the junta would confer an official license to practice.

Complaints about the illegal practice of medicine were heard, weighed, and referred to the appropriate authorities (who generally responded halfheartedly or not at all). In 1909, the faculty retained the old Protomedicato's judicial function, and elected an agente fiscal who could initiate investigations and lay charges against illegal practitioners.[37]

A good deal of time was taken up with cases of legal medicine assigned to individual members, but whose findings had to be ratified by the board. Delegates to international conferences were nominated or their reports were heard, and projects for medical and public health reform were called for or proposed — for a school of pharmacy, obstetrics, or nursing, for improvements in urban sanitation, and so on. Extraordinary sessions were convoked during times of epidemics or other pressing public health or professional concerns. Physicians might be appointed to visit an area stricken by an epidemic outbreak and take emergency measures if necessary. In the case of the 1899 yellow fever epidemic in Alajuela, an entire team of physicians was dispatched to make an exact determination of the disease as well as to take over the allegedly bungled containment operation of the local authorities and district physicians.[38]

A Code of Medical Ethics, adopted late in the life of the Protomedicato through the reforming impetus of the short-lived Costa Rican Medical Society, was ratified by the Faculty of Medicine. It was only occasionally invoked: in 1896, the board censured two doctors from the capital, one of the old school and the other of the new, who had put their portraits beside newspaper advertisements recommending Scott's Emulsion, on the grounds that this practice was "against Medical Ethics and professional decorum" — a rather harsh reproach for endorsing cod liver oil, but perhaps reflective of a drive to prevent the profession's image of objective integrity from being tarnished by commercial endorsements.[39]

Medical Education

The statutes of Costa Rica's new Faculty of Medicine, Surgery, and Pharmacy contained vague references to it serving as the foundation of a future medical school — indeed, the function had been inherently attached to official medical bodies since the earliest days of the Protomedicato, embodied in the term facultativo (which is synonymous with medical doctor). Any interest in establishing a medical school was complicated by the closure of the University of Santo Tomás in 1888. The university, which formerly hosted haphazard efforts to develop medical education, had finally succeeded in graduating three bachelors in medicine in the 1870s. Its demise was part of an education reform that sought to concentrate resources at the level of primary and secondary training and left the College of Law as the only postsecondary institution in the country. No medical school was on the immediate agenda, although within five years of its founding the faculty had successfully sponsored a college of pharmacy and school of obstetrics (subjects I will return to in a future chapter).[40]

In this, Costa Rica went against a continental trend. The latter half of the nineteenth century was a time of great expansion in medical education throughout Latin America, motivated by the consolidation of national and regional identities and institutions, a need for more practitioners, and the demand of the respectable middle classes for respectable postsecondary training for their children. In Argentina, the 1852 reform of the medical school coincided with the consolidation of the federal state and initiated a takeoff in the training of native practitioners. In 1867, a new medical school was founded in Guayaquil, a booming second city with a poor public health record and historic shortage of physicians, and was consolidated over the following twenty years. The medical school of Montevideo dates from 1876, and that of the University of Córdoba was inaugurated in 1877. In Peru, the shock of losing the War of the Pacific led to a general modernization of institutions, including the "refloating" of the Faculty of Medicine at San Marcos, as Marcos Cueto puts it.[41] A similar process was at work in Central America, where in the 1880s a thoroughly reformed medical faculty was reopened in San Salvador and a new institution inaugurated in Tegucigalpa, Honduras. In Nicaragua, the university in Granada began to offer medical instruction (to emulate the academy in the archrival city of León). By the end of the nineteenth century, Costa Rica was one of only four Latin American political territories without the capacity to graduate physicians (Panama, Paraguay, and Puerto Rico were the others).[42]

What effect did the absence of a local medical school have on the shape of Costa Rica's professional community? One of the main results may well have been that Costa Rica, despite its small number of practitioners, had a more up-to-date, intellectually flexible, and research-oriented medical establishment than did countries *with* medical schools. For example, in 1889, when the Ecuadoran government contracted Gustavo von Lagerheim of Hamburg to train Quito doctors in bacteriology (he apparently brought the first microscope to be known in the country), the doctor received a chilly reception from the highlands medical establishment and left in a huff in 1892. In Brazil and Cuba, medical instruction remained under the sway of a traditionalist cabal, and posts were passed down through clientelism and nepotism.[43] Julyan Peard cites Gilberto Freyre's withering critique of the Bahian medical school prior to 1880 in which he claims that instruction subordinated "scientific study to the study of classical literature, oratory, elegance, and purity in speaking and writing, to debate over questions more grammatical than physiological, and to dissecting problems closer to the pathology of literary style than to human anatomy."[44] Dain Borges concludes that the Brazilian medical faculties "existed to transmit ideas more than to invent them" — a determination of passive transmission within the academy essentially shared by Nancy Leys Stepan and Peard. Even after the changes wrought by republican politics at home and the revolution in bacteriology abroad, students received "homeopathic doses of practical experience in anatomy and microbiology [and a] bounty of experience in the scholastic mode."[45] Marcos Cueto confirms the same for Lima, where despite efforts at reform and the creation of a chair in bacteriology in 1895, "science did not displace the ornamental and memory-based education that reined in the University."[46]

All of Costa Rica's physicians and surgeons had studied outside the country, and all of the leading lights in the profession had received training in centers of medical science. Especially for the first generation of returning native practitioners, there was no need to err on the side of tradition in order to curry favor with a stagnant old school. Furthermore, the eclectic array of institutions in which they had studied prevented any particular orthodoxy from taking hold. For example, many Latin American university medical programs were beholden to the curriculum of the Paris Medical Faculty — the case of Buenos Aires being the most extreme — and a fervent commitment to orthodox clinical medicine retarded the expansion of teaching into the laboratory-based domains of cellular biology and bacteriology. In Costa Rica, new medical ideas seem to have been discussed, tried out, and incorporated without great obstacles. This may have been a case of the "advantage of backwardness" playing itself out in medical culture, allowing a direct and unfettered implantation of a relatively advanced model of scientific activity among physicians and surgeons, at least in the capital city.[47]

One should not be too sanguine about this. For one thing, almost all of Latin America's scientifically ambitious physicians either studied in Europe or traveled there to complete their training after graduating from the local universities. The great Brazilian microbiologist and public health reformer Oswaldo Cruz was only exceptional in doing his postgraduate training at the Pasteur Institute: hundreds of Brazilian students studied medicine in Montpellier, Brussels, and Louvain in the nineteenth century, and many more did further studies or residencies in Europe after graduating at home. The numbers of Argentine medical students in Paris reached the point that in 1901, a group of nineteen was able to found a "Centro de médicos argentinos."[48] This was a product of state policy as well as personal choice and wealth. The liberal modernizing regimes began to endow the bright lights of national medicine with scholarships to study abroad.

The very policy, however, underscores the obstacles to medical modernization in many countries, for it was part of a state strategy to circumvent the institutional bottleneck of the local universities and traditionalism of the local medical establishments (the case of Cruz and his bacteriologic institute is the best known).[49] On their return, many of these scholarship students found their métier in institutions of research and experimental practice that were outside the traditional university structure, typically within the network of national or municipal public health facilities. In Peru, the distinguished bacteriologist David Matto was unusual in finding a place inside the university, though many other Peruvians who had studied abroad on state fellowships returned to work in the national department of health or Lima's municipal hygiene facility.[50]

Did Costa Rica's lack of a local medical school mean less practitioners? If one compares Costa Rica to Ecuador, it would seem that it did not. Despite the Andean country having two schools of its own, professional growth rates were about the same as in Costa Rica. Between 1863 and 1909, the numbers of physicians in Ecuador roughly tripled, from 81 to 236; in Costa Rica, they grew at a slightly faster rate, from about 30 in 1864 to 106 in 1914.[51] While the popularity of medicine grew enormously at Peru's University of San Marcos between 1854 and 1868, the proportion of students enrolled in the discipline moving from 7 to 31 percent, there were still only 78 medical students in the latter year, and between 1857 and 1899 the number of physicians graduating in any given year was never more than 20.[52] Julyan Peard's figures for enrollments in the Bahia and Rio de Janeiro Medical Schools between the 1860s and 1889 show that graduation rates among those who matriculated in medicine fluctuated between 10 and 20 percent, and the numbers of medical graduates from both faculties combined averaged only 110 per year.[53]

Of course, the fact that to become a physician in Costa Rica meant undertaking an expensive sojourn abroad all but guaranteed that practitioners would be from a higher social standing than those in a country where candidates could study at home. Native Costa Rican practitioners were a homogeneous lot in terms of class, race, and gender. The country's first female physician, Jadwisia de Picado, was a Polish immigrant who had married a native practitioner during their student years in Europe. She incorporated in 1902, thirteen years after Cecilia Grierson became the first Argentine woman to receive a medical degree, and fifteen after Brazil graduated its first woman physician. Picado's incorporation was fair and uncontested; her exam was approved and the faculty voted unanimously in favor of her incorporation, without her sex being officially raised as an issue. Given the apparent lack of strong opposition to the idea of female practitioners among the all-male Costa Rican medical establishment, a local school would likely have allowed more women to pursue the career. As it was, the first Costa Rican–born woman to complete medical studies abroad did not return to practice until 1923.[54] As for class, the upper-crust origin of most Costa Rican native practitioners certainly shaped their approach to medicine but it did not translate into resistance to reform of the profession or medical practice during this era. And had there been more from a lower-class background, they would not necessarily have been more radical. Julyan Peard notes that the Bahian medical school was well stocked with sons of the petite bourgeoisie, but concludes that this lower social standing actually made them more conformist since any reformist impulses might have jeopardized their opportunities for social climbing.[55]

Neither did the absence of a medical school prevent the development of a small community of medical scientists. This was promoted by professional association, and by the reorganization and modernization of hospital facilities. The Faculty of Medicine maintained a reading room with a number of leading medical publications and generous hours (although the board chastised physicians for their failure to make proper use of it). A wave of enthusiasm swept through the capital's doctors in 1899, and a weekly series of "open conferences" was planned, with each physician in the country invited to speak in alphabetic order. Again, though, it was attended largely by the elite practitioners of the city. The talks were published in the *Gaceta Médica*. The success of these informal talks led to an effort by some of the younger recruits in the capital to form an Academy of Medicine and Natural Sciences, another common phenomenon in Latin America, though the Cuban and Brazilian academies were much earlier. Only physicians joined, however, and the enthusiasm ran out after four months, and with it the academy.[56]

The *Gaceta Médica* itself was a prime manifestation of the crossing of professional and scientific purpose, and the fact that the journal was published monthly for over twenty years demonstrates that the medical profession had achieved a certain mature strength by the turn of the twentieth century. The journal had high standards, establishing itself as a quality compendium of professional business, clinical, and surgical case studies, articles on national medical and public health initiatives, translations of international articles of importance, and reports on new pharmaceuticals, techniques, and technologies. The gazette was part of a notable increase in medical publishing in Costa Rica. A grand total of six books on medicine had been published in the country between the arrival of the printing press in 1830 and 1895; over the following fifteen years, along with the publications in the gazette, at least twenty-four medical treatises were published. They included a translation of Ronald Ross's work on the cause, prevention, and treatment of malaria, William C. Gorgas's work on mosquito eradication to prevent yellow fever, textbooks for the School of Obstetrics, a three-volume manual on sanitary policing by the German-trained Roberto Cortés, as well as the three prizewinning books noted above.[57]

Surgery that was in local terms experimental, was the preserve of a small circle of highly trained men who pioneered new techniques in the surgical department of the capital's hospital. The atmosphere appears to have been more collegial than competitive. Durán, for instance, happily stepped aside to allow Tomás Calnek the honor of performing the country's first ovariotomy (1891) and hysterectomy (1895), both of which ended well for the patient (similar operations were undertaken throughout Latin America on roughly the same schedule). Unusual cases of surgery would become the object for clinical seminars. As part of the lecture series organized by the faculty in 1899, Gerardo Jiménez Núñez presented the case of a young female orphan operated on at the hospital for a complicated wound to the thoracic cavity. He used hospital charts and files documenting the amounts and appearance of urine and feces before and after the operation, changes in patient temperature, and other vital measurements. The four-hour session ended with a lively discussion between Jiménez, Calnek, and the hospital's surgery residents, Federico Zumbado and Elías Rojas. The talk was also the basis of a paper published in the *Gaceta Médica*.[58]

Marcos Cueto has observed that the positivist intellectual milieu of fin de siècle Peru generated a "scientific nationalism" that sought to elucidate hitherto ignored material realities, leading to research such as that which discovered the germ that caused Verruga Peruana.[59] A similar ideological context motivated a trio of San José's leading doctors to carry out experiments on one of their country's most common afflictions in 1894–1895, even though the bacteriologic laboratory they had created at the Hospital San Juan de Dios was still "in diapers" (as one physician later put it).[60] Durán had observed that among the patients he saw in the hospital, there were a large number with chronic anemia who did not respond to standard treatment, and whose condition was accompanied by odd heart palpitations and noises. Going over some back issues of the *Lancet,* he came on a report of Edoardo Perroncito's 1880 discovery that hookworm infection was the cause of an outbreak of severe anemia in the Italian laborers digging the St. Gotthard tunnel in Switzerland. The workers' symptoms were much like those he was observing, and he mentioned his suspicions to the hospital surgeon, Calnek. A patient under Calnek's care who exhibited these symptoms died soon after, and the young surgeon intern Gerardo Jiménez Núñez practiced an autopsy under the direction of his two senior colleagues and found multitudes of hookworms in the esophagus.[61]

Durán and Jiménez realized that these symptoms corresponded to the condition called *cansancio* (weariness), a debilitating fatigue common in parts of rural Costa Rica. Some physicians had speculated that the condition was due to poor water supplies, while others attributed the symptoms to a form of malaria. The two confirmed their hunch with an expedition to Puriscal, where cansancio was particularly endemic, discovering ancylostoma eggs in the fecal matter of many sufferers. They began performing autopsies regularly on patients who had perished while suffering acute anemia at the capital's hospital, and repeatedly found that their digestive tracts were infested with hookworms. They then undertook systematic fecal exams on all patients with these symptoms and treated those who tested positive with thymol, the vermifuge used by Perroncito during the 1880 outbreak. In February 1895, Durán submitted his findings to the Guatemalan Faculty of Medicine (Costa Rica's faculty and its gazette were still a number of months from birth). He and Jiménez began to map hookworm infestation in Costa Rica based on the geographic origins of the sufferers examined in the hospital (probably the country's first attempt at medical geography).[62]

Though he made no mention of it, Durán's instincts might also have been nudged by knowledge of Herbert Prowe's discoveries in the late 1880s that ancylostomiasis was endemic to El Salvador and Guatemala. It is less likely that he would have been aware of Otto Wucherer's 1868–1871 articles in the *Gazeta Médica da Bahia* concerning his discovery of ancylostoma in autopsy subjects who had been suffering from *cansanço,* a severe tropical anemia.[63] In his classic study of the discovery of hookworm disease in the United States, John Ettling remarks that "by 1875 [when Durán finished his medical studies in England] European physicians with a respectable grounding in parasitology and certainly all European zoologists knew about hookworms and accepted them as the cause of a severe anemia characteristically found in warmer climates."[64] Unfortunately for Wucherer, Prowe, and Durán, a generalist's knowledge of parasitology prevented them from refining their discoveries and perhaps winning international acclaim, for they had actually uncovered a different species of hookworm than that identified by Perroncito in Europe. Charles Wardell Stiles would get the credit for discovering *Anchylostoma americana* in 1901.[65]

It is worth comparing the project of the Costa Rican generation of reformers with the formation of the Tropicalista School of Bahia some fifteen years earlier, for it underlines the latitude enjoyed by young men like Durán and Ulloa—of a breadth that would have been enviable to the Brazilians. It also highlights the fact that scientific ambitions were shared by many medical practitioners on the periphery who wished to achieve according to standards they considered international. Julyan Peard locates the beginnings of the Tropicalista School in the initiative of John Paterson, a Scot resident for many years in Brazil, to hold an informal fortnightly gathering of interested physicians to discuss their own cases as well as reports in the latest medical literature. The group's access to the marginalized Santa Casa hospital was central to their ability to cultivate a nucleus of world-class scientists, "a means to centralize the Tropicalistas' otherwise isolated research efforts, and a place where like-minded doctors could experiment with new surgical methods and therapies." Also crucial was the founding of their own journal, a "vehicle for publication and discourse."[66]

There are striking similarities between this crucible and the forge that generated Costa Rica's first nucleus of scientifically driven physicians—not least the fact that among the Brazilians' first scientific breakthroughs was Wucherer's discovery of ancylostomiasis in 1866. Both groups defined themselves through a youthful critique of an antiquated medical establishment, and grew out of gatherings to share clinical experience and scientific knowledge. In each case, a group identity was institutionalized by gaining access to a charity hospital where they had free rein to transform the facility into a research center and by founding a journal. There are notable differences as well. Costa Rica's scientific nucleus came somewhat later and its central promoters were nationals. It was correspondingly more formal in its aspirations, though it never established a "school" as such, and it did not boast quite such brilliant lights as Paterson, Wucherer, and Nina Rodrigues. But most crucial for the evolution of Costa Rican medicine and public health, the San José physicians were not a group of resident aliens and avant-garde greenhorns marginalized from professional power in a somewhat decadent regional center; they were members of the national ruling class who occupied the profession's most important positions in the capital city.

Though it may not have registered with the world's leading medical journals, the Costa Rican discovery was impressive given the nascent state of research in the country. It reveals the rare ambition of a core of physicians who were eager to illuminate the national health through an engagement with the international scientific community. Costa Rica, then, like its larger Latin American counterparts, must be put on the map of peripheral countries that developed small, but highly original and motivated vanguards of medical research. As we will see in a later chapter on the campaigns to eradicate hookworm, the greater significance of this early triumph in Costa Rican medical research lay in its applications, an area in which the country's experience was extraordinary indeed, and placed it at the forefront of Latin American — and even global — public health.

It is tempting to characterize this drastic transformation of Costa Rican elite practitioners as a process of medical decolonization. The foreign, mostly European practitioners who had dominated medicine and pharmacy in San José were displaced. A powerful coterie of native-born physicians equipped with advanced learning and a strong spirit of reform created a professional as well as political space for elite medical practice, and understood their role in terms of the progress of the nation on the nation's terms. Yet clearly, the main result of young nationals assuming a directive role over the reform of medicine was a more rapid and efficient implementation of models of professional association along with medical and surgical practices associated with the United States and Europe. Like all decolonization processes in the modern world, this one was paradoxical. The progress and national well-being promoted by the new national community of doctors was not incompatible with the exigencies of local and foreign capital, a model of medical commercialism and professional monopoly, and the ideologies that prevailed in the imperial metropoles. Throughout Latin America, this second wave of physicians would itself reproduce "colonizing" projects within its national borders. Nevertheless, this generation did create the first network of national medical institutions and establish the first coherent agenda of national health concerns. As we will see, in both areas doctors maintained a great degree of autonomy from the state, the ruling class of cafetaleros, and foreign interests like the United Fruit Company.

4

Conventional Practice: New Science,

Old Art, and Persistent Heterogeneity

Sometime in 1896, Dr. Francisco Fonseca called at the house of Dr. Carlos Durán and asked if his colleague would accompany him to the outlying town of Desamparados to give an opinion on a two-year-old girl under his care who was bedridden with fever. Fonseca had initially diagnosed laryngitis, prescribing an emetic and the application of heat pads to her throat, but when the girl's condition worsened, he hastened to consult the experienced surgeon. A half-hour horseback ride brought them to the patient's house, where they found the child suffocating. Durán intubated and, after examination, diagnosed diphtheria. He returned the next day to inject her with antitoxin and take a throat swab, which he dropped at the hospital lab on his way home. The head of the lab, Dr. Emilio Echeverría, quickly made a positive analysis. Durán returned periodically over the next nine days as the girl's health improved, continuing the injections until he saw her up and playing on the patio.[1]

On the one hand, the episode reveals the simultaneous extremes of simplicity and sophistication that might characterize a physician's practice in late-nineteenth-century San José. Fonseca was willing to call impromptu on the country's preeminent physician, and a former president of the republic, with reasonable expectation of assistance despite the considerable inconvenience of the consultation. This suggests an easy collegiality without unbridgeable separations of rank, though the fact that this young "country doctor" had graduated four years earlier from a German university underscores the cosmopolitan elitism that knit this community together. The mode of transport (Durán was more commonly seen traversing the streets of the capital in a sleek black fly) and the bucolic setting of the patient's home show how short was the distance between the heart of medical power in the country and the bedside of a farmer's ailing child.

Yet that medical power was sophisticated, capable of emergency intervention, knowledgeable diagnosis, rapid bacteriologic analysis, and delivery of a new therapeutic arsenal. The promising experimental results of Pierre Paul Emile Roux's diphtheria antitoxin had only been announced in 1894, and the commercial marketing of it had begun shortly before Durán began using it. Though on a world scale Durán was not avant-garde in his treatment — the public health departments of New York and Boston were using diphtheria antitoxin systematically by 1897, and a serum was being produced in a private Havana lab by 1899 — he was quite up-to-date. Medical time was assuming its modern dimensions in Costa Rica: from experimental findings presented at a scientific congress in Budapest to common treatment at the bedside of a young child in a semirural town on the Latin American periphery took only two years.[2]

On the other hand, the case was selected for publication in the *Gaceta Médica* and its facts arranged in order to reproduce the romance narrative of modern medical science triumphally saving the lives of innocent sufferers. It was an ideological representation of Costa Rican medical practitioners as they should be and the ability of medical science to deliver on its promises. In the normal course of events, physicians still had little in their therapeutic arsenal that could effect such dramatic "cures," the contact between the average sufferer and average physician was hardly so transparent or common, and Costa Rican physicians as a group were far from a homogeneous and effectively functioning group. By the nineteenth century's end physicians and surgeons, led by a new generation of Costa Rican nationals, had come to establish clearer criteria for professional incorporation and staffed a network that was approaching countrywide extension. Nevertheless, the process itself generated a new set of divisions within the medical profession.

Those occupying the lower, and most populous, echelons of the category of médico — doctors from previous generations, other countries, and the provinces — in general those with less prestigious and somewhat suspect educational backgrounds, might be hard-pressed to differentiate themselves from certain groups of empirics, let alone from titled pharmacists and dentists. The bacteriologic revolution and dramatic new surgical procedures might have been the pillars of the new professional legitimacy being proposed by the positivist medical elite, but the average general practitioner did not necessarily incorporate them into his work immediately or tout court, nor see them as the foundation of a holy war on popular medicine. Given the rapid growth in the number of physicians at the end of the nineteenth century, some of whom now had to establish practice in the rural areas where the demand for official medicine was often weak, a few compromises with the medical beliefs and practices of the potential clientele might have to be made.

New Professional Geography

Between 1870 and 1910, the corps of medical doctors became large enough to develop internal stratifications of geography, social stature, professional eminence, and generation. The four variables were intrinsically related. The period may be divided into two phases of roughly equal lengths. Between 1870 and 1890, Costa Rican physicians and surgeons became younger on average, and their composition changed drastically in terms of nationality and place of study. The spatial distribution of practitioners remained roughly the same, and the numbers of those calling themselves doctors practicing at any one time grew rather slowly. Nevertheless, many of these doctors in the provincial areas in the 1864 data were licensed empirics who were replaced by fully qualified practitioners over the subsequent two decades (see table 2).

Between 40 and 45 percent of licensed practitioners lived in San José, and another 40 to 50 percent practiced in the other three principal towns of the Central Valley (with slightly fewer in Alajuela than in Heredia and Cartago). There was a single district physician, sustained by a government subsidy, in the port of Puntarenas, the northern border town of Liberia, and with the opening of the Caribbean coast to railroad construction and banana cultivation after 1880, the new port of Limón. The rate of incorporation of practitioners did rise considerably over the two decades: forty-eight practitioners incorporated in the decade of 1870 alone, which was almost as many as had practiced in the previous fifty years combined. But the two decades corresponded to the retirement of the first wave of physicians, pharmacists, and empirics whose numbers had peaked in the 1850s (and who still accounted for

Table 2. Number of Costa Rican physicians
and place of practice, 1864–1914

	1864[a]	1883	1892	1904	1914
San José	17	15	18	30	43
Alajuela/Cartago/Heredia	16	17	21	20	25
Puntarenas/Limon	4[b]	2	2	7	9
Guanacaste	1	1	1	4	7
Other	—	—	—	20	22
	38	35	42	81	106

a. includes licensed empirics

b. only Puntarenas

Sources: República de Costa Rica, *Censo general de la República de Costa Rica (27 de noviembre de 1864)* (San José: Imprenta Nacional, 1868), 91–95, *Censo de la República de Costa Rica* [1883] (n.p., n.d.), 85, and *Censo general de la República de Costa Rica (1892)* (San José: Tipografía Nacional, 1893), 73; GMCR 8, no. 5 (1904), 75; and Rockefeller Foundation Archives, record group 5, series 51, box 7, folder 103, Rockefeller Archive Center, North Tarrytown, N.Y.

the bulk of the 1864 statistics). The renewal of the profession occurred through natural displacement, which seems to have made for a relatively smooth transition to a national and professional body of physicians.

This picture changed abruptly in the seven years after 1892 when seventy-seven new medical doctors incorporated. Over the course of the decade the total number of doctors practicing in the country more than doubled, from forty-two to about one hundred. Some of this increase was accounted for by an influx of medical practitioners of Cuban and Spanish origin, escaping the wars of independence while also taking advantage of an 1850 treaty between Spain and Costa Rica that apparently gave nationals of either country the right to have their credentials automatically recognized in the other. These new immigrants did not have to undergo examination or certification by the Costa Rican faculty. Their arrival coincided with the expansion of the network of town doctor posts. The sympathy the refugees enjoyed, as well as the political influence of older Cuban immigrants, helped many of them win government appointments as district physicians.

The Cuban refugee physicians also just preceded another wave of

Popular Medicine to Medical Populism

young nationals returning to practice after their studies abroad. This generation was not so lucky as the 1870s' one of Durán and Ulloa. The plum postings and practices available in the capital were already dominated by their still relatively young and quite dynamic predecessor generation. The bottleneck coincided with an economic recession brought on by a drop in the price of coffee between 1897 and 1906, complicating any hopes for an expansion of consumer demand for medical services in San José. This set the stage for a nationalist backlash against the "Cubans," which was also a displaced anxiety about the lack of opportunities in the capital where the arrival of newly trained young nationals had led to a doubling of the number of doctors in San José over the final seven years of the century.[3] In 1900, soon after returning with a prestigious degree in medicine from Strasbourg, Vicente Láchner Sandoval complained in nationalist, Darwinian fashion that one hundred physicians in a country of scarcely three hundred thousand had made "arduous the native doctor's struggle for existence." He echoed a widely held view when he not only blamed the Cubans who monopolized the office of town doctor for "making it difficult today for native sons to get one of these posts" but accused them of being little more than curanderos with false titles.[4]

In 1864, there had been 1 licensed medical practitioner (including licensed empirics) for every 3,171 Costa Ricans, and in San José 1 for every 1,257 residents. This ratio had fallen nicely in physicians' favor as their number remained roughly the same, while the population almost doubled: by 1892, it was 1 to 6,253 for the country and 1 to 2,300 for San José. Then, in the space of eight years, the ratio returned to midcentury levels, shooting up toward 1 to 3,000, and in the capital reaching 1 to 1,250—a change that left young physicians like Láchner Sandoval feeling desperate.[5] The late-nineteenth-century glut seems to have been a common phenomenon in Latin America. Dain Borges and Julyan Peard both note the growing competition among physicians in Bahia at this time, equating it with a rise in the number of graduates from the medical schools.[6]

In terms of spatial distribution, two significant trends mark the period 1890–1910. After the 1894 reform and expansion of the network of town doctors, most cantonal centers acquired a medical practitioner: Puriscal, Paraíso, Palmares, Juan Viñas, Esparta, Aserrí, Nicoya, and so on. For the first time, Costa Rica had a web of rural practitioners that

Conventional Practice

extended into most areas of settlement and accounted for about 20 percent of the country's physicians. At the other pole, the number of doctors residing in San José doubled (while the number in the three other principal towns languished), and the capital maintained its statistical concentration of practitioners. This was despite the rapid expansion of the rural network and a growing number of physicians in the country's two booming ports, Puntarenas and Limón, each of which now had three, four, or five practitioners at any one time.

Professional Hierarchy

The expanded, more strongly organized, and truly countrywide community of physicians had a basic four-tier hierarchy. The professional, political, scientific, and commercial elite of the Costa Rican medical profession were the doctors of the capital, San José. To be a physician in San José was to occupy a profession of great social distinction. It suggested that you came from a respectable family, had traveled and studied in the centers of Western civilization, had an excellent income and access to the halls of power, and pursued a noble science that promoted the interests and well-being of the nation. Entrance to this elite tier was not automatically extended but the pattern of membership was clear enough in the 1870s and 1880s. It followed roughly the course taken by Durán and Ulloa. One grew up the son of a reputable family, pursued medical studies in Europe or the United States, and employed social influence on returning to gain an appointment to the Junta of Charity, hospital directorate, and professional and political office. One then undertook sophisticated surgical, clinical, and laboratory work as well as promoted institutional reform while building up private practice in a favorable environment of stable numbers of practitioners, growing municipal populace, and economic prosperity. It should be remembered that the members of this generation were first-comers; occupying the elite tier was made easier because they themselves invented it, and there were few established native practitioners to confront. Professional association was so outmoded it had to be re-created, the hospital had yet to assume any modern shape, and the young nationals wielded intimidating new theoretical and surgical weaponry.

Incorporation to the elite tier became more difficult toward the turn of the twentieth century—a pattern visible in the larger cities of Cuba and Brazil as well. Borges and Peard argue that as the number of physicians rose sharply at the end of the nineteenth century, the increased competition made patronage and social background ever more important for winning university, hospital, or government health posts, which were requisite for building a lucrative practice. In Cuba, nepotism was particularly manifest and actual medical dynasties were established.[7] The strictures of patronage and genealogy were not as pronounced in Costa Rica but they were felt, and apprenticeships grew longer.

Gerardo Jiménez, for example, followed very much in the footsteps of Durán, but his ascent was not nearly so vertiginous. Born in 1869, the same year that Durán left for his studies in Europe, Jiménez studied at Guy's in the early 1890s. Returning in 1895, he volunteered to work in the laboratory at the hospital and was lucky enough to play a role in the discovery of hookworm disease. He received the coveted nomination as surgical resident in the hospital the following year, and three years later won appointment as head of surgery. Having built up a private practice in the satellite town of Guadelupe, Jiménez became active on the board of the faculty, and with his brother, an engineer, wrote an extensive tome on hygienic water and housing that won the faculty prize in 1901. Unfortunately, the prize was awarded posthumously after Jiménez suffered an untimely death at the age of thirty-two, just as he was on the verge of professional preeminence.[8]

Others did not fare so well professionally (though they had better luck on the vitality front), despite having the right credentials and showing a good deal of hard work. The angry young Láchner Sandoval was the son of a German musician and educator who had immigrated to Costa Rica in the 1850s. Láchner Sandoval journeyed to the land of his father's birth for medical studies and began his Costa Rican apprenticeship even while a student in Strasbourg, appointing himself German correspondent to the *Gaceta Médica*. He translated into Spanish long and complex articles from German medical journals, and explained Wilhelm Conrad Röntgen's discovery of X rays (he provided the first plates seen in the country). Returning in 1900, he threw himself into laboratory research at the hospital, focusing on the national parasitology that had earned Durán such acclaim, and helped to identify the presence in Costa Rica of *Balantidium coli*. He continued to translate German medical literature, participated actively in the faculty board, and even took on the job of editor of the *Gaceta Médica*. Still, as he made clear in his highly personalized essay on the history of public health in Costa Rica, written in 1900, no professional postings opened up for him in the capital and he could not make a go of it in private practice (one obstacle may have been the absence of a criollo family pedigree). In 1901, deciding to try his luck in the second tier, Láchner Sandoval resigned his position on the faculty board, left San José, and established a practice in Alajuela, the major town with the least number of medical practitioners. Even here the going was not easy, and within a few years he was on the move to a more peripheral post as a town doctor.[9]

If the life of a physician in San José at the dawn of the twentieth century was a privileged one, it was also extremely full and difficult. An upper-crust background and a medical title from the right place were not enough to qualify for professional eminence or successful practice. One also had to demonstrate public spirit through pro bono work, remain active in professional institutions, and display a commitment to scientific inquiry, however rudimentary. One morning or day per week had to be reserved for free consultation for poor patients in the office and invariably a free visit to an orphanage or other charity institution. If one was lucky enough to be a chief or consulting physician or surgeon at the hospital, daily rounds had to be made or surgery performed, again for no remuneration.

A successful practitioner would almost certainly have at least one public or private institutional contract, either with an elite school or as a doctor of prisons, venereal prophylaxis, or military barracks. Some physicians held down posts with the municipal health department; others, in times of epidemiological emergency, might find themselves delegated to a rural area to investigate or to assume the direction of the public health response. Some doctors taught courses—in hygiene at the city's two secondary schools, or in more specialized subjects at the schools of pharmacy or midwifery that opened their doors in the late 1890s.

At least one evening a week would be dedicated to the meeting of the faculty board or Junta of Charity. One had to keep abreast of developments in the field, and pursue scientific research and publication. And to really cap a career, sitting as a congressional deputy would take up a minimum of two months a year, while an appointment as a minister would involve much more. All of these roles were, of course, above and beyond actual private practice. To be a physician in the capital was a full-time calling requiring no mean dedication. That it took its toll on private life is suggested by the fact that of the twenty native Costa Rican physicians in the capital city in 1904, only eight were married, while ten were single, one was divorced, and another separated.[10]

Why was it worth it? It allowed those from the respectable classes to earn, maintain, consolidate, or raise their social stature. Most seem to have had a genuine fascination for the art and science of medicine, and a belief that they were at the vanguard of a noble civilizing mission. Finally, the capital's doctors made a good deal of money on top of the family wealth that most already enjoyed. In 1914, Henry Carter of the Rockefeller Foundation estimated that physicians in San José made "between $3,000 and $20,000 gold" per year.[11] Even the lower end of this range was a respectable sum in turn-of-the-century San José, and the upper end compared favorably to what little is known of physicians' earnings in other parts of Latin America. The premier practitioner in Costa Rica earned two times what his counterpart did in Arequipa, Peru in 1907, and four times the best-paid physicians of La Paz; his revenues from practice probably rivaled the enviable salaries enjoyed by the medical elites of Chile and Buenos Aires.[12]

The leading physicians from the provincial capitals made up the second rank of medical practitioners. Though geography and a slight remove from the center of things kept them from the absolute pinnacle of the profession, they certainly shared class membership with their brethren from the national capital. Among the doctors of Alajuela, Cartago, and Heredia, it was not unusual to find names of oligarchic pedigree like Peralta, Dobles, and Volio. A perfect example is José María Jiménez Oreamuno of Cartago, who made the classic career pilgrimage of a physician from the provincial upper crust. Born in 1849 to one of the oldest and most distinguished families in the country, the son of a physician who was twice president of the republic, brother of a man who would be president on three occasions, he was sent to finish secondary school in Guatemala in the 1860s. Rather than continue on to study medicine at San Carlos as the previous generation of Cartago physicians had done, he moved to Philadelphia to get his medical degree at Jefferson College (Carlos Finlay's alma mater), graduating in 1870. Jiménez did a clinical tour of duty in the hospitals of Pennsylvania and then returned to Cartago, where he became one of the founders of the city's

Conventional Practice

hospital, served as district physician of Cartago during the early years of his practice, and became the official doctor of the elite boys and girls colleges of San Luis Gonzaga and the Bethlemite nuns. He was the physician of choice among the eminent families of the old colonial capital, and also served in the municipality and as a deputy in the national congress. His U.S. training set him apart from his predecessors in Cartago, as did his frequent visits to Europe and the United States, where he made efforts to update his knowledge of medicine.[13]

Others of this tier, like Juan Flores of Heredia, who had studied and interned in New York prior to incorporating as a physician in Costa Rica in 1869, were even able to occupy the leading political posts of the profession. Flores was president of the Faculty of Medicine in 1899 and then minister of the interior in 1903. One might include in this second tier immigrant physicians who arrived with impeccable credentials and references, and whose reputations preceded them. Many of the foreign physicians mentioned earlier in the San José census of 1904 fit this category, as did the Cuban gynecologist, Luis Ros Pochet. After practicing in New York, he briefly established himself in Costa Rica in the late 1890s and immediately enjoyed the respect of his Costa Rican colleagues. The same could be said for Benjamín de Céspedes, who had made a reputation as the author of a book-length study of Cuban prostitution. Céspedes participated actively in the profession, won the faculty prize in 1900 for his book on infant hygiene, presented to the faculty the first-ever project for a national sanitary code in 1902 (which was not adopted), and combined government appointments with a lucrative practice in Heredia and later Limón.[14]

Costa Rican physicians from less eminent social backgrounds occupied the third tier. Dr. Alberto Borbón, born in San José in 1860, is said to have pursued his dream of a medical career by studying in Guatemala "with scarce financial resources" prior to incorporating in Costa Rica in 1887. Not surprisingly, in 1899 he was practicing outside the city proper as the district physician for Santa Ana and Escazú. This was, to be sure, one of the more sought after town doctor posts due to its proximity to San José, but it left him outside the medical establishment of the capital. He was never a member of the faculty board, and the municipal census of 1904, five years after his death, found his widow, five children, and three grandchildren living without servants. The family was now maintained by two sons — one who worked in retail, and another who had reproduced the career of his father (unfortunately, the place where he studied medicine is not registered in the faculty records, which in itself suggests a place of little prestige). Other nationals from lower social backgrounds who pursued medical studies likely did so close to home, and were among the twenty-six physicians of the period who graduated in Guatemala, El Salvador, or one of the two schools in Nicaragua.[15]

The fourth and lowest tier was comprised of foreigners, many of them with dubious credentials, who worked in the more peripheral town doctor posts. Of the twenty-two town doctors who filed regular reports in 1899, ten of them had received their medical titles in Cuba and Spain. Five of the remaining nine had studied in Nicaragua and two in Guatemala (meaning they were almost certainly Costa Ricans or from other Central American countries). Teófilo de Barrios, who was named to the Cañas and Bagaces district physician post in 1894, was a Nicaraguan exiled after the fall of the conservative regime in 1893, and described in his 1900 obituary as "a member of one of the most politically influential families of Central America."[16] Láchner Sandoval's accusation in 1900 that Cubans dominated these posts was, therefore, somewhat exaggerated. But he was not alone in attacking the quality and legitimacy of the largely immigrant body of town doctors. The Faculty of Medicine fought hard against the government's interpretation of the 1850 treaty throughout the 1890s, and often stalled certification of Cuban practitioners by questioning the consular authentication of diplomas, even though they eventually had to back down. The battle was only won in 1900 when the Spanish government refused to act equally in the case of a Costa Rican professional who wished to practice in Spain, forcing the government in San José to interpret the treaty more stringently.[17]

Urban Practice

Regrettably, no records are available to serve as the basis for a detailed reconstruction of a doctor's practice, either urban or rural, and almost all the available evidence comes after 1895 when occasional clinical notes were published in the *Gaceta Médica*. It suggests, however, that elite physicians and surgeons in San José had incorporated laboratory analysis into their everyday practices, kept themselves up-to-date with emerging diagnostics, procedures, and therapies, and in trying them out, weighed and debated the results among one another.

Most of the consultations recorded in the *Gaceta Médica* were, for obvious reasons, exceptional. They nonetheless indicate some procedures that had become a routine part of practice. In 1900, a twelve-year-old boy traveled some distance with his parents to the Desamparados office of Roberto Fonseca, on the semirural outskirts of San José. The boy had been bitten by a snake and was in poor condition. Fonseca, only two years from graduating in medicine from Montpellier, determined to inject a serum developed by a local colleague and reported excellent results. The entire procedure was handled on the spot, within the routine of the office, and many consultations probably fit this pattern.[18]

Durán's clinical notes on the use of diphtheria antitoxin record that six of the eight encounters were house calls, and twice children were brought to his office (the nature of the disease would have tended to promote a greater number of house calls). Durán had his consulting room in a special section of his home, and this appears to have been the norm for established city physicians. Though Durán lived in a wealthy neighborhood a few blocks east of the city's central plaza, by the nineteenth century's end there was even a section of San José just to the north of the hospital where a cluster of seven physicians maintained their offices, five of them within a four-block area.[19]

In an 1899 case, a nineteen-year-old soldier, recently stationed on a Pacific island penal colony, could not beat a fever despite his family's administration of a saline purgative and small doses of quinine, and he visited Dr. José María Soto Alfaro's office. Soto Alfaro resorted to the age-old routine of taking the young man's pulse and checking his urine, but he also took his temperature. Soto Alfaro's colleague, Antonio Giustiniani (also a member of an important cafetalero family), in discussing other cases of suspected yellow fever, referred to "the thermometer that I apply almost automatically." The soldier's case also reveals how common it was for doctors to call in a colleague in difficult or confusing cases, as Soto did with Giustiniani in this instance. The two oligarchs discounted yellow fever, and treated the patient with champagne tonic, ergot, lemonade, and an unspecified bichloride.[20]

When a young French cabinetmaker had a recurrence of a hernia getting out of a cold bath in 1896, he called for Soto Alfaro to pay a house call. The doctor tried to reduce the hernia through a warm bath, the application of a poultice, and taxis, but without success. He then called in Dr. Elías Rojas for help. Seeing that the patient's condition was worsening, they determined to anesthetize him and operate on the spot. After considering the man's lodgings, though, they discarded the notion "because the room was not conducive to an operation, neither from the point of view of comfort nor from that of hygiene." They transported him to the Hospital San Juan de Dios and now sought assistance from another colleague, César Borja. After elaborate aseptic procedures including repeated hand washings, cleansing of the wound, and the sterilization of instruments, the three operated using "the well-known procedure of Professor Tillaux," achieving excellent results even though the case had become complicated by infection and a ruptured testicle.[21]

Doctors were ready to perform minor surgery on the spot during house calls, and arrived with ether or, in cases of obstetrics, chloroform at the ready. In 1901, Juan Flores of Heredia was called to the bedside of a sick and feverish woman who had recently given birth attended by a barrio midwife. He immediately called in a colleague, and they anesthetized the patient with chloroform, examined her, performed a curettage, injected her with antistreptococcal serum (a product of the Pasteur Institute then in experimental use, but that proved ineffective despite high hopes), gave her an intrauterine bath, put her on a diet of broth and milk, and ordered the room to be ventilated and cleaned. The woman enjoyed a complete recovery.[22]

Vaginal examinations were common if the patient was from the upper or middle classes. The gynecologist Luis Ros Pochet, one of the country's first specialists, reported that between March and December of 1896, ninety-two women of all ages had consulted him "with trouble in their genital organs."[23] In the same year, Soto was called by a midwife to assist a woman who had been in labor for three days (again, he would finally bring in a colleague prior to taking any action). He notes that he practiced a uterine exploration "in the presence of the patient."[24] Doctors probably used some screening device, practiced vertical touching, or simply averted their gaze unless they were alone and the patient was anesthetized. In the rural towns, physicians had more difficulty in this respect. Carlos Pupo Pérez, district physician in Escazú, remarked in 1904 that a woman suffering from severe puerperal fever, "following the advice of 'one who knows' [the midwife who had attended her] categorically refused any kind of genital examination," although here a more fundamental questioning of physician authority was also clearly involved.[25]

It would seem, however, that physicians did not attend childbirths unless something serious went wrong. Though wealthy women might have a physician in attendance throughout the birth, the practice of obstetrics was still dominated by the midwife, and there were a number with foreign training and faculty certification who attended the well-to-do of San José in the 1890s. Even though doctors complained vociferously about the ignorance and perilous practices of the average midwife — in 1901, Flores claimed there was not a single one in Heredia who was not "ignorant" — taking over the time-consuming and delicate oversight of labor was not on their agenda.[26] Most of their reports on interventions in cases of difficult childbirths in the cities suggest that they at least had a working relationship with midwives, although doctors were increasingly adamant that these female practitioners needed better education and were anxious about the possible undermining of their medical authority. Instead of taking direct control of the birthing process, physicians began to achieve indirect control by opening a faculty-run school of midwifery in 1899, a subject I will broach in a subsequent chapter.

While still rudimentary, specialization was occurring by the end of the nineteenth century. Aside from the specialists in surgery, the city acquired its first oculist in the early 1900s, the Spaniard Juan Arrea y Cosp. The young oligarch Calderón Muñoz cultivated a specialty in pediatrics, and a general trend toward gynecology can be observed in the thesis topics of a number of native practitioners incorporating near the turn of the twentieth century, such as Teodoro Picado's 1898 University of Geneva dissertation "L'atresie cicatriecelle du vagin." The Cuban gynecologist Ros Pochet made explicit reference to "the exercise of our specialty," and the case notes he published in the *Gaceta Médica* in 1896 confirmed that a profitable market was opening up to those who could address the formerly taboo complaints of affluent girls and women.[27]

Psychiatry was initially the exclusive preserve of the foreign directors of the Asilo Chapuí, adjacent to the hospital. The first to hold the post was Maximillian Bansen, a Prussian who had studied medicine in Berlin and then served for a year as the assistant to the director of the Orates Stephansfeld Asylum in Alsace prior to emigrating to Costa Rica in 1876. Bansen was not well liked by his colleagues due to an arrogant and aloof personality, and there were few tears shed when he died suddenly on a trip to the fatherland in 1901. He was succeeded in the direction of the Chapuí by another German, Theodore Prestinary, who also served as the hospital's resident "alienist" until his death in 1912.[28]

Most of the leading doctors of the day seem to have tended toward the general practice of medicine and surgery. Private practice consisted of a mixture of office consultations, planned and unplanned house calls, management of a dispensary, surgery — occasionally in the home of the patient, but increasingly at a hospital — and if possible, a paying, part-time public position. As a representative of the Rockefeller Foundation reported in 1914, the physicians of San José augmented their regular earnings through "connections with drug stores from which they get a rebate, or [they] dispense their own medicines."[29] Yet a medical doctor would be less likely to represent him or herself as head of a pharmacy than had been the case in San José in the 1850s. The forging of a medical identity had shifted away from this commercial domain and toward the institutional site of the hospital.

The Hospital Comes of Age

Not until the waning days of Costa Rica's colonial era was a small hospital established in Cartago by Friar Bancos, and the project did not last more than a few years. As Paulina Malavassi has shown in an innovative thesis, even the concerted efforts of two late-colonial governors to create a leper colony foundered, and after independence the new polity could barely muster the fiscal and political wherewithal to establish a single institution of medical charity and public health. The government finally opted for the construction of a rudimentary leprosarium in 1833, though this was decided at the expense of creating a hospital.[30]

In 1845, as part of an ambitious plan to create a school of medicine, the hospital project was rekindled and a Junta of Charity created to see it into being. The first massive edifice of the Hospital San Juan de Dios was finally built in the 1850s after the archbishop entreated the faithful to contribute materials and labor to build this temple of beneficence. It went virtually unused, and came to function as a giant but sparsely

populated municipal jail and madhouse as well as a refuge for a smatter-
ing of destitute individuals. The Hospital San Juan de Dios did not really
open as a permanently operative institution of medical beneficence
until 1864, when a special tax to maintain it was put in the hands of a
board of charity made up of eminent citizens. It finally opened with
twenty beds, but with no regular medical staff; there was an informal
agreement that "from time to time doctors Frantzius, Espinach, and
Cruz Alvarado would visit the sick." The hospital did not gain a sure
administrative footing until the arrival of a congregation of the Sisters
of Charity in 1873, yet even so it remained essentially a home for the
chronically infirm, aged, or indigent.[31]

Costa Rica was distinct from most Latin American countries in remaining so long without a hospital institution. On the other hand, it
telescoped three hundred years of hospital history into a few decades,
reproducing in miniature the transformation of the Latin American
hospital from charity hospice and asylum to a facility designed to
achieve short-term medical and surgical results along with what Guenter Risse calls a "site for development of professional agendas, notably
clinical training and research."[32] In Costa Rica, as elsewhere in Latin
America, the key decade for the updates, redesign, and expansion of
hospital facilities was the 1880s.[33]

In the late 1870s and early 1880s, Durán was instrumental in establishing a stricter admissions policy that barred paupers and those with
chronic diseases (a separate Asilo de Incurables was established in
1881). He created an accounting regime as well as a system for gathering information on each individual patient. The hospital's ward system,
based until then only on sex, was transformed in order to separate those
with infectious diseases from other patients, and the position of a medical intern was created. Mortality rates began to fall, from just over 25
percent of those admitted in 1875 to 7.5 percent in 1881, and the
average length of stay fell by one-third, from sixty-two to forty-two
days.[34]

By the mid-1880s, Durán was at the center of a hospital coterie of
leading young physicians and surgeons of the city, including Ulloa,
Calnek, Martin Bonnefil, Federico Zumbado, and Daniel Nuñez (also a
graduate of Guy's). New statutes were written, internal differentiations
were established between general medicine and surgery, internships
were increased, residencies were instituted, a reform of nursing was

undertaken, and separate wings were erected for foreigners and children. New operating theaters were built, modern sewage facilities installed, anesthetic and aseptic procedures were introduced, and a bacteriologic laboratory was created. Around the operating table, in the lab, making rounds on any given day, testing theories, were a group of seven or eight well-trained, ambitious but collegial men.[35]

Aside from a superintendent and two residents, one in surgery and another in general medicine, the hospital work of San José's physicians was done as an ad hoc charitable duty prior to 1898. Of course, doctors had their own clinical and laboratory-based reasons for assisting in the hospital, and this type of charitable work raised their stature, and thus in the long run, their earnings in private practice.[36] In 1898, ten formal positions were created for physicians and surgeons. The old job of superintendent was preserved, as were the residencies. Two chief surgeons, two assistant surgeons, and a consulting surgeon were named, along with two chief physicians and a consulting physician. Only the chief surgeon was to receive a salary, but the formal appointments were crucial status markers that could help determine the course of a career. The first list of appointees was a "who's who" of the leading practitioners of the capital, most of whom have already appeared on these pages: Durán, José Varela, Jiménez, Zumbado, Soto, Rojas, Rafael Calderón Muñoz, Calnek, Bonnefil, and Núñez.[37]

Rounds became regular and mandatory for all officeholders. Tighter discipline was established in the wards, a system of patient cards introduced, and hospital statistics kept with greater rigor. Pathology became a regular function of the residents. Some effort was made to reform nursing on the wards (the Sisters of Charity performed more administrative and maintenance roles than actual nursing). From an average of five hundred patients a year treated or operated on in the hospital between 1889 and 1895, the number approximately doubled between the latter year and 1909. The most notable change was a gradual shift from a large preponderance of male patients to gender parity, from men accounting for 80 percent of patients in 1890 to 52 percent in the latter year.[38] Most patients were from the domestic service, artisan, or lower-middle-class ranks of the capital city, and the most common ailments were dysentery and other gastric illnesses, malaria, and problems requiring routine surgery.

In 1900 Láchner Sandoval, fresh from his German studies, described

the Hospital San Juan de Dios as a complex in which the original building had been gradually dismantled and replaced with a more modern
pavilion system: in the general medicine section, there were two for
women, one for men, and one for "foreigners"; there was one for men
and another for women in the surgery section; a pavilion was set aside
for servants and supplies; and another housed the Sisters of Charity.[39]
Mortality rates continued to drop from about 10 percent in the late
1890s to 3 percent in 1909. Typical of the transformation of popular
attitudes toward the hospital throughout the West during this era, in
1903 the residents Rojas and Giustiniani wrote that "every day the
needy are more and more convinced that in the hospital they will receive better treatment than anywhere else, and as a result today they
approach the doors of this asylum of charity with greater will than
before, to seek relief from their pains."[40] Doctors, meanwhile, were
more likely to intern their well-to-do patients in the hospital, especially
for surgery, where they were separated from the indigent.

Hospitals were much slower to develop in the rest of the country. An
infirmary had been established in Puntarenas as early as 1852, the Hospital San Rafael reflecting the importance of that Pacific port town in the
growing coffee trade, even though it must have remained rather rudimentary, and was given over primarily to providing shelter for sailors and
other common travelers stricken with fever. Early in the twentieth century, the Puntarenas hospital was overseen by a professional nurse (still a
rarity in Costa Rica) who had trained in Philadelphia, and the patients
were visited daily by the town doctor.[41] Similarly rudimentary hospital
facilities began to open in the older principal towns after 1880: in Cartago and Liberia in 1880, Alajuela and Limón in 1884, and Heredia in
1888. In 1891 efforts to establish hospital facilities marked the municipal ambitions of Grecia and Palmares, new, flourishing town centers on
the agricultural frontier. The funding obstacles were immense, and the
projects were often delayed indefinitely. For example, the local elites in
San Ramón announced their intention to build a hospital in 1886, but
did not inaugurate the building until twenty years later. In the mean-
time, residents donated furniture and beds for makeshift infirmaries
that were attended by women volunteers.[42]

In 1903, the Costa Rican government contracted with the United
Fruit Company to jointly manage a new hospital facility in the port of
Limón (to be built at company expense), though the facility seems to

have been all but taken over by the company. The local Junta of Charity found it cheaper to send patients who were not employees of the company by rail to San José's Hospital San Juan de Dios for treatment—a source of constant complaint by hospital administrators in the capital. The company's elaborate medical section, malaria treatment campaigns, and controversial policies concerning worker eligibility for hospital coverage were central to the development of medicine in the Caribbean coast banana enclave, although little is known about them.[43]

Rural and Port Practice

In 1900, Carlos Aragón was the town doctor for the second circuit of Alajuela province. He was a graduate of the medical program at the University of El Salvador who had only just incorporated in the Costa Rican faculty. Aragón resided in Grecia, the largest town on the northwestern rim of the Central Valley. During the trimester of October to December—the height of the rainy season—he visited eleven "satellite" villages within a six-kilometer radius of Grecia. Over the course of these three months, he submitted twelve certified reports on matters of legal medicine (for the most part, probably death certificates) and vaccinated hundreds of schoolchildren with results he claimed were satisfactory.[44]

This doctor's quarterly journey through the smaller towns of the district in some ways recapitulated the more familiar tour of the parish priest: his medicines and touch a comfort to the indigent, his attempts to certify and explain recent deaths a modern ritual of last rites, his vaccination of the schoolchildren a first communion. The visits gradually wove the modern state into the fabric of life of the Costa Rican village. But the town doctors were not simply impositions from above. Especially here in the recent settlements of the Central Valley's agricultural frontier, communities banded together to influence public medical matters in their area. Often residents of larger towns, soon after acquiring parish or cantonal status, collectively petitioned the central government to establish a town doctor post. Inevitably, fifty or more signatures would be affixed (usually only of men, but occasionally the women of the town would addend their own petition). In 1895, for example, taking advantage of the announcement that the system of town doctors would be expanded, the principal residents of Naranjo,

Conventional Practice

some ten kilometers further west of Grecia, requested that the government in San José reconsider its decision to append the canton to the circuit of the town doctor in Grecia and grant Naranjo a public physician of its own. The request probably originated with the local elites — who dismissed out of hand the ability of traditional curanderos to effectively treat the ill — but interest in having a town doctor extended far beyond one or two leading families and local officials.[45]

Nor did towns passively accept those the central government named to the position. On a number of occasions residents petitioned to replace their town doctor, usually because it was felt that the physician was not attentive in performing his public duties. In 1895, some seventy men from the coffee district of Santo Domingo de Heredia, an area dominated by prosperous small farmers, including some who were illiterate (which at the time was uncommon for men in this area, suggesting that some of those petitioning were humble folk), demanded the removal of Dr. Julio Corvetti from his post. Their claim that the doctor was often absent when serious injuries needed attending was confirmed by the alcalde, who added that Corvetti frequently ignored the request of the authorities to keep them informed of his whereabouts.[46] In another instance large numbers of citizens from Liberia, the principal town of the northern Guanacastecan frontier, backed up by the municipality, demanded the resignation of their town doctor, Rodolfo Alvarado, because he had launched a campaign to become a member of the national parliament. They refused to run the risk that party preference might interfere with the impartial treatment inherent in the office of the public physician: "It is undeniable that for a town doctor to live up to his delicate duty, he must remain absolutely removed from any question and from any group who might awaken in him and foment unjust and dangerous hatreds against a great portion of those whose health and life he is obligated to preserve."[47]

The role of the district physician was not an easy one, then, embroiled as it was in local politics, and burdened with an unrealistic range of duties and great local expectations. The nature of the job would have varied a great deal according to the circuit covered, political economy of the district, and training, dedication, and demeanor of the individual practitioner. Nevertheless, if there was one basic function that all town doctors tended to fulfill, it was vaccination. The office had been created in 1850 with systematic vaccination in mind. Since an 1884 decree making the procedure obligatory, town doctors had been averaging three thousand vaccinations per year. Our doctor in turn-of-the-century Grecia, Carlos Aragón, vaccinated 862 individuals in the three-month reporting period, meaning he would have equaled the average had he vaccinated at an equivalent rate in each quarter.[48] With the tripling of town doctor posts after 1894 (and assuming that all were vaccinating at this rate), by 1900 the vast majority of Costa Rican children between the ages six and fourteen would have been vaccinated. Even Láchner Sandoval, so critical of the quality of the district physicians, admitted that vaccination had become general and effective by the late 1890s.[49]

This was a major public health success, one that stands out all the more if one recalls that in 1904, a major metropolis like Rio de Janeiro could explode in its famous "revolt against the vaccine." The uprising was motivated by a complex matrix of forces, and was only triggered by the autocratic modernizing style of the Rodrigues Alves regime.[50] Yet Sidney Chalhoub has recently shown that a deep strain of "vaccinophobia" in Afro-Brazilian culture was fueled in many cases by the actions of the vaccination brigades of the liberal state. In Chile, too, there was great resistance to the house-to-house mandatory vaccination in the working-class *conventillos* of Santiago during the 1880s, and persistent evasion of physicians made the campaigns ineffective.[51] Throughout Western Europe and the Americas, there were a variety of popular beliefs about the dangers of vaccination, among them the fear that syphilis was spread through arm-to-arm vaccination.[52]

The macabre consequences of a successful popular struggle against vaccination tout court (rather than, say, against the style in which it was implemented) were all too evident in Rio, where the mandatory vaccination law was never enforced after the revolt of 1904: four years later, the city experienced one of the worst outbreaks of smallpox in its history and over nine thousand died from the disease. In Chile, smallpox claimed over thirty thousand lives between 1879 and 1887.[53] In Costa Rica, by contrast, after the countrywide epidemic of 1852 that helped spur the government to institutionalize the office of town doctor, subsequent outbreaks of smallpox were localized and less virulent, and the populace suffered only periodic, confined outbreaks after the disease appeared briefly in three locales in 1891.[54] A 1902 outbreak in Ipis met a swift emergency response, with eight physicians sent in to vaccinate en masse. The fact that the government had to print and post throughout

Conventional Practice

the region notices threatening stiff fines for those who could not present a certificate of vaccination to police authorities shows that rural Costa Ricans, too, exhibited some aversion to the procedure. This, however, was counteracted in many regions by the support given the office of the town doctor by prominent members of the communities.[55] In any case, the comparison with other countries underlines the early success of the Costa Rican state in making basic public health measures part of the routine ritual of government throughout the country. The town doctors were the main protagonists in this process in the rural areas. The successful extension of public primary education into many rural communities by the 1880s also made it easier for the town doctor to perform mass vaccinations.

Aside from vaccinating systematically, attending to emergencies of childbirth or injury, and performing legal medical duties (including the issuing of death certificates), district physicians were supposed to act as higienistas at large, denouncing unhealthy practices and sites of pollution, engaging in basic epidemiological mapping, and warning the government of the outbreak of infectious disease in their jurisdiction. Residents might call on them to pass judgment on whether or not a local coffee processing plant was polluting the water supply — potentially a highly explosive intervention. Finally, the town doctors were also supposed to fulfill a somewhat modernized version of the ancient charitable charge: treating the indigent and providing them medicines gratis. To qualify for such charity, residents had to apply to the *jefe político* of the area for a certificate of indigence, though it is unclear whether there may have been a stigma attached to such a petition that would have made the request unpalatable. The only references to the process are complaints by some town doctors that the political bosses of their areas dispensed such certificates willy-nilly, even to those who should have been paying for treatment. District physicians counted on supplementing their salaries through private consultations, but they constantly complained that false certification of indigence, on the one hand, and the cut-rate prices of the curanderos on the other, made significant private practice impossible.[56]

By the first decade of the twentieth century, though, the salaries of the district physicians were not insubstantial. Posts in the more rural areas of Guanacaste or Limón, where the tradition of the curandero was deeply entrenched, were made more attractive with salaries in the range of 3,000 colonies per annum. Middle-range salaries for posts on the periphery of the Central Valley like Aragón's paid 2,280 colones per year, and such places tended to be staffed by the less-elite-trained doctors. The lower-end salary of 1,800 colones a year applied to offices in the agricultural districts that were closest to the provincial capitals; generally these were the most desirable because their prosperity promised a greater private clientele and allowed the practitioners continued contact with city life. A post like this could attract the Swiss-trained public health reformer Carlos Pupo Pérez in the early 1900s, and later Mauro Fernández, the son of an important family of the San José oligarchy. This range of base salaries was relatively good. The top scale was approximately the same as that paid to a deputy in the national legislature or the director of San José's elite secondary school in 1892, a quarter of the salary earned by the president of the republic in the same year, four times more than the average wage of an artisan, and about twelve times more than the wage of an agricultural laborer. Considering supplementary earnings from private consultation and the dispensary, a town doctor could do relatively well by 1910.[57]

Between 1900 and 1910, the professional squeeze in the capital combined with a nativist backlash to nationalize the circuit of town doctors. The thirty district physician posts had been all but cleansed of the Cuban, other foreign, and lower-class national usurpers by 1908. Only seven of those who had been town doctors in 1899 still held posts, and only one of these had a Cuban degree. Five of the new crop did have Cuban or Spanish degrees, but at least one of these was a well-regarded physician who had immigrated directly from Spain, and another was Céspedes, who served as the official doctor of Limón. Of the rest, fourteen had incorporated as physicians in Costa Rica since 1900, and their degrees came from the United States (four), Germany (three), France (two), England, Belgium, and Switzerland. Láchner Sandoval himself was finally ensconced as district physician in the booming sugar district of Juan Viñas, and vocal young reformers from respectable backgrounds like the U.S.-trained Mauro Fernández, the Swiss-trained Carlos Pupo Pérez, and the French-trained Carlos Alvarado also held posts.[58]

The rapid transformation of the town doctor from foreigners with dubious credentials to dedicated young nationals trained in elite universities was almost as dramatic as the nationalization of the profession after 1870. A number of forces beyond xenophobic nativism and academic presumption promoted this change. First, the postings came with guaranteed minimum salaries, and these were gradually raised in order to attract candidates to locales that were undesirable because of their isolation, the general poverty of their inhabitants, and the belief that those who could afford to pay for a healer would continue to prefer the services of the local curandero.[59] The period was also a time of self-conscious nation building by Costa Rican intellectuals. Beginning in 1885, a popular national hero was rescued from the oblivion of the 1856–1857 war against Walker; significantly, Juan Santamaría, the hero in question, was a humble agricultural laborer from Alajuela. A series of national monuments were erected, and the campaign against Walker was reconstructed as a surrogate war of independence. Rather tardy by Latin American standards, a small coterie of writers began the classic costumbrista task of observing and recording the lore of the folk, reworking it, and projecting a homogenized version of it back to the people in the guise of a national culture. Whereas many of the physicians of the mid–nineteenth century had been dedicated naturalists, the young physicians of the fin de siècle were driven by nationalist impulses that included the romance of discovering the country folk and bringing civilization to them in the form of the great new medical truths.[60]

Young district physicians could hone their independence and clinical experience away from the critical and competitive eyes of their elder urban colleagues, paying their dues and fulfilling a heroic national mission in the process. In short, the post of district physician became part of a ritual of youth and apprenticeship—a sort of medical *compagnonnage* involving a classic pattern: a journey away from the city, an immersion in the rustic world of the periphery while acquiring skills, followed (hopefully) by reincorporation.[61]

The main outcome was that by 1910, Costa Rica's district physicians were no longer characterized by dubious or outdated medical qualifications and simple charity-oriented work for the poor. A significant number were highly trained doctors in search of a mission of national importance. The existence of this impressive cadre on the periphery would allow the state and Faculty of Medicine to plan a precocious national public health campaign against hookworm disease in 1907. By that year, it might be said that the post of town doctor had been promoted from fourth- to third-division medicine. Not all town doctors were at ease in the role of modern physician, and a 1909 report to the Faculty of Medicine underlined how many were still without a microscope or the knowledge of how to use it. Here the record would have varied according to the generation of practitioner. The younger ones were quite at home with microscopy and up-to-date on medical techniques.[62] They also participated actively in a national scientific dialogue with their colleagues, sometimes based on their experience as district physicians. In 1904, Pupo Pérez used his notes on sixteen cases of puerperal fever in Santa Ana and Escazú (on the distant rural periphery of greater San José) to evaluate the Pasteur Institute's antistreptococcal serum, and concluded correctly that it was not demonstrably effective. His paper also revealed that he performed minor surgery in patients' homes, often in extremely marginal conditions. In one instance, he had a family member administer ether; in another, he had to postpone an operation until the following morning because the family was too poor even to own a candle. During the dry season, he frequently had to water down the dirt floors prior to examining or performing surgery on a patient, otherwise any movement would raise a cloud of dust.[63]

The district physicians in the two principal ports were not rural physicians per se, although their circuits included the rural hinterland. They were paid more handsomely than their country counterparts— 4,320 colones per annum to the official doctor of Limón in 1908 (enough to attract Mauro Fernández that year, and later Benjamín de Céspedes), and 3,780 a year to the port doctor in Puntarenas.[64] Limón in particular had become the main outlet for the United Fruit Company's rapidly growing banana exports, and the post of district physician involved delicate diplomacy (probably erring on the side of corporate compromise, given the economic consequence of imposing a quarantine and the enormous political clout of the company). It also made the occupant a member of the elite in a cosmopolitan enclave boomtown, port, and railroad terminus—one that served as a way station for prominent travelers from the United States, Caribbean, and heartland of Costa Rica itself. Indeed, during the heyday of the banana economy, medical practice in Limón could become a route to national and international professional preeminence. Emilio Echeverría, a graduate of Columbia University's medical school in 1889, and who trained at London's School of Tropical Medicine in 1904, would become director of United Fruit's medical department between 1906 and 1912. Three years later, he was elected president of the Faculty of Medicine.[65]

Puntarenas remained a key port throughout this period, still shipping the majority of the country's coffee exports and receiving numerous travelers. A portrait of the district physician there, Spencer Franklin, comes to us from George Palmer Putnam, a U.S. publisher and travel writer who passed through in 1912. Franklin, a U.S. as well as U.S.-trained physician who had occupied the position since immigrating in 1909, met Putnam's boat to inspect the passengers and crew for contagious disease. Putnam spent the day with Franklin. He claimed that the locals called Franklin "the doctor who rolls up his sleeves" ("*el doctor arremengado*"), and saw him justify this by attending to a stream of patients in the office he maintained in his home. He also had adjacent to his office "a little work room [that] was the scene of several operations" along with a dispensary with a full-time attendant who apparently kept himself busy with prescriptions throughout the morning. According to Palmer, "No walk we took was free from interruption by some one who wished medical advice."[66]

Franklin made his rounds at the local hospital, its fifty beds half occupied, many by sufferers of hookworm infection. "As the doctor enters the clean, bare wards every inmate who is able to do so, rises." Franklin then chatted cheerfully in Spanish with each patient, and one old man with heart trouble, described as "something of a gay Lothario," was given a friendly lecture. The doctor advised him that "a man with your heart simply must give up plural wives." Franklin's good cheer complemented a prosperous practice: on top of his salary of 4,000 colones a year (about $2,400), Franklin also clearly had a thriving private practice, and his total earnings must have rivaled those of a leading physician in the capital. The town doctor of Puntarenas was certainly a member of the local elite, as Palmer found out that evening while accompanying him to a band concert in the plaza.[67] But he was part of a dying breed. Not only was the foreign doctor of unknown academic and social background on the road to extinction, the alien practitioner in general was becoming a rarity: as the Rockefeller Foundation's first

Costa Rican mission leader, Dr. Henry Carter, put it in 1914, "Doctors are a close corporation and do anything they can to keep foreigners out of the Country [*sic*]."[68]

There is not enough evidence to explore the degree to which the late nineteenth century in Costa Rica was a time of epistemological confrontation "on the ground" between practicing physicians espousing the new bacteriologic vector of biomedicine and curanderos maintaining the humoral worldviews of popular curing. But it is worth noting that among the European-trained medical elites of San José, there were devout Catholics such as Rafael Calderón Muñoz, and that the modernized Hospital San Juan de Dios retained its Catholic spiritual mission. As much as it sometimes clashed with them, in practice biomedicine could also coexist with other levels of belief about healing, and one should cease to expect practicing physicians to be epistemologically consistent and monochromatic. Jaime Benchimol has provided a lively re-creation of the efforts of the hygienists of Rio to wed bacteriology with miasmism in the 1880s.[69] Even among physicians actively engaged in scientific practice and debate, then, there was a tendency to try to combine or smooth over conflicts between different medical epistemologies and adopt potentially conflicting theories according to which hats were being worn.

Marriages of official and popular medical practices were no doubt common among rural doctors. Discussing Argentina, Ricardo González Leandri cites the case of a young physician who in 1897 successfully established himself in a rural area of the province of Buenos Aires by appropriating certain practices and stylistic touches from his curandero competitors.[70] A fascinating window on hybrid practice, also established by a provincial district physician, is that of Manuel Núñez Butrón in 1930s' Peru as analyzed by Marcos Cueto. Núñez Butrón's "medical *indigenismo*" was a clear case of self-conscious medical eclecticism by an individual practitioner motivated by cultural and humanitarian concerns. The Lima- and European-trained medical doctor, appointed district physician in his native Puno, incorporated both scientific and magical conceptions of disease (without resolving the tension between them) in order to create a brigade that could carry out basic sanitary work in highland indigenous communities. The brigade even included sorcerers and herbalists who "without renouncing their beliefs completely, nevertheless accepted some of Núñez Butrón's methods."[71] As the next chapter shows, such a selective acceptance and incorporation of conventional medical beliefs and methods was characteristic of a broad range of popular practitioners in late-nineteenth-century Costa Rica.

5

Other Healers: Survival,

Revival, and Public Endorsement

In 1900, Vicente Láchner Sandoval, a young Costa Rican physician recently returned from studying in Germany, wrote an opinionated historical essay on local medicine and public health for a fin de siècle tome celebrating the country's progress. He noted that under the liberal modernizing regimes of Generals Tomás Guardia and Próspero Fernández (1870–1885), licenses to practice medicine were regularly granted to empirics "without the government demanding from them any proof whatsoever" of their medical abilities—and despite vociferous protests from the physicians who sat on the Protomedicato. Worse, lamented an indignant Láchner Sandoval, even after this practice was definitively abolished by the Protomedicato in 1887, the medical profession's efforts to bring before the courts curanderos whose treatments had harmed and even killed patients were inevitably thwarted because "these delinquents have never lacked the protection of someone of high stature or the 'educated classes'—or even the same authorities charged with guarding the public health—to help them escape from the hands of justice."[1]

By the time of Láchner Sandoval's complaint, the medical profession was a political force to be reckoned with and was actively trying to make de facto its de jure monopoly over the legitimate practice of healing. Yet not only were Costa Rican physicians far from achieving professional homogeneity, they still had difficulty differentiating themselves from pharmacists and dentists, who were reluctant to assume a subordinate role in the official medical hierarchy or have the application of their medical knowledge subject to formal restrictions. The booming export economy of the late nineteenth century and a growing populace, especially that of San José, created a larger market for specialized medical services. This benefited physicians, but it also attracted to the country a variety of unorthodox and irregular medical practitioners who competed with them.

In the 1890s, along with the unprecedented influx of conventional practitioners came doctors of unconventional medicine, especially homeopaths, who were articulate and forceful in claiming scientific authority and legitimacy. The liberal government of Tomás Guardia sponsored the building of a railroad from the Central Valley to the Caribbean coast, and this brought large groups of Afro-Antillean and Chinese workers. The subsequent banana boom in the Caribbean province of Limón lured tens of thousands more Antilleans prior to 1914. As a result, the practice of Chinese and Afro-Antillean medicine was established in Costa Rica by the end of the century. Meanwhile, in the cities and towns of the Central Valley, empiricism thrived.

Paradoxically, despite the political and ideological influence of physicians at the apex of the liberal state, police and politicos were at best conspicuously reticent to persecute and prosecute unlicensed practitioners, carrying on a long tradition of tolerance. Indeed, as an exasperated Láchner Sandoval underlined, many a "charlatan" was actively supported by influential Costa Ricans and the state found a variety of mechanisms to reinvent licensed empiricism despite the protestations of professionals. The rise of the medical profession did not lead to the suppression of rival healers but rather to a largely vain effort to contain a greater number and variety of rivals than ever — an effort undermined at many turns by the public power itself.

The Subordination (and Insubordination) of Pharmacists

The inability of medical doctors to incorporate pharmacy as a compliant junior partner in the new medical monopoly was probably inevitable, but it created a territorial problem. I have already touched on the uneasy and commercially competitive relationship between pharmacists and physicians that dated back to the mid–nineteenth century. Nevertheless, the twelve licensed pharmacists in the late 1850s, all of them foreigners, had been invited to join the medical association created in 1858, and pharmacists with recognized credentials were considered full members of the medical elite. In 1895, when pharmacists were included in the new Faculty of Medicine, Surgery, and Pharmacy, there were only seventeen men with recognized titles to practice pharmacy, and they were still all of them immigrants.[2] The School of Pharmacy was successfully created two years later under the aegis of the faculty. With the first graduating class of thirteen in 1900, the number of licensed pharmacists in the country nearly doubled in one fell swoop, and what had been a profession made up exclusively of immigrants was thoroughly nationalized in the space of a few years: between 1902 and 1905, twenty-four Costa Ricans graduated from the school, and twenty more between 1906 and 1910.[3]

Soon after the first graduation in 1900, a tension was apparent between the two basic constituencies of the joint professional body. It was evident that within a few more graduating cohorts, pharmacists would have a voting majority in the faculty. In a heavy-handed move to preempt this eventuality, physicians moved in 1902 to nullify pharmacists' votes on certain issues and proposed procedural changes that would ensure a junior partner status for pharmacists within the professional association. Using just such tactics, they struck down a law that physicians had to staff their dispensaries with a titled pharmacist or cease to sell medicines. A separatist movement quickly formed among the pharmacists, and that same year they split off from the Faculty of Medicine to form their own association, the College of Pharmacists.[4]

While they never explicitly styled themselves as medical practitioners, pharmacists maintained that they had a duty to help the sick and the right to provide medicine to patients at their discretion. If physicians would not cease to play the role of pharmacist, why should pharmacists avoid acting as doctors? The center of San José was still the site of the most important pharmacies. In their advertisements, large concerns like the Botica Francesa (which also manufactured and sold its own medicines throughout Central America) made no bones about their experts' ability to provide drugs for specific ailments, from hookworm disease to kidney infection. The proprietress of the Botica Francesa, Amparo López Calleja, cultivated a reputation as a skilled healer, in part on the basis of the popularity enjoyed by her father, a Cuban independence leader and empiric who had provided medical services free to the people of San José after going into exile there in the 1870s, and who became a "veritable popular idol."[5] This uneasy and, in practice, poorly defined division of powers continued to characterize professional relations between physicians and pharmacists, which remained tense throughout the period of my study. But despite a rather unresolved official status, for common and chronic health concerns pharmacists considered themselves and were considered by the public to be knowledgeable general practitioners of conventional medicine.[6]

A similar process was at work in dentistry during Costa Rica's belle epoque. A handful of dental surgeons had practiced in the capital city since the 1850s and had been included in the group of legitimate medical practitioners as defined by the Protomedicato. In 1892, there were six in San José (including Céline Durval, who a year earlier had become the first female practitioner to have her credentials recognized by the Costa Rican Protomedicato).[7] By 1898, there were eleven dentists offering modern services in San José. Maximiliano Fischel, for example, advertised himself as an "American dental surgeon [and] graduate of Philadelphia," and offered "all the latest advances: porcelain and gold crowns, partial and complete dentures, gold, tin, silver, and cement fillings. . . . Extractions under anesthetic, cures of the gums." Prices, he promised, were modest, and the work was guaranteed.[8] Yet still in 1895 a foreign dental empiric could operate openly in the capital, "dressed illegally in *frac* and sporting some medallions and decorations," and "followed by a large crowd who admired the . . . way he grasped the sufferer and, after applying his miracle liquid to the molar, in a flash pried it out with his fingers or the point of a stick." The jocular reportage of the leading newspaper suggests that the quacksalver's transgression against the medical profession was not a grave concern of public opinion.[9]

New Competitors

The second half of the nineteenth century also saw a new breed of unorthodox practitioners try to gain official recognition as legitimate medical professionals, led by homeopaths, chiropractors, osteopaths, and psychologists. In Costa Rica, only homeopathy made a strong run at the medical establishment. It did so rather late by Latin American standards, reflecting both the country's small and peripheral market as well as the fact that homeopathy was the largest nineteenth-century unorthodox "sect."[10] Homeopathy was developed in the early 1800s by the

German physician Samuel Hahnemann, who was dismayed by the inefficacy of traditional cures and began a series of pharmaceutical experiments. These led him to what became the homeopathic law of *similia:* the proposition that "like cures like" — that "disease could be cured by drugs which produced, in a healthy person, the symptoms found in those who were sick."[11] Small doses of medicines (sometimes infinitesimal) that induced mild symptoms similar to a particular disease would cure the disease, and this approach was appealing to many who reacted against the excessive treatments that characterized conventional medical therapeutics of the day.[12]

Hahnemann had attacked even vitalistic regular medicine for its tendency to treat symptoms as though they were isolated from one another, rather than understanding the organic combination of symptoms for each disease and treating them comprehensively (as he claimed his own drug regimen could do). He also alleged that the ultimate cause of disease was unknowable to medical science, in that it was a disturbance in the vital self. Latin American homeopaths often reproduced this critique, attacking "allopathic materialism" for viewing the body as a mere machine and proposing that homeopathy sought to rehabilitate the lost harmony of the changed organs in accordance with the more vitalistic understanding of the divine condition, "stamped by God on his creations."[13] This epistemological struggle was difficult to separate from a struggle to break down the medical monopoly of conventional practitioners.

But the challenge of homeopathy did not necessarily come from outside the medical profession. In Brazil, a thesis on homeopathy was presented at the Rio Medical Faculty as early as 1836, and there were a number of efforts in the 1840s to establish schools of homeopathic medicine along with homeopathic drugstores. By the end of the decade, despite the emergence of a number of highly respected practitioners, it had fallen afoul of the medical establishment and been relegated to the margins of the profession. Still, it had managed to take root as a permanent part of the medical culture of the country, and practitioners — including some physicians — continued to demand official recognition for the discipline as a legitimate form of medical science. The unorthodox discipline emerged in the rest of Latin America a decade or two later.[14]

Hahnemann had interpreted Edward Jenner's breakthrough in vaccination as a confirmation of his "law of similars," and it is worth speculating that the growing popularity of homeopathy throughout Latin America was spurred by the increasing familiarity of the populace with the logic of smallpox vaccination. It might also have had to do with the mild nature of the diluted drugs and homeopathy's general rejection of "heroic treatment" — that is, the use of medicines with powerful physical effects and side effects. Homeopathic medicine chests first became available for sale in San José pharmacies in the early 1860s, and their popularity may have been fueled by the massive use of heroic drugs during the cholera epidemic of 1856 as the basis of unsuccessful treatments.[15] Though homeopathy was obviously known in Costa Rica by the mid–nineteenth century, it was only at the beginning of the twentieth century that practitioners made a run at the medical establishment, by which point their conventional opponents had already established a powerful professional bastion.

Costa Rican physicians did not respond to homeopathy with blanket hostility, however. In 1900, Teodoro Picado, a physician, wrote in a series of articles on "professional obligations" in the *Gaceta Médica,* the official organ of the Faculty of Medicine, that physicians were permitted to attend to a request from a homeopath for joint consultation as long as no theoretical debates ensued and the diagnosis conformed to "classical therapy." The medical faculty also offered to recognize homeopathic degrees as a basis for incorporation, but only if practitioners could pass the same exams as the "allopaths." Similar stands were taken by the Mexican and Brazilian professional bodies. Homeopathy was widely tolerated, and some of its practitioners were held in high regard by physicians.[16]

Nevertheless, many homeopaths did seek to undermine the legitimacy of conventional medical theory and practice, and this occurred in Costa Rica as well. Practitioners of this unorthodox specialty had been known since Hahnemann's first efforts for the evangelical zeal with which they mobilized a populist, but science-based critique of the monopolism and intellectual pretensions of physicians. The prestige that conventional medicine had acquired through its association with bacteriology presented a new pillar that had to be demolished. In 1905, Gregorio Quesada published a sustained assault on allopathic medicine in Costa Rica as simply one alternative among many legitimate approaches to modern medicine. The upstart homeopath questioned the scientific standing of physicians, arguing that the "modern microbists" were heirs to a long tradition of pseudoscientific nonsense that had also once been considered absolute truth, but that turned out to be mere dogma (humoralism, Brownism, antiphlogism, and so on). "True, today they do not bleed every patient like they used to (with the exception of his or her pocketbook), and drugs are handed out in smaller sizes to make them less disagreeable," yet he pointed out that the profession was still far from consolidating a scientific mastery over the field of human health. In the short run, the search for complete acceptance was in vain, though in 1905 the city directory registered two practitioners in San José under the ambiguous category "Homeopaths (doctors)."[17]

In Brazil, homeopathy had overlapped with another form of unorthodox medicine: spiritism. In 1858, a group of physicians who practiced homeopathy and the laying on of hands, and gave free treatment to the poor, embraced the French magician and spiritist Allan Kardec's *Book of the Spirits* (1857). Kardec's brand of spiritist healing reproduced many of the theories of Anton Mesmer concerning the magnetic, fluidlike aura that surrounded the individual, which was a counterpart to the physical being and reflected illness in the body. The Brazilians created their own hybrid practice of Kardec's theses, an eclectic combination of healing that included passes to discharge magnetic fluids and realign disturbed currents, personal counseling, and drug prescriptions (usually homeopathic).[18] Elsewhere in late-nineteenth-century Latin America, spiritism and animal magnetism would combine with traditional folk healing, becoming familiar throughout the continent and playing an enormous role in redefining popular conceptions of healing.[19] There is little evidence of powerful spiritist healing currents in Costa Rica. Again, however, the influence can be read in the title of the first Costa Rican study to touch on aspects of psychology, *The Will of Microorganisms,* published in 1905 by the enfant terrible, educator, and social philosopher Roberto Brenes Mesén. In a later publication, Brenes Mesén maintained that mysticism would have to be part of the developing inquiry into the human mind and will because it was "an instrument of research into the truth."[20]

Conventional Irregulars

Most of the evidence available on curanderos and empirics between 1880 and 1900, the period I have identified as the liberal *reforma médica,* comes from two physician-led campaigns against the unlicensed practice of medicine. The first was announced in an 1886 circular referring to stipulations in the new Penal Code (of 1880) and urging local authorities to suppress any curanderos operating in their area. The timing probably reflected the fact that the coterie of positivist reformers known as the Olympians were coming into their own following the death of General Próspero Fernández in 1885. Bernardo Soto, the young lawyer who replaced him as president, had refreshed the cabinet with generational and ideological cohorts like Durán. The cases reported during this crackdown provide a glimpse of curanderos in the agricultural districts. The second campaign against curanderos was unleashed in the years 1893–1895, corresponding to the crystallization of the new professional body of physicians and the vertiginous rise in the number of trained doctors incorporating in the country. Unlicensed practitioners were warned in the newspapers of the day that they would no longer be tolerated and would face stiff fines or jail sentences. The available records of prosecutions during these years come from San José, and though this does not necessarily mean that the efforts of the authorities were confined to the capital, it is a distinct possibility given the market concerns and political power of the doctors of San José. Two clear trends emerge from these two rounds of prosecutions. First is the sense that the most notorious — and hence likely the most popular — irregulars in both rural and urban areas had incorporated important elements of conventional medicine into their practices. Second is the fact that official action was half-hearted.

In March 1886, the governor of Puntarenas rounded up five popular healers in and around the port, and another one in the town of Esparta that lay inland on the road to San José. Three were described as curanderos and another three as apothecaries (boticarios), who "although it can't be said in all rigor that they practice the trade of the curandero, it is known that in this district there are many poor people who, not having resources to buy medicines, visit their establishments so that they might be prescribed and given them free of charge." The governor also noted that one of those who might be considered more properly a curandero, don Vicente Rodríguez, was practicing the office "by virtue of an accord of August 1883 with the executive power" and asked the minister of the interior whether that authorization made Rodríguez exempt from the new law.[21]

The attempt at a crackdown had something of a reverse effect. Given that the central government was not accompanying this with any effort to extend certified medical services, the rural populace moved to request the legitimation of their newly criminalized curanderos. Later that same year, for instance, in October 1886, a petition was made to the minister of the interior by some fifty residents of San Ramón, a major new center born of agricultural settlement on the northwestern edge of the Central Valley. They requested that since the cash-strapped government had recently suppressed the town doctor in the district, the empiric Manuel María Guerrero might be allowed to heal people in cases of emergency without fear of being prosecuted as a curandero. Guerrero, whose experience included acting as a dispensary attendant (boticario) for "notable physicians," had "saved the lives of two mothers and their fetuses by his rapid and opportune interventions without charging a single cent."[22] Guerrero fits the profile of those arrested in Puntarenas: the town apothecary, he apparently had a conventional if informal apprenticeship in the employ of a physician that had allowed him to develop some surgical skills. The outcome of the petition is not known, but in the early 1890s two other empirics operated openly and semi-officially in San Ramón (which was still without a physician), among other activities performing autopsies on a regular basis in order to issue death certificates.[23]

For its very mundanity and conventionalism, it is also worth looking at the case of a foreign quack from the era who had a particular and well-publicized specialty. In 1890 a Spaniard, "Dr." Abel Murillo, set himself up in Costa Rica, and without making any attempt to get authorization from the Protomedicato, began to advertise himself in newspapers and handbills as a specialist in curing tapeworm. The painter Antonio Jarquín came on one of these ads in a downtown rooming house, and reading its description of symptoms that corresponded to tapeworm (general ones like stomach-, head-, and backache) and much impressed by the drawings of various tapeworms that accompanied the text, decided he was so afflicted and sought Murillo out. Murillo examined Jarquín by taking his pulse, poking an ophthalmoscope in his left eye, and pronouncing him sick with tapeworm. He then charged him the considerable sum of thirty colones for two separate "medicines" that were essentially purges in pill form (with other patients, Murillo had written out prescriptions that were filled in a San José pharmacy).

He was convicted of the unlicensed practice of medicine and fined fifty-five pesos, probably significantly less than he had earned during his stay in San José.[24] Two years later, he was arrested in his new home, Curridabat, on the outskirts of San José for the same routine; again he was fined, this time sixty pesos, and happily paid up.[25]

This is not to say that all irregulars fell within the boundaries of conventional practice. For one thing, not enough is known about the activities of even these empirics to make a final judgment on their approach to medicine. It is difficult, moreover, to ascertain with confidence whether the records correspond to the actual range of unlicensed healers. There were popular healers on the Costa Rican landscape who were more clearly marginal in social position and medical powers. Pedro Martínez, for one, was detained by the town doctor and a police official in Heredia in 1884, charged with a combination of vagrancy, being a public nuisance, and practicing medicine without a license. Martínez was a thirty-two-year-old former carpenter, sometime criminal, and itinerant mystic who wandered through the Central Valley, Bible in hand, dressed in outlandish robes, a blue sash, and purple shoes, declaiming religious prophecy and impersonating John the Baptist. He claimed that he no longer practiced medicine, yet it was alleged that he continued to heal and provide medicines in return for food.[26] Though Martínez is a more radical figure in which irregular medicine, criminality, vagabondage, and religious mysticism all overlap, his was an uncommon case.

The empirics cited during the crackdown on the unlicensed practice of medicine between 1893 and 1895 were all from the new popular barrios of San José, places like Peor es Nada (literally, "Better Than Nothing") that were growing up in the capital city.[27] These women and men were members of the community, and like their clientele, often claimed to be artisans by trade. They treated common internal medical complaints and chronic ailments — stomachaches, rheumatism, and so on — and they did so with a fairly ordinary therapeutic arsenal of herbals, although they had incorporated some key stylistic elements of the modern conventional physician's practice.

In 1893, a leading physician, Jenaro Rucavado, denounced Petronila Vargas for the illegal practice of medicine. Vargas was well-known to artisan families in the popular barrios of the capital. Though Vargas herself had not delivered the baby, she had prescribed herbal remedies to a woman suffering after a harsh delivery, charging the sum of two pesos for the consultation (probably about half what a physician would charge). The curandera was illiterate, but her daughter, who accompanied her on her visits, was not, and the girl had written the prescription for the medicine on a scrap of paper. Thus, the curandera was incorporating into her practice the physician's prescription signifier, a scrawl on paper (the prescription would have been filled at a pharmacy, which would then have paid Vargas a commission).[28]

The case is echoed in striking fashion by that of Ramona Barboza Meléndez, charged two years later. She frequently diagnosed patients in her house for common complaints like stomachaches, and prescribed medicines such as ointments and linseed powder. Interestingly, Barboza Meléndez was also illiterate and had her son write out the prescriptions, which were filled at the pharmacy next door, the Botica de la Fe. Barboza Meléndez apparently charged only one peso for a consultation (though in one instance the medicines cost forty pesos, part of which would have gone back to her as a commission). There seems to have been little difference between this type of common female urban curandera of the 1890s and her male counterparts, except that she may have been more likely to attend to the delicate complaints of the fair sex.[29] Barrio pharmacies normally had close associations like this with nearby curanderos and curanderas, and filled these informal prescriptions as a matter of course. Needless to say, in this case the pharmacist, León Duberrán, denied any knowledge of the affiliation even though he did agree that the medicines in question came from his shop.[30]

One of the unlicensed barrio apothecaries in turn-of-the-century San José was the Guatemalan Carlos García Granados, prosecuted in late 1895 for vending drugs without a patent and for substituting ingredients in a prescription written by the physician Gerardo Jiménez. Jiménez had prescribed potassium iodine, some quinine compounds in pill form, and a mercurial pomade to an artisan who went to García Granados to have it filled. The druggist instead prepared a potion, labeled "Costa Rican Pharmacy," that had none of the prescribed substances and some pills containing rhubarb rather than quinine. One might speculate that the physician and the irregular practitioner had conflicting beliefs about what were appropriate medicines for the illness in question. Nevertheless, García Granados proved to have fulfilled a lengthy apprenticeship in a Guatemala City pharmacy run by a titled

Other Healers

professional and had spent a year in the same city staffing the dispensary in a physician's office. As in the great majority of cases to be found in the historical record, this "irregular" had significant conventional training.[31] Furthermore, as should now be apparent, legitimate and illegitimate practitioner webs intersected and overlapped with some frequency: titled pharmacists prepared medicines prescribed by curanderos; apothecary empirics prepared (or substituted alternatives for) medicines prescribed by physicians; empirics trained under the auspices of physicians and pharmacists, and might see their status change from unlicensed to licensed (or tolerated) based on that apprenticeship, especially if they had public opinion behind them.

Ethnicity and Popular Medicine

As for the fate of indigenous healers in this era, the privatization of communal lands, plundering and abolition of religious brotherhoods, and encroachment by mestizo farmers contributed to a gradual process of involuntary *mestizaje* in all but a few countries. Indian groups who had long lived within the political order of Hispanic America came under intense pressure as liberal states consolidated. Little is known about how they endured this assault, how their practices might have changed as a result, or the degree to which medical interaction with neighboring mestizo communities was affected. Strong indigenous medical cultures, however, survived this onslaught in Guatemala, Peru, Bolivia, and Mexico at least. The Kallawaya of Bolivia, though persecuted by the authorities during the liberal era, continued to make their annual circuit of herb gathering, curing in far-off lands, and trading medicine for goods. They were even invited to Panama during the failed French effort to dig a channel across the isthmus due to their skill at treating malaria, suggesting that indigenous healing practices were not simply fighting a vain rearguard action.[32]

Indigenous groups who had managed to survive in the more difficult to dominate areas beyond the frontiers of Hispanic settlement now came under genocidal assault, most notoriously in southern Argentina and Chile as well as northern Mexico. A similar process was reproduced in Costa Rica, where the Guatusos-Malekus in the north were subject to the grotesque private conquest of rubber tappers, turned into slaves for sex and labor or sold into domestic service. The renewed evangelical efforts of the Costa Rican church after 1880 brought impoverishment and cultural decimation in the guise of missionary mercy to the Guatuso, and also to the Bribri people in the southern region of Talamanca.[33] The banana boom on the Caribbean coast furthered the disaster for the latter in the 1890s. In 1875, when the U.S. ethnographer William Gabb entered the area he observed three different types of Bribri shaman, including an awa, who he likened to a doctor who addressed physical maladies. When another anthropologist visited the Bribri in 1917, no medical rituals of any kind were being performed as far as he could tell, though there was still a shaman responsible for burial rituals.[34]

It seems unlikely, therefore, that native indigenous medicine posed much of a commercial or ideological threat to Costa Rican physicians as the nineteenth century progressed, though it probably continued to inform the practices of some popular healers. Moreover, although indigenous medical cultures experienced a period of pronounced crisis and disorientation, in such places, too, they survived, and their practices were even revalued through incorporation into the medical marketplace. In the 1950s, the anthropologist Doris Stone remarked that the Bribri and Cabecar curanderos of Talamanca were regaining their prominence in neighboring mestizo communities after a period of decadence. Part of their renaissance was due to the flow of Hispanic patients who came to consult them because of the rising cost of patent medicines offered by *los chinos*.[35]

The railway labor migration of the 1870s and 1880s introduced Chinese medicine into Costa Rica as many thousands of indentured Chinese laborers arrived to build the line. A small portion of them settled in Costa Rica, especially in the retail and service sectors of secondary towns, and helped a tiny trickle of further immigrants get into the country despite restrictions on Chinese immigration starting in the 1890s.[36] Although little is known about its practice in Costa Rica, Chinese herbal medicine rapidly became popular in Cuba after the arrival of the first indentured laborers from China in the 1840s.[37] In Costa Rica, by the 1920s the subsecretary of health would complain of the "numerous Chinese, black, and other curanderos who exercise their quackery with the tacit consent of the authorities."[38]

The revival of African-based medicine, beginning in the 1870s, was the single most significant event in the country's popular medical culture during the late nineteenth century. The renaissance was a result of the large number of Antillean laborers, initially from Curaçao, and then later from St. Kitts and especially Jamaica, who were brought in by the companies that constructed the railroad to the Caribbean port of Limón. Many thousands of them stayed after the line was finished in 1890, to tend their own farms, and increasingly to work in the plantations, transport networks, and dock facilities of the burgeoning banana enterprise that would eventually become the United Fruit Company. Antilleans were far and away the largest immigrant populace in Costa Rica between the censuses of 1883 and 1927, and between 1900 and 1913 alone some twenty thousand Jamaicans and smaller numbers of other West Indians migrated to Limón.[39]

Richard Sheridan has studied the African-based medicine of eighteenth- and early-nineteenth-century Jamaica. As with many of the world's medical currents, healing, magic, and religion were tightly clustered, and can only be separated for analysis at the risk of missing the point. Nonetheless, practitioners had an elaborate knowledge of medicinal herbs, practiced both curative and preventive health as well as an array of minor surgical techniques (especially bonesetting), knew of inoculation, and engaged in light bloodletting. There were two basic types of West Indian medical practitioners, Obeah and Myalist, roughly equivalent to "bad" and "good." The Obeah practitioners were sorcerers who could cure illness (and cause it through a deep knowledge of poisons) and help those suffering from bad spirits or curses (or inflict the same). Myalism was a religious sect of African origin that reconstituted itself in Jamaica, and according to an observer of the 1840s, is "in many ways the antithesis of Obeah": practiced in the open and only beneficent in its purposes. Initiates to the cult acquired a strong grounding in herbal medicine.[40] The spread of Afro-Caribbean healing among the mestizo populace of the country's heartland may have originated in the construction camps along the railway line, where large numbers of migrant mestizo workers found themselves in an insalubrious and unfamiliar region, away from local medical traditions and in close proximity to Antillean crews.[41] Whether or not the rapid spread was assisted by a collective memory of black and mulatto healers of the late colonial period remains for further research.

In her study of United Fruit and labor in Limón province, Aviva Chomsky has documented the presence of two traditional healers who played murky, but allegedly crucial leadership roles in the 1910 strike of Afro-Antillean workers against the company. After the crackdown on the strike, J. Washington Sterling, described as an "obeah man," was charged by Costa Rican authorities with practicing medicine without a license and was expelled from the country; another even more mysterious figure, known only as Francis and labeled a "brujo," or sorcerer, disappeared (appropriately for a sorcerer).[42] If Sterling indeed practiced Obeah, he did so while running a drugstore and practicing medicine of a conventional nature, albeit without a license.

In transcripts from Sterling's trial, Septimus Keeval, another English subject resident in Limón who described himself as a "doctor" (médico), claimed he had been called to attend to a former patient of Sterling's, Mary Watson, who the accused had given various bottles of medicine. She later died. Together with a police officer, Keeval had gone to Sterling's shop and found in the back room "an operating table, . . . a stethoscope, an ophthalmoscope, a tooth extractor, and a doctor's bag; tools that only doctors use." Keeval also contended that Sterling made house calls around Limón on a bicycle.[43] Thus, to the degree that Sterling practiced Obeah (asserted but never explored in the trial), he evidently combined it with the conventional general medical practice of pulling teeth and office surgery, and his instruments show that he was, at the very least, intent on *representing* himself to his clientele as conversant in the use of standard clinical instruments.

The Obeah man had also been charged previously for an illegal operation on a woman patient in Limón. Keeval and other authorities accused Sterling of being an abortionist, purporting to have "the evidence of two persons, the wife of one whom he killed, and the other ruined by an illegal and brutal operation on her womb," presumably in places in Jamaica and Nicaragua where Sterling had also practiced medicine illegally.[44] Sterling had unspecified medical titles and had made a considerable effort to try to acquire a license to practice from the Costa Rican Faculty of Medicine — without success.

The case of Sterling shows that one must be careful about presuming a fundamental or unbridgeable separation between conventional medicine and ethno-medical practice, and remain attentive to their possible eclectic recombination. It also offers further evidence of the degree to which popular medicine was becoming conventional, and the extent to which conventional practice was becoming popular. This could make it

Other Healers

133

more difficult than ever for licensed practitioners to distinguish themselves from their unlicensed rivals. As a result, there is also a possibility that the portrayal of Sterling as an Obeah man may have allowed medical authorities to distinguish themselves more clearly from a relatively conventional, yet unlicensed and unschooled practitioner by associating him with medical sorcery and taboo procedures like abortion. Unfortunately, the case does not allow one to gain a precise idea of how involved he was with either.

The Limits of Professional Policing and the Return of the Licensed Empiric

By and large, physicians were frustrated in their efforts to have authorities crack down on both new and old types of irregular practitioners, even during this sustained and focused campaign promoted by a dynamic new professional association in the 1890s. Petronila Vargas was initially convicted and fined sixty pesos in 1893, but this was reduced to only ten pesos after an appeal to the governor of the province.[45] Ramona Barboza, arrested in 1895 and again in 1897, admitted that she had once been a curandera, but was no longer practicing. Despite overwhelming evidence that this was a fib and that she had a thriving practice in the barrio, she mounted spirited challenges by creating alibis and was exonerated on appeal twice by San José's principal police agent.[46] Given the unquestionable political power of physicians, why was enforcement and punishment so lax?

It is difficult to answer this with any precision because the issue involves the shadowy zones of informal tolerance and unspoken political culture, but fragmentary evidence points to a number of reasons. At a very basic level, police and judicial authorities might hesitate to persecute unlicensed medical practitioners because they or their loved ones sympathized with the individuals in question or unconventional medicine in general. In 1864, Father Juan Corredor eluded prosecution for illegally practicing medicine thanks to the sympathy of other powerful clerics, the governor (whose sister the priest was treating), and "many distinguished families of Cartago."[47] In the 1880s, a politically influential Chilean physician, José Joaquín Aguirre, called on the country's Supreme Court to take more severe action against quackery, only to discover that three of its four judges normally consulted curanderos rather than physicians.[48]

At the most dramatic level, government agents were attuned to the potentially volatile response of any official persecution of irregular healers. David Sowell's work on Miguel Perdomo Neira, a popular Andean healer and surgeon of the 1860s and 1870s, has shown that the rivalry between popular healers and biomedical monopolists — and between the followers of each — could all too easily acquire overtones of ideological and class conflict. Due to his well-publicized association with the secret arts of indigenous healing, the Catholic faith, conservative ideology, and the plight of the poor, Perdomo Neira was perfect for channeling popular resentment against the modernizing liberals in the guise of the scientific medical elite of Bogotá. Though I am reading between the lines of Sowell's work here, the Colombian authorities appear to have treated the incendiary healer with care, even in the face of rioting by his followers.[49]

The popular healer was always a potential lightning rod for rebellion, particularly if questions of subordinate ethnicity or class coincided with the practice of any form of alternative medicine, and charismatic popular healers were at the center of some of Latin America's most serious nineteenth-century rebellions. During Brazil's Maranhão uprising in 1839, it was "the Negro Cosme, considered a witch doctor," who organized thousands of runaway slaves, had himself declared emperor, and ended up offering the most serious rebel challenge to central authority. In Mexico, the faith healer Teresita, the Saint of Cabora, provided spiritual fortification for the people of Tomóchi in their resistance to a punishing Porfirian modernism. Another charismatic healer rebel, the thaumaturge Antônio Conselheiro, led the people of Canudos in their tragic backlands confrontation with the forces of Brazilian state positivism at the end of the century. When in 1912 another messianic curandero, José María, began organizing armed followers in the Contestado region of the Brazilian backlands, his rapid liquidation by Canudos-wary authorities only sparked a new uprising equipped with a new cult.[50] The prosecution of Washington Sterling by Costa Rican authorities in 1910 was, in this sense, a serious risk since he was apparently both a political dissident and an irregular healer. Still, in that instance the strike had been decisively crushed and the politically dangerous moment had passed; the attack on Sterling was a mopping-up operation to ensure that he would not be there to serve as the focal point for any future rising.

The general tolerance of Costa Rican authorities toward unlicensed healers might best be understood in terms of two complementary vectors of political pragmatism. First, officials were all too aware that outside the major towns and cities, most sufferers had no alternative but to appeal to an irregular healer — and even within cities and towns many were without the means to consult a physician or surgeon. This can be pointedly demonstrated by referring to an unusual case from 1867, when the residents of Puntarenas petitioned the government to license a local empiric in order to break the stranglehold of the new town doctor, Francisco Alvarez. Faced with a populace not accustomed to paying for a regular doctor, Alvarez was allegedly refusing to provide free medical services and medicines to the poor (as his office obliged him to do) while threatening serious legal action against any irregular practitioners. In this way, according to the petition, he was seeking to maximize his potential clientele by ensuring that any sufferer who could possibly pay for his services would do so, even though this meant leaving the poor and indigent without the possibility of any attention whatsoever. Whether or not the charges were true, the government showed itself sympathetic to the request of the residents and licensed a local apothecary as an empiric in medicine who might provide services at a lower fee.[51]

The state action was uncommon in that it meant licensing an empiric to operate in the same jurisdiction as a licensed physician. But it reveals the pragmatic acceptance of the inevitability of the curandero. This is connected to the second point of political pragmatism: the incorporation of empirics into the network of public power in places where physicians could not represent official state medicine. The state not only had a keen interest in avoiding association with professional efforts that might be interpreted as forcibly depriving the suffering common people of any medical comfort, it also needed to associate itself with whoever was considered a legitimate medical authority in areas that were outside the ambit of the medical profession. Rural empirics, in turn, became increasingly familiar with the basic biopolitical and clinical dimensions of medicine.

The granting of empirics' licenses had continued unabated through the 1870s and 1880s. In 1887, a year after their crackdown on curanderos, the physicians on the Protomedicato abolished the licensing of empirics and revoked all outstanding licenses. This period of more intense policing was followed by a gradual return to the status quo, and by 1889 the doctors on the Protomedicato were compelled to tender their collective resignation in protest when the police refused to prosecute a particularly notorious charlatan.[52] The prohibition on licensed empiricism was maintained, however, and sealed by a resurgent medical profession. The police campaign of the 1890s against the unlicensed practice of medicine in the capital city was unusually sustained. A number of trials ended with warnings and then, on reincidence, moved to increasingly large fines.[53] But the will to impose rigorous standards and police them soon faded again, and as Láchner Sandoval's article of 1900 demonstrates, governments quickly found ways to circumvent the restriction on licensed empiricism.

The most controversial episode in this regard had to do with the doctors who filled the expanded network of town doctor posts in the 1890s. Láchner Sandoval echoed a widely held view when he insisted in 1900 that the Cubans were little more than curanderos with false titles.[54] They might be viewed instead as the licensed empirics of the age of medical monopoly. When the web of town doctors was expanded in 1894, the posts remained quite undesirable to the majority of native practitioners who were still enjoying a buoyant market in the main towns. The base salaries offered could not rival the possible earnings of private and public practice in the larger centers, and it was unclear whether rural people would consult physicians rather than curanderos. The state was likely relieved to have an influx of Cuban practitioners. Their credentials may not have been impeccable, yet it was after all a long-established tradition to grant empirics' licenses for practice in peripheral areas. By adhering to a naive reading of the treaty with Spain, the government was able to circumvent the Protomedicato's 1887 abolition of the licensing of empirics for rural practice.

The Cubans of the 1890s were evidently not scientifically driven allies of the new medical elites of the capital city. Neither were they necessarily such quacks as Láchner Sandoval made them out. Ross Danielson has observed that many legitimate practitioners are thought to have abandoned the interior of Cuba, especially during the worst fighting of 1895–1898. He notes, however, that among the "forces of the Liberation Armies were included their barbers and bleeders, and, no doubt, a supply of folk healers."[55] In either case, their style of medicine was probably more attuned with the healing culture of the rural areas of Costa Rica in which they came to operate. Further research will likely find that they served as important bridges between the popular medicine of the rural areas and the new medical styles, beliefs, and practices finding form in the cities.

The basic fact remained that the incipient state bureaucracy needed to register deaths and their cause, gather legal medical testimony, and receive the most reliable possible information about the presence of disease in the country. If physicians could not take up residence in all those areas of the country where the state required these functions to be performed, whether for reasons of lifestyle or due to the absence of a market for conventional medicine, then the state would appoint in their place or tacitly tolerate the most likely candidate. If this had the effect of melding certain strains of popular medicine with official medical culture, so much the better. In 1922, the new subsecretary of hygiene, Solón Núñez, would report that 80 percent of the death certificates during the year had been issued by empirics.[56]

In 1900, one Cuban physician of impeccable credentials resident in Costa Rica, Benjamín de Céspedes, won the Faculty of Medicine prize with a manuscript titled *Infant Hygiene*. In it, the renowned medical reformer denounced "women empirics . . . who bring sterility and death to all homes," and wrote with particular alarm about the ideological warfare that midwives carried on against doctors. He claimed that no matter what the circumstances of the birth, midwives refused to call for a physician; indeed, they were more likely to describe to the patient the horrors of the "facultative intervention, with its iron instruments, forceps, chloroform, and so on with the object of influencing the victim in favor of their barbarous services."[57] Yet as far as can be ascertained, the Costa Rican archives contain no records of prosecutions for the illegal practice of midwifery. Curiously, the healer who was potentially the physicians' worst enemy, and whose knowledge and practice often expressed an explicit, epistemological challenge to modern medicine, was the most tolerated of all underground practitioners. As Céspedes's book went to print, however, the medical profession was moving to sublimate its rival.

6

Midwives of the Republic

When Luisa González's mother went into labor in 1912 she was attended by Mariana, an old woman who was *comadrona* of La Puebla, San José's poorest barrio. The midwife and her ministrations would have been familiar to women throughout Latin America, and they would not have seemed out of place a hundred and fifty years earlier. The overworked woman, bags under her eyes, entered the ramshackle home "discreetly," dressed head to toe in a black fichu, smoking a cigarette, and carrying one bottle of alcohol and another of honey. She lit a candle in the mother's room and began earnestly to say a prayer to San Ramón Nonato, a thirteenth-century Catalan thaumaturge who was the patron saint of pregnant women. The prayer urged San Ramón to give protection to the humble woman; to intercede with God and Christ so that "this tiny creature enclosed in the dark cell of the womb be conserved in life and health"; and to help the midwife "come out of this trance to offer a new being at the feet of the Lord." The prayer ended in an oration from the Litany of the Saints, "Kyrie eleyson, Christe eleyson. Pater de Coeli Deus, miserere nobis."[1]

Actually, by the time Mariana slipped wearily across the threshold of this household of humble artisans, she was already something of a relic. Over the first three decades of the twentieth century, the traditional *partera* was gradually supplanted by the schooled and licensed midwives, or *obstétras*, who had been graduating from the Faculty of Medicine's School of Obstetrics since 1902. By 1950, the majority of Costa Rican children were brought into the world by female hands trained in a rigorous clinical program and, in the final instance, subordinate to the authority as well as oversight of a physician.[2]

This medicalization of childbirth was the product of a complex intersection of historical forces. It was partially propelled by a new state interest in taking over the patriarchal function formerly located in the patrimonial household and applying eugenic principals to the improvement of the populace.[3] This concern meshed nicely with the professional interest of physicians, whose monopoly and ideological authority were mocked by the continued prevalence of the partera. But the new obstetric midwives were not simply molded from above to become tools of a eugenic and patriarchal state, as some authors tend to portray them. In Costa Rica, the training of these young women was also promoted from below, in many instances by municipalities on the agricultural frontier distressed by maternal and infant mortality and attempting to acquire learned medical practitioners for the town. Just as communities had mobilized previously to petition the state for public schools as well as appealed for the central government to assign them a town doctor or license a local empiric, they now offered scholarships to young local women to learn the art and science of midwifery. Moreover, the women themselves were of the popular classes, seizing an opportunity for guaranteed public employment on graduation from a prestigious program in the capital. The midwives from the School of Obstetrics were the first Costa Ricans to graduate from a formal program of medical science inside the country, and they left the institution imbued with a scientific identity and charged with an exalted national mission.

Parteras

During the nineteenth century, as they had during the colonial period, most Latin American midwives learned the art through a lifetime of apprenticeship. The vocation was often hereditary, "a desolating routine, acquired from mother, sister, or relative," according to Mexican surgeon Antonio Serrano's 1805 report to the viceroy.[4] Luz María Hernández Sáenz suggests that in addition to being hereditary, midwifery was a widow's specialty: of twenty-four women listing their occupation as midwife in Mexico City's census of 1811–1812, fifteen were widows.[5]

Though medical and governmental elites in Latin America considered empirical midwives racially suspect and prone to religious oration along with magical ritual, even the unschooled midwife was understood to be knowledgeable about the body and, in the absence of titled practitioners, was called on to provide legal medical testimony on female anatomy, especially in cases of rape, incest, or defloration.[6] In 1835 in Guanacaste, the most isolated region of Costa Rica, in the face of the alleged rape of a ten year old, the alcalde ordered that "the child be examined by two wise women [*mujeres inteligentes*] to determine the gravity of the assault." The women charged with the task, Juana Arias and Trinidad Zúñiga, subsequently gave testimony on the state of pubescence of the victim and the signs of assault.[7]

Midwives with formal schooling and title were rare. Nevertheless, as the independent era dawned, republican governments throughout the region inherited from their Bourbon predecessor an interest in midwife education. Elite families also demonstrated a greater interest in having births attended by trained midwives, some of whom were male, and sometimes by surgeons. Latin America enjoyed a significant influx of foreign, particularly French, midwives beginning with the arrival of women with titles from the Paris Medical Faculty to work in the court at Rio de Janeiro. Many of them set up schools on their arrival, or were specifically invited for that purpose.[8] The male midwife was not nearly so common in Latin America as he was in England and even the British Caribbean. Still, by the late eighteenth century some surgeons did specialize in obstetrics, like the three comadrones practicing in Caracas (all foreign).[9]

Costa Rica also experienced this transformation of midwifery. Even an outpost like San José briefly boasted the presence of a man midwife, Mateo de Urrundurraga, in 1824. A Frenchwoman, Madame Gallimé, delivered the children of San José's elite families between 1835 and 1838 when she was invited by the president of Ecuador to open a school for midwives in Quito. She returned to a much more prosperous Costa Rican capital a decade later to offer her services as a midwife and *modista* (presumably, a makeup and fashion expert) to a new stratum of cafetaleras.[10] For those who could afford the schooled midwife and wished to have her over the traditional practitioner, childbirth became, if not divorced from religion, then certainly less mystical, more technical, and more physiological. It might be said that the first two-thirds of the nineteenth century was the first phase in the "medicalization" of parturition in Latin America.

But it should be noted that popular manuals on childbirth were available in Latin America from the early 1700s, and even illiterate midwives might have had the opportunity to absorb new knowledge and techniques from such books.[11] The process quickened in the nineteenth century as a result of the arrival of schooled midwives from Europe and the establishment of a great number of formal programs in obstetrics, including in provincial *liceos* and *colegios,* in addition to the opportunities they offered local parteras for apprenticeship. Though their status might have remained low, as Silvia Marina Arrom suggests for the case of the growing number of *parteras recibidas* in Mexico City, the number of Latin American midwives who had received some formal schooling expanded considerably over the first two-thirds of the nineteenth century.[12]

Judith Leavitt has shown that by the mid–nineteenth century in the United States, physicians had begun to enter the birthing room as a normal part of practice, for the most part at the behest of the mothers themselves.[13] There was certainly increased interest in childbirth among physicians and surgeons throughout Latin America from the latter part of the eighteenth century onward. But in the estimation of Guatemala's medical luminary Narciso Esparragosa, who experimented with birthing instruments in the 1790s, women's sense of honor impeded the male practitioner's ability to attend many births — a complaint echoed in other parts of the Americas.[14] Physicians and surgeons remained on the margins of childbirth; standby healers of last resort, their intervention was only legitimate when parturition threatened to become something else. This may have begun to change in the second half of the nineteenth century as doctors' use of forceps became more sophisticated, and the use of chloroform (employed in obstetrics in Brazil as early as 1848) brought women relief from pain and made them oblivious to shame.[15] Nevertheless, in Costa Rica the vast majority of births were still overseen by a midwife between 1870 and 1910 despite the rise of the professional male practitioner documented in the preceding two chapters. In the country's first census of 1864, twenty-four women listed their occupation as comadrona. They were present in all of the country's administrative units: eight in San José, four or five in each of the other three provinces, and one or two in Puntarenas and Guanacaste (the census does not allow for any greater geographic precision).[16] There were undoubtedly a great many more women adept in assisting at births, but the twenty-four who registered themselves as midwives evidently derived their primary social identity and significant resources from the regular practice of the art.

These women were artisans of a special kind. Luisa González's portrait of such a midwife emphasizes that they were integrally involved with the community, and that their knowledge of herbal medicines and birthing techniques was interwoven with religious and magical belief as well as ritual. Mariana, the empiric midwife, "at that time a respectable and leading figure" in the barrio, directed the entire birthing process "with great mastery." Meanwhile, the extended family and some female friends attended on the midwife and mother, while Luisa's grandmother oversaw operations in the kitchen, among other activities boiling large pots of water (I will return to the importance of this in a moment). Five hours later, when the birth had taken place without difficulty, all the women in the house gathered to recite the same prayer and thank the Lord. The bloody sheets and water were removed from the room, and the liquid poured on the herb garden, to augment the curative power of the medicinal plants. The father began to bury the placenta in the garden, at which point an argument broke out over how best to dispose of it, for the afterbirth could serve as the active ingredient in a variety of powerful charms and had a market value of five colones—one- to two-days' pay for a male artisan of the era. The midwife sat down to an enormous lunch, though whether or not she was paid in coin is unfortunately not recorded, and finally convinced the family to give her the placenta so that she could "make a gift of it" to the barrio wisewoman. The midwife then left the honey and alcohol for the mother to take together to "clean her mistreated womb."[17]

In 1901, a physician in Heredia described one woman in labor who had been given "some profoundly mysterious concoctions" by the comadrona. Three years later in a rural area outside San José, another young physician noted that he had been to see a woman many days into her labor and found that the midwife had given her "*zapayola* enemas, applied poultices, and poured hot urine over the womb." The reports, both from complicated deliveries, offer further glimpses of the manner in which midwives might combine herbal medicine with magical ritual.[18]

The wisewoman referred to by Mariana, the impressive Doña Dorila, was an older woman, also apparently widowed, who presided over the daily *tertulias* of the barrio women (semiformalized group discussions on the patios or over laundry). She was expert at interpreting their experience through recourse to tales and legends that she told with great skill. She also had a notebook, "like a casebook, with the prescription [*la receta*] for concoctions, rites, beliefs, interpretations of dreams, lists of aphrodisiacs, prayers, etc." The book, bound in blue and gold fabric, was "the great fount of her rich experience, which earned her many colones a month." Principal among her arsenal were special admixtures and prayers to maintain the love of a male partner or to keep him from straying sexually; one of Luisa's aunts had a potion that she sprinkled each day over the marriage bed and claimed was the reason for her bliss.[19]

Dorila had once been a laboring woman of La Puebla like the others, but had developed an expertise that let her live comfortably—indeed much more comfortably than most. She was not stingy: "her generous and believing heart" was responsible for regular donations at the altar of the parish church, and for outfitting for their first communion the poorer children of the barrio who would otherwise have been unable to fulfill the ceremony with dignity. Luisa González was a communist educator looking back askance and aghast at the ignorance that allowed the people of the barrio to be exploited—including by one another—and writing in an age when feminist celebrations of the woman healer were not yet fashionable. Yet she cannot find it in her to doubt the enormous role that this wisewoman played in relieving the general suffering of the women and children of La Puebla, giving them hope, and grounding their lives and experience in a rich lore and belief system.[20]

Of course, Dorila was a sorceress. Though there were surely others like her throughout the country, it is worth noting that La Puebla was originally the outlying village of the blacks and mulattoes of San José: the description of this wisewoman is perhaps a portrait of the syncretic fate of African shamanic medicine after 150 years in an increasingly Hispanicized mestizo culture. Her semiformalized function as a group therapist, complete with interpretation of dreams, is striking in its overtones (her literacy even allowing her to jot down notes in her magically decorated "casebook").[21]

As the medical profession began to gel in the 1870s, its members adopted the Bourbon disdain for the untrained midwife, and also began to conceive of her as an ideological and practical rival.[22] In 1882, as part of the ambitious early reform of medicine promoted by Durán and Ulloa, a school of midwifery was opened in the capital under the auspices of the community of physicians and surgeons, but it withered on the vine when not a single woman enrolled.[23] While midwifery was not aggressively criminalized by the liberals, technically it could have been prosecuted under the new laws against the illegal practice of medicine, and the art was forced underground: no women dared declare themselves comadronas in the censuses of 1883 and 1892.

A modus vivendi continued to exist, and as physicians made clear in case notes published in the *Gaceta Médica*, midwives facing insurmountable difficulties would often seek out a doctor. Still, in 1901, Juan Flores reported a case from Heredia where after a second day of difficult labor, one woman's family began to suggest to the midwife that a doctor be called, "but the comadrona was opposed, saying that all was going well and that the only thing we physicians did was operate to earn more money." After the third day, the family finally overruled her and called Flores in, and he used his forceps to extract a dead fetus.[24] As his experience shows, for all their paternalistic disdain for the common midwife, physicians were not in a happy position vis-à-vis childbirth. Because they were generally only called in as a last resort, their task was relatively thankless for it would almost inevitably end with a dead infant or mother. There was the prospect of taking over the birthing procedure, but as Irvine Loudon has nicely summed up the problem of obstetrics for the modern physician, delivering babies was "time-consuming, badly paid, hard, tiring and worrying work."[25] Rather than take the position of physicians in the United States, Costa Rican doctors, like their Latin American counterparts, continued to seek a more continental solution to managing obstetrics, and their efforts finally gained momentum at the century's end due to the confluence of multiple interests and rise of a particular national anxiety.

The New Context: Scientific Childbirth as Auto-immigration

In the 1890s, a racist malaise began troubling the constitution of Costa Rica's elites. The master social pathology driving the anxieties of national decline in fin de siècle France and England was the dwindling birthrate (especially as measured against that of Germany). In the United States, it was a panic over the drop in birthrates among Anglo-Saxon, middle-class families, who were said to be committing "race suicide" (a term made famous by Theodore Roosevelt, borrowing from the noted sociologist E. A. Ross).[26] In Costa Rica, in the words of an early-twentieth-century minister of the interior, it was "the well-known

high rates of infant mortality." These were rates that progressive reformers considered both unnecessary and the reason that the country
was forced to accept racially undesirable immigrants to satisfy labor
needs.[27] In fact, the rate of infant mortality was high, hovering at about
three hundred per thousand from 1890 through 1914 (such a rate was
not unusual in Latin America, though it was far higher than countries
like Argentina and Cuba that were considered medically advanced).[28]

Political leaders and nationalist intellectuals felt that the country
suffered historically from a shortage of labor, and efforts to overcome
the lack with European immigrants had never prospered. The majority
of those who did arrive after 1870, most of them to work on the railroad
and later in the banana industry, were Nicaraguans, Chinese, and by far
the largest group of immigrants between the censuses of 1892 and
1927, anglophone West Indians of African heritage, mostly from Jamaica.[29] This worry was formulated in explicitly eugenic terms — terms
that meshed easily with the language of public health. The new immigration law of 1897 barred Chinese, Arabs, Turks, Syrians, Armenians,
and Gypsies on the grounds that they were "harmful [*nocivos*] to the
progress and welfare of the republic" since "because of their race, their
habits of life, and their nomadic spirit, which is unadaptable to an
environment of order and work, they would be for the country a cause
of physiological degeneration and propitious sources for the development of idleness and vice."[30]

Physicians were greatly influenced by this malaise, and they contributed to it as well. Just such a fear that the Costa Rican race was degener-
ating had provided the context for Durán's original research on cansancio in the mid-1890s. It was also behind the higienista effort to pass a law
on venereal prophylaxis, and to submit prostitutes to regular inspection
for venereal disease and, if found infected, medical incarceration. After
some excellent historical research on the subject, it is still a mystery how
this fantasy was sustained throughout the West since the refusal to include any systematic treatment of infected males made the discrepancy
between goals and methods utterly ludicrous according to the contemporary medical knowledge on the transmission of venereal disease.
Donna Guy has pointed out for the Argentine case that this "dubious"
aspect of higienista practice was upheld through the confident bluster
of male physicians despite the evidence. Allan Brandt, for his part, has
argued that venereal epidemiology in the United States was "socially

constructed" on a bifurcated notion of women as either good or bad, innocent or fallen, and in which a unidirectional mode of transmission with only one possible ultimate source was posited.[31] But because the maintenance of the system was illogical even on its own terms, ultimately symbolic associations were what justified its perpetuation. As much as anything, the creation of a salon for venereally diseased prostitutes in San José's hospital, and the appointment of a physician to oversee it, was a distorted mirror image of the state's—and medical profession's—growing interest in regulating the reproductive capacity of the healthy female components of the national organism.

Immigration anxiety and public health had formed a strange bond—one described by the great positivist reformer of the liberal period Cleto González Víquez after he assumed the presidency in 1906. In an address to Congress, he contended that "to bring immigrants is to augment the population with elements that do not always turn out to be useful, and which in any case come to share the disadvantages of cities and towns without hygiene; to sanitize towns is to augment and improve the indigenous [sic] population, which for reasons of climate, customs, language, and other circumstances, is the most desirable populace." González Víquez would later apply the revealing label "auto-immigration" to this program to increase the quantity and quality of the Costa Rican "race" through a state commitment to public health.[32] The nineteenth-century liberal Argentine nation-builder, Juan Alberdi's famous dictum *"gobernar es poblar"* — "to govern is to populate" —was here sublated: to govern was to sanitize.[33] The transformation of midwifery was central to this new state commitment to the public health.

Establishing a school of midwifery had been on the medical profession's agenda since the abortive effort of 1882. A second attempt in 1897 petered out when a mere three women enrolled, only one of whom was able to stay the course.[34] But in this context of panic over infant mortality and eugenic concern for the vitality of the national organism, the targeting of midwifery acquired greater urgency. That Benjamín de Céspedes would compose a treatise on the *Hygiene of Infants* in Costa Rica reflects this urgency, as does the professional association's decision to award it the Faculty Prize in 1899. The work expressed Costa Rican physicians' disrespect for the traditional midwife — the *mujeres empíricas*—and laid much of the blame for infant mortality at her "most grotesque and pernicious practices," while insisting that midwives were involved in other crimes against reproduction, especially abortion.[35]

The New School for Scientific Midwives

A school of midwifery was finally established with limited success in 1899, when ten women enrolled. This class included three mature widows — evidently experienced midwives seeking to improve their knowledge and status — who were the only ones to graduate, the rest withdrawing after "tiring of their studies." In 1900, the newly renamed "School of Obstetrics" was placed on firmer ground when agreement was reached with the Junta of Charity to fund a lying-in hospital, the Maternidad, intended to assist the most indigent mothers while also serving as a clinical facility for the school. In the same year, eligibility was restricted to those between the ages of eighteen and thirty who had completed primary school. The restrictions were obviously aimed at excluding mature midwives from using the school for upgrading skills and status as well as concentrating on the training of more malleable young women students. Also in 1900, the municipal government of San José created a number of scholarships for humble students from the city and outlying districts, with the likelihood of employment as town obstetrician on graduation.[36]

The scholarships attracted some inspired candidates. Mercedes Bonilla Chacón, a single twenty-eight year old, summed up their appeal: "Finding myself in extreme poverty, this would be a means to honestly satisfy my necessities, while at the same time carrying out a public service that demands not a few sacrifices." Unfortunately, she was from too marginal a background to find the requisite guarantor, and her application was rejected.[37] Emiliana Calvo Rojas, an unmarried eighteen year old from La Unión in the province of San José, applied for a fellowship in 1903, but was turned down because she did not live in the municipality. After gaining acceptance to the School of Obstetrics, however, she decided to attend anyway, and astutely convinced the powerful lawyer Alberto Echandi, who was guarantor of another student who relinquished her fellowship and dropped the program, to ask that the stipend be transferred to her. Calvo Rojas graduated from the arduous two-year program and returned to her home district to practice. One of her letters of reference, from the principal of her primary school, had described her as a student who "reaped the affection of her teachers with her love of study, her application, and her good behavior."[38] The School of Obstetrics offered this young woman from rural Costa Rica a chance to prolong those budding intellectual yearnings, and the prestige of a title and profession.

The Faculty of Medicine and Surgery asked all municipalities to consider a fellowship program, and by the following year six of the students enrolled, "coming from all points in the republic," and were maintained in the school by municipal fellowships worth between twenty-five and fifty colones a month — a fairly tight stipend, but enough to squeeze by.[39] It is interesting to compare these fellowships with those created by the central government in the 1890s to encourage working-class girls from the capital, and girls from the provinces, to study at the Colegio de Señoritas, the new teacher-training school in San José. As Bonilla's letter of application makes clear, some of the candidates for the School of Obstetrics shared a motivation with their normal school sisters: the greater prestige and salary guaranteed by specialized secondary study for women. The normal school, however, was not open to women who had already begun their career as teachers and wished to upgrade their credentials; fellowships were available only to younger girls (from eleven to sixteen) who were continuing on directly from primary studies. Hence the appeal of scholarships to the School of Obstetrics for women like Isaura Marín, a twenty-eight year old from Naranjo who with municipal backing left her teaching job to pursue training as a midwife.[40]

By 1903 San José was offering seven fellowships, Alajuela and Puntarenas two each, and Cartago, Barba (just outside Heredia), Liberia, and Naranjo (on the periphery of the Central Valley) one each, and more cantons joined the program later in the year.[41] The fact that stipends for studying obstetrics were provided by the always cash-strapped municipalities suggests how valuable a trained midwife was in the eyes of local elites. It is interesting to find in an 1895 petition to the central government from fifty male residents of Naranjo requesting that a town doctor be assigned to the town, a popular referent for González Víquez's notion of auto-immigration, though one with humanitarian rather than eugenic overtones. They criticized the shoddy attention of curanderos, and insisted that the best way to increase the population and supply laboring arms to agriculture as well as industry was not to foment immigration but to "free from the grip of death so many children [they claimed, two of every three born] who die for lack of physicians."[42] Given this concern among local elites, it is not surprising that six years later, Naranjo was among the first rural municipalities to sponsor a midwife. Midwifery, in this sense, became another form of licensed empiricism in areas where physicians were scarce or absent altogether.

A leading member of the Faculty of Medicine, Francisco Rucavado, was commissioned to write the textbook for the new school. The text certainly stressed that midwives strictly defer to physicians in all irregular or unusual births and in the prescription of medicine, and that they ban superstition from the birthing room. But to portray the training as mere indoctrination would be wrong. Rucavado's texts, which were amply discussed and emended in sessions of the Faculty of Medicine board, complemented a rigorous two years of theoretical, clinical, and practical study imparted by three doctors. The illustrated textbooks, which were based on his lecture notes, encompassed 320 pages of analysis, without any attempt at popularization, in physiology, the physiology and anomalies of pregnancy, embryology, anatomy, and antisepsis.[43]

The scientific tone of the school was not put on, nor were exams a mere formality. First-year students had to pass four arduous oral exams in anatomy, antisepsis, embryology, and the physiology of pregnancy. In a good year like 1903, the examination committee failed four out of fourteen students. Other years, half the class failed at least one subject and between the lines of the faculty reports one can always read a few shattered hopes. Those who survived the first year were more likely to complete the program, though they had to pass a second round of oral exams, assist in two dozen births, and oversee five on their own in the Maternidad.[44]

By the beginning of 1903, three more graduates were providing services in San José and nineteen students were enrolled in both years of the program. Pleased with the development of the School of Obstetrics, the Faculty of Medicine announced that henceforth birthing women would not be attended by "empiric comadronas" but by "*doctos obstétricos* [obstetric doctors]."[45] The use of the term was not patronizing. It should be remembered that this school was the only outlet for the teaching impulse of Costa Rican physicians, and they willingly brought a scientific spirit to the classes — one that was reciprocated. In 1902, the students of the School of Obstetrics encouraged their clinical professor, Marcos Zúñiga, to lecture on a new theory of the formation of the placenta. The results of his research, brought together first in his lecture notes, were deemed worthy of publication in the *Gaceta Médica*.[46]

The students took their scientific mission seriously. A series of articles appeared in 1902 in the *Gaceta Médica* written by "the students of the School of Obstetrics." They had decided to answer the editor's call for more submissions for the journal — one that was notably not heeded by the majority of physicians and pharmacists in the faculty. One article, "Our Methods of Nourishing the Child," cited essays from the German medical literature on programs to provide poor children with sterilized milk, reviewed statistical data to support the superiority of breast-feeding (including a chemical analysis comparing breast with cow's milk), and advanced an ideal schedule for feeding.[47]

The young women dedicated the article to the memory of their classmate, the unfortunate Isaura Marín who had died just before presenting her final exam. "Her soul, inspired by the glow of science and protected by the rule of Minerva, was so close to reaching the pinnacle of her aspirations," they wrote. The School of Obstetrics had obviously achieved a Costa Rican first: female bonding in a scientific circle. There can be no doubt that the students were self-conscious of this: they declared their classmate part of the "superior intellectual life" of the country. In so doing, of course, they inscribed themselves in the same category.[48]

Their initiation into professional and scientific life was crowned during a special gathering of the faculty board. On the evening of 16 March 1903, "in solemn session, the Faculty of Medicine conferred the title of obstetrician on the students of the School of Obstetrics of Costa Rica." Following a sober discourse by the eminent, German-trained Dr. Pánfilo Valverde, president of the faculty, who again invoked the magic incantation of "professionalism," the young women swore an oath and received a diploma accrediting them as "midwives of the republic."[49] At the time, this was the most prestigious academic graduation ceremony in the country after that of the College of Law, and the medical doctors who conferred the title on these women were among the most august and powerful members of Costa Rican society.

The Transformation of Childbirth

By 1904, there were eight graduates of the School of Obstetrics practicing in Costa Rica, six of them in San José, one in Alajuela, and one in

Barba. The number had almost tripled by 1906 to twenty-two, with ten in the capital (and two more on the immediate outskirts of San José) and the rest spread throughout the republic. The numbers grew steadily until by 1927 there were eighty-six schooled midwives in the country. These women health professionals rapidly transformed birthing after 1900. Prior to the turn of the century, all but a handful of elite women in the provincial capitals (who could turn to a foreign-trained midwife or physician) gave birth with the assistance of friends or the traditional midwife empiric. Fifteen years later, the kind of birth witnessed by Luisa González in her poor San José neighborhood in 1912 was becoming much less common, particularly in the capital.

Let us look at the 1914 report filed by the wonderfully named América Villalobos, a graduate of the School of Obstetrics, and employed as town midwife by the municipality of San José to assist poor women's births in the western and most populous working-class half of the capital. In the first two months of that year, she oversaw the delivery of eleven children in the homes of humble women. She was also attending births during the same period for families who could pay for her services. In the same year, there were at least nine other schooled midwives practicing in San José, and one hundred indigent women gave birth in the Maternidad under the care of a physician and obstetric midwives-in-training. Let us assume that Villalobos delivered one hundred children a year (sixty under the municipal program and forty as a private practitioner). If her professional sisters of the capital delivered roughly the same number of infants over the course of the year, and those born in the Maternidad are added, then 1,100 of the 1,860 children born in San José in 1914 (59 percent) were delivered by a midwife trained in obstetrical science rather than a traditional comadrona.[50]

Outside the capital, of course, the portion was much smaller, with twenty-five obstetricians practicing, and probably able to attend many fewer births due to a less concentrated population in some of the areas. Nevertheless, even assuming an average of sixty births per midwife per year, that means that nearly 10 percent of all Costa Rican births were attended to by a trained midwife as early as 1914. By 1927, when the number of obstetricians reached eighty-six, they would have attended to roughly 25 percent of births nationally. Graduates of the School of Obstetrics might also have been disseminating more contemporary medical knowledge to their unschooled colleagues (the water-boiling procedures of the González household suggest such transmission; recall that the first graduates of the school were elderly widows just like Mariana). Moreover, Rucavado's obstetrics textbook, at a mere two colones a copy, might have made its way into the hands of the more autodidact of midwife empirics. Whether by these routes or some other, at least basic notions of asepsis were incorporated by even the most "traditional" practitioners of the art. In 1927, a leading Costa Rican scientist observed an indigenous midwife deliver a child in a village on the isolated Osa peninsula. She cut the umbilical cord with a pair of scissors, but only after burning them with alcohol so that they would be "sterilized" (the term was hers).[51]

It would be nice to know a great deal more about the practice of the obstetrical midwives, particularly the degree to which they worked with the new philanthropic agencies, such as the Asilo de Infancia (established in 1905 by the Catholic Damas Vicentinas) and Gota de Leche (created in 1913 by eminent women of the merchant-planter class), that were attempting to promote hygienic and modern mothering techniques among the urban poor. Both groups did work with Jadwisa de Picado, Costa Rica's lone female physician of the era and, like many early women doctors in Latin America, a devoted infant higienista.[52] And while it is apparent that the midwives of the republic enjoyed official stature, nothing is known of how they were received by birthing women of the popular classes accustomed to the discreet arrival and mystical liturgies of elderly widows like Mariana.[53]

In an article on infanticide in late-nineteenth-century Buenos Aires, Kristin Ruggiero focuses on the increasing employment of certified midwives, many of them Italian immigrants, by the Public Assistance Office. Ruggiero argues that these midwives became "gyneco-police," part of a network of police intelligence mobilized by the liberal state to maintain gender discipline among working-class women, and so were ultimately plugged more into male than female networks.[54] Trained midwives, just like *normalistas* and the school nurses who became the first generation of Costa Rican social workers, did become willing standard-bearers of liberal civilization. Many of them working-class women themselves, they ended up policing, controlling, and inspecting their sisters with techniques and ideals imparted from a patriarchal state. As Celia Davies points out, however, they might also become "mother's friends," and given the findings of Judith Leavitt, one must pause before assuming

Midwives of the Republic

that working-class women in childbirth would not have chosen the schooled obstetrician in close contact with a physician over the traditional midwife.[55] Finally, as Seth Koven and Sonya Michel have remarked, "Maternalism served women as an important avenue into the public sphere" in Western Europe and the United States, and I would add, in Latin America as well.[56] These midwives of the republic were part of a broader process of "maternalizing" the public sphere — in this case literally — one that complicated the liberal construction of an exclusively male public sphere. In this sense, they must be considered part of the same field of "new women" led by certified schoolteachers, many also of working-class and rural backgrounds, who challenged the liberal patriarchy on a variety of fronts in the 1910s and 1920s.[57]

It is notable that in the census of 1927, the eighty-six women "obstetricians" registered were classed under the "liberal professions," while nurses (almost half of them men, and still mostly untitled) were grouped under "services" beside much less prestigious occupations.[58] The stature of the midwives of the republic would be reduced only over the subsequent twenty years. The success of the School of Obstetrics was key in finally anchoring the Faculty of Medicine's project to create a school of nursing, after three ill-fated efforts (the first, in 1899, designed to accompany the school of midwifery; another in 1907; and a further one in 1917). In the early 1920s, the two schools were at last effectively combined into one Escuela de Enfermería y Obstetricia, with an option for students to do an extra year of study and become nurse-midwives.[59] Nurse-midwives would henceforth operate more directly under the control of a physician, in hospitals and the rural health clinics that proliferated in the 1930s and 1940s. Not coincidentally, the same years also saw a parallel stripping of directive roles from women philanthropists and reformers as the state took more formal and centralized control over the sprawling, semiautonomous philanthropic network of maternalist institutions by creating the National Child Welfare Board, dominated by leading male political figures and physicians.[60]

7

Hookworm Disease and the

Popularization of Biomedical Practice

Among the medical literature generated by Costa Rica's late-nineteenth-century wave of oligarch physicians were two popular health pamphlets written by Juan Ulloa, commissioned by the Faculty of Medicine in 1898 in the face of epidemic outbreaks of whooping cough and scarlet fever. Ulloa pioneered a genre that would soon become a staple of Costa Rican public medicine, "departing from the usual technicalities, to try to explain myself in more simple terms that will be understood by all the social classes."[1] Less than two decades later, in 1915, after a difficult three-hour horseback ride from Puntarenas to a district lab in the small village of Miramar, a visiting physician working for the Rockefeller Foundation was surprised to be greeted by hand-painted signs reading (in Spanish), "Please don't spit on the ground," "Campaign against Ancylostomiasis," "Avoid Typhoid Fever." Dr. John Elmendorf noted that a laboratory set up under the auspices of the Rockefeller Foundation's antihookworm program had become the temporary focus of activity in the village. The building that housed the lab was decorated with educational placards demonstrating common sanitary measures and the life cycle of the hookworm, and with clinical pictures of patients in different stages of the disease. Elmendorf was infected with the general enthusiasm of the populace.[2]

Though Elmendorf probably imagined otherwise, such intense, grassroots participation in public health work in an isolated jungle village was not something the Rockefeller emissaries could have manufactured on their own in such a short period of time. When the foundation's inspectors and microscopists came to set up the lab, the inhabitants of places like Miramar had at least two decades of experience with outsiders arriving to convert them to the new medical faith. Like most of their compatriots, they had bared their arms for district physicians or vaccinators general and had been raised with the hygiene counsel of their village schoolteacher. They were also treated for hookworm disease during the first, autochthonous Costa Rican campaign that ran from 1907 through 1914. Such prior, indigenous initiatives set the stage for the dramatic success enjoyed by the Rockefeller campaign in this, its first Latin American host country.[3]

Scholars of Rockefeller international public health have often proposed that the imperial colossus penetrated the neocolonial periphery with a novel and alien medical and public health epistemology and technology. Working with unidirectional assumptions about the cultural flows of imperialism or privileging the role of political economy, many such studies also take the Rockefeller Foundation as their principal historical subject. Once the perspective shifts away from the grand institutional or geopolitical unities of the foundation or the United States — and particularly if the experience of public health officials, healers, and sufferers in host countries comes into view — it is possible to develop a more nuanced picture of the biomedical interaction between center and periphery.[4]

For one thing, in the Costa Rican case, local medical practitioners preceded Rockefeller philanthropy in both research on hookworm disease and the development of public health campaigns to treat it. The success of the foundation in Costa Rica would have been impossible without their prior efforts and the foundation adapting its mission to a preexisting public health plan of local making that focused on working through the extensive network of primary schools. As important, the antihookworm propaganda and treatment of ancylostomiasis involved medical practitioners retraining the entire populace in a new set of ideas and beliefs about disease and its cure. They did so through repeated, intimate contact with sufferers — encounters that combined gentle and not so gentle persuasion with a calculated translation of the new biomedical approach into terms intelligible and appealing within popular medical culture. While this did involve some conflict between official and popular medical culture, the predominant encounter ended with the negotiated consent by peasants and workers to this radical corporeal intrusion by the public power.

During the first Costa Rican antihookworm campaign, the principal agents in this popularization were the district physicians. The more totalizing second phase of examination and treatment, directed by the Rockefeller Foundation, was accomplished without the town doctors, and largely without the direct participation of physicians at all; public health technicians were transformed into officially sanctioned curers — a process that once again reinvented the licensed empiric. The medicalization of everyday life that took place in the Costa Rican countryside after 1907 was not primarily the work of the medical profession but of agents of public health and social medicine — microscopists, inspectors, and teachers — the vast majority of whom had little or no formal medical schooling.

This is not to say that physicians were cut out of the picture of health in Costa Rica during this era, though for reasons discussed in more detail in the following chapter the profession as a whole suffered a certain decadence. Rather, these two decades saw the advent of a new type of medical luminary — the physician specialist in social medicine and public health, concerned more with technocratic than professional power and a believer in statist centralism over a professional monopoly with public jurisdiction. If Durán and Ulloa were exemplary of the first wave of nationalist oligarch physicians, between 1910 and 1930 the tenor of social medicine would be defined by the figures of Louis Schapiro and Solón Núñez — the first a native of the United States, and the second of ordinary social and radical ideological roots.

Peripheral Precedence

Medical scientists in a number of Latin American countries had discovered the endemic nature of hookworm disease in advance of Rockefeller medicine men: Wucherer in Brazil (1866), Prowe in El Salvador (1887) and Guatemala (1889), Durán in Costa Rica (1895), and Roberto Franco in Colombia (1905).[5] British public health experts had long been aware of the disease in the tropical territories of the empire.[6] But Guatemalan and Salvadoran officials decided the affliction was not serious enough to warrant a public health campaign (although some work was done on army troops); and the appeals to government by Brazilian and Colombian physicians were unheeded, or died on the tables of the legislatures.[7] What distinguished Costa Rica from all these cases, and what made it unique in Latin American and world terms, was

that its physicians and public health activists had the political wherewithal to create a national treatment campaign. Their motives were
broadly similar to those that led the Rockefeller Foundation into the
crusade against the hookworm in the U.S. South.

The treatment of hookworm disease was an especially good vehicle
for educating the popular classes in fundamental notions of medical
science and hygiene. To begin with, the pernicious parasite was peculiarly suited to serve as a stand-in for the "germ" in germ theory.[8] The
worm was microscopic (though large ones were just visible to the naked
eye) and yet looked monstrous when magnified. It also left an itching
sensation at the point where it entered the body in the soft tissue between the toes. The hookworm was thus an excellent example by which
to substitute a basic logic of humoral medicine with a basic notion of
bacteriology. The *identity* of a disease was not the ensemble of symptoms
experienced by the sufferer as a particular illness (hence, cansancio,
or weariness, the name by which the affliction was known throughout
Latin America); rather, it was the invisible organism that entered the
body and provoked such symptoms (hookworm disease).[9]

Even better, there was a "cure" for hookworm disease — that is, an
effective method of purging the worms from the host body through the
ingestion of a powerful, but simple and cheap vermifuge made from
extract of thyme, followed up by a jolt of Epsom salts.[10] So hookworm
treatment could also promote the idea that scientific medicine prof-
fered specific cures. Expulsion of the worms from the body relieved in
short order the anemic exhaustion that was the disease's most common
symptom. The patient felt noticeably better within twenty-four to forty-
eight hours — he or she felt "cured" — and so the entire procedure was
an effective dramatization of the basic ideas and promise of modern
medicine. Meanwhile, the recurrence of hookworm disease could be
easily prevented through the adoption of a number of elementary sanitary habits, and this made it ideal for promoting the tenets of public
health.

Obviously, those who advocated treatment campaigns were aware
that a question of political economy was involved: hookworm disease
was associated with low productivity in workers. Juan César García has
argued that creating a healthier labor force was the principal factor
motivating microbiological research in late-nineteenth-century Latin
America, and he identifies the Costa Rican hookworm discovery and

treatment program as part of this pattern of applied oligarchic science. According to García, physicians like Durán and Ulloa, members of the Costa Rican ruling class, engaged in research and promoted treatment in order to improve the health of coffee pickers so as to further their own profits as well as those of their class peers.[11] Recently, scholars have been less inclined to see the "health is wealth" justification in such instrumental terms. The economic motives that led ruling groups to embrace certain medical or public health strategies are still acknowledged, from the maximum vitality and reproduction of the labor force, to the greater investment, trade, and European immigration that it was thought would come with more efficient sanitary measures. Moreover, as Marcos Cueto puts it, bacteriology allowed public health ideologues to pose the question of "avoidable disease" and allege that potential wealth was being wasted by not taking action.[12] Yet these motives were both complemented as well as contradicted by civilizing projects that drew their inspiration from cultural concerns and racist fears, and often from institutional impulses toward the consolidation of state power for its own sake.

Like much of Costa Rica's incipient scientific activity, research on hookworm disease had to justify itself in terms of its benefit to export agriculture (especially given that the discovery of the disease coincided with a prolonged crisis in the international coffee economy).[13] But the most endemic zones of hookworm disease in Costa Rica were, in actuality, precisely on the Pacific littoral, outside the coffee and banana zones, and the mechanistic model of coffee oligarchs treating their workers does not explain why Durán and company fought so hard to help sufferers in those areas. To take a counterfactual example that reinforces the point, Christopher Abel has shown that between 1905 and 1911, Colombian hookworm researchers "argued forcefully that more than 90 percent of coffee and sugarcane workers and their families were infested by the debilitating parasite" and yet were unsuccessful in getting state support for a treatment campaign.[14] Indeed, economic assertions were rhetorical tools used by physicians and progressive reformers looking to overcome the reticence of politicians stuck on laissez-faire.

Like Durán's initial research on hookworm disease in the mid-1890s, the campaigns were also motivated by beliefs about the destiny of the nation, attainment of modernity, and as much as anything else, purity of

Hookworm Disease

the race. In a 1901 update on hookworm, Durán's codiscoverer Gerardo Jiménez noted the perceived physiological degeneracy of the "people of the [Pacific] coast and lowlands" — their "differences in color and vigor, and their indolence" — as compared to the "well-developed, properly colored, active, and industrious settler of the central highlands." These negative aspects of the peasant of the Pacific littoral had always been attributed to "climactic influences, poor diet, and decadent variations of our race." The discovery of hookworm disease calls all that into question, and provides a clarion call to address this grave disease that can be "so easily cured" in order to "procure the growth and improvement of our population." This manner of seeing the racial dimension of cansancio was reproduced over the next six years and had not changed substantially when Mauro Fernández gave a lecture on the scourge to the National Agricultural Society in 1907.[15]

At a meeting in August 1907, with Durán presiding, the Faculty of Medicine resolved to recommend to the government, "as a hygienic and humanitarian measure of immediate benefit for our people," that two young physicians receive funding to tour the "infested zones" of the country to measure levels of hookworm infection and treat the sick.[16] In February 1908, the government of Cleto González Víquez agreed.[17] The renewal of interest in a treatment program corresponded to the accession of the old Junta of Charity cohorts, González Víquez and Durán, to their respective presidencies. Durán, now head of the body responsible for the national public health, had an opportunity to attempt a more ambitious project based on the findings of his own pioneering research. González Víquez, for his part, had a long history of pushing sanitary and medical reform as a member of the Junta of Charity, but also as a councillor and mayor of San José's municipal government. Among his substantial and wide-ranging intellectual activities was the translation in 1904 of William Gorgas's work on mosquito control and yellow fever prophylaxis. González Víquez's first tenure as president of the republic was marked by a series of ambitious social policy projects, including the building of modern water and sewer works in the major cities, the completion of a panoptic penitentiary, and a new police and penal code.[18] The hookworm program, however, was a radical departure in that of all the public health and other social policy initiatives of the liberal era, this was the only one to develop a specifically rural locus (though it should be emphasized that the liberal

educational reform was highly successful in promoting primary education in the rural areas).

The two doctors chosen for the exploratory tour were Luis Jiménez
and Carlos Alvarado. The first was from a prominent family, a graduate
of the University of Pennsylvania (1902) who had charted out a career
for himself in the tight confines of the capital's medical community by
becoming a specialist "epidemic expeditionary" and the director of ad
hoc projects. Alvarado, his junior partner, had only returned from
studying in France the previous year. A tour of the country to continue
the high-profile research of the patriarch of Costa Rican medicine and
further the interests of the nation was a perfect opportunity to prove his
mettle.[19] Jiménez and Alvarado undertook five expeditions during the
dry season of 1908. They covered most secondary towns and their surrounding areas in the Central Valley, the Pacific littoral, San Carlos, and
Guanacaste (notably they did not go to Limón province, the banana
enclave of the United Fruit Company), accumulating data on the extent
of hookworm infestation in the different zones and treating over five
thousand people for hookworm disease.[20] Almost imperceptibly, they
initiated an important shift in the framing of hookworm disease.

Durán and Gerardo Jiménez had originally determined in their
1890s' experiments that cansancio was a problem that affected the
darker, "zambo" peasantry of the Pacific coastal plain. Jiménez maintained the same through 1901, when he argued that hookworm infestation occurred only up to seven hundred meters above sea level; although he knew there was some infection in the Central Valley, he felt
that it was relatively rare.[21] As late as Fernández's 1907 lecture to the
agricultural society, the same presumption was being made. In Luis
Jiménez and Alvarado's tour, and through the manner in which they
presented their results, the disease was made "national" — it would no
longer be used to determine a subracial gradation within the Hispanic
populace; while hookworm *disease* might be concentrated on the Pacific
littoral, all poor, rural Costa Ricans suffered hookworm *infection* to one
degree or another, and purging them of the parasite would return all to
an identical level of purity.[22]

In August 1908, the Faculty of Medicine named Luis Jiménez and
another contemporary young medical reformer, Carlos Pupo Pérez, to
organize and head up a new bacteriologic lab at a salary of seventy-
five colones a month.[23] The government, still headed by González

Víquez, approved a generous appropriation of twenty-five thousand colones (ten thousand U.S. dollars) to combat the hookworm over the summer of 1910.[24] The timing was excellent for maintaining momentum and enthusiasm, for over the Christmas–New Year's break of 1909–1910 (the beginning of Costa Rica's summer), the country was host to the Fourth International Sanitary Conference of the American Republics (the organization that held the conference was the precursor of the Pan-American Health Organization). In his keynote address, Durán extolled Jiménez and Alvarado's work as among the country's greatest medical triumphs, and the two later presented the results of their research to the hemisphere's public health potentates.[25]

The treatment program of 1910 to 1914 was decentralized in comparison to the later Rockefeller approach. Though the results varied greatly according to the degree of dedication of individual district physicians, the scale of the operation was impressive. Luis Jiménez and Pupo Pérez served as coordinators and laboratory directors in San José, while the town doctors took stool specimens in their jurisdiction, especially from schoolchildren, and sent them to San José for analysis. Positive samples were identified and district physicians sent the corresponding number of standardized treatment packets of thymol and Betamaftol, purchased in large quantities from the Botica Francesa. The initial reluctance of the town doctors was partially overcome in 1911 when they were promised one colon for each person deemed by the lab to have been cured of hookworm affliction. At its height, the transportation and mail network of the country was turned into a fecal distribution system, with thousands of specimens coming into the lab each month.[26]

Popular hygiene literature was also distributed. Besides the pamphlet version of Fernández's 1907 conference, twenty thousand single sheets with the title "El Cansancio" were distributed by district physicians. The page contained a description of the disease, its side effects, mode of transmission, and method of treatment, and explained that prevention required the construction of a privy. It also contained a blowup of the hookworm and its eggs, designed as a view through a microscope.[27] Large landowners who employed significant numbers of laborers were enlisted to administer medicine en masse, but this apparently did not have happy results.[28]

The antihookworm program immediately became the vehicle for the first truly national dialogue among physicians, and it got rather prickly at times. One debate was between the remaining traditional country doctors and the young turk scientists. At the outset of the campaign some district physicians, like Narciso Barberena of San Mateo, begged off adding tests for hookworm infection to their duties, informing the minister of the interior that infection rates in their districts were insignificant. Jiménez was able to counter Barberena's claim by citing statistics gathered during his 1908 expedition, showing that he had treated four hundred hookworm-afflicted people in San Mateo in ten days.[29]

There was also a debate provoked by the fact that district physicians with scientific training did not simply want to follow the orders of the two directors in San José. Citing studies of the antihookworm commission in Puerto Rico, Vicente Láchner Sandoval, the town doctor of Juan Viñas, called into question the standard doses established by Jiménez and Pupo Pérez. He also insisted that sending specimens through the mail to a central laboratory was unsatisfactory, and that the role of the town doctors should be expanded, with a subsidy to create their own laboratory facilities. Durán was called in to arbitrate the dispute, diplomatically siding with Jiménez. Mauro Fernández, meanwhile, who had taken over for Pupo Pérez as a district physician of Escazú, was a strong critic of the system, anticipating the scheme that Luis Jiménez would initially propose to the Rockefeller Foundation, one akin to that presented in the original report: special treatment teams headed by physicians working systematically in designated areas.[30]

District physicians also devised or suggested new methods and techniques for the campaign. Mariano Figueres, the official doctor of Santa Ana, had begun a complete census of his area and was attempting to gradually sample all residents to achieve complete eradication. In December 1913, the district physician of San Antonio de Belén, Miguel Dobles, recommended that since it was still "an incredible mystery for many common people [*personas del pueblo*] the idea that there are beings invisible to the eye, and that they are the ones that cause so many types of disease," it was time to begin "public conferences and to show these people with microscopes the truth of the theory of microbes and microscopic parasites." In both cases, they anticipated methods later implemented by the Rockefeller-sponsored antihookworm mission.[31]

The laboratory examined sixty thousand specimens during its four years of operation, and the program picked up momentum: in 1913, its final year, 22,600 Costa Ricans received attention for the disease, even though the appropriation was exhausted by August.[32] The response of rural people to the campaign was initially skepticism and resistance to the medicine, but some district physicians began to provide evidence of a change in attitude. The official doctor of Desamparados maintained that by July 1911, six months into the campaign, many people were voluntarily presenting him with stool samples on the word of people who had been "cured," and who rapidly felt better, more agile, and "ready to work."[33]

Nevertheless, Jiménez and Pupo Pérez grew discouraged by indications that those successfully treated exhibited a high rate of reinfection, and they came to the conclusion that the treatment program had to be complemented by a stronger prophylactic component — the building of latrines in particular. They also understood that at twenty-five colones a shot, many of the most afflicted were unable to afford to build their own toilet facilities even if they had wanted to. When the government of Ricardo Jiménez turned down their request for a greater budget appropriation to add latrine construction to the antihookworm work, Luis Jiménez and Pupo Pérez briefly considered abandoning the treatment program altogether and dedicating all the resources to subsidizing privy construction.[34] Before they could get too pessimistic or strike out on a new course, the Rockefeller medicine men came calling.

Imperial Interface

The methods of the International Health Commission's battle against the hookworm were far from established in 1914. Just as the methodology had changed drastically over the five years of work in the U.S. South, so would it evolve greatly in Costa Rica, in part based on the experience of the prior local campaign. Henry Carter, who set up the Costa Rican office, began in May 1914 by asking Luis Jiménez to prepare a proposal on how to integrate the previous system with the Rockefeller mission. The ideal project Jiménez dreamed up, with the Rockefeller millions very much in mind, involved a central station for San José and environs along with six teams of microscopists and sanitary inspectors in the more endemic zones of the country, each one under the direction of a physician. The major cost came from his most radical proposal: recalling the crisis of prophylaxis they had run into during the initial campaign, he suggested that a whopping seven thousand U.S. dollars per month be spent over four years to ensure that everyone in Costa Rica have a latrine at the end of that time.[35]

Jiménez's proposals were not taken up, and he lost his own position when the new government of Alfredo González Flores decided to terminate the Costa Rican program and let the foundation take complete control over all antihookworm work. Pupo Pérez and Mauro Fernández, who had been involved in the prior local program, did serve as Costa Rican subdirectors of the Rockefeller office during its first two years of operation. Carter suggested rehiring Jiménez in some capacity, but it did not work out.[36] It is worth speculating that Jiménez blew his future in imperial health by embracing an approach to eradication that was too mundane in its sanitary engineering practicality. The Rockefeller Foundation was not about to become a systematic builder of toilets. "Disease eradication" had to be glamorous in some way to be palatable to the directors in New York.

This had been the source of a tense relationship between Charles Wardell Stiles (the discoverer of *anchylostoma americana* and the man who convinced the Rockefellers to get involved in antihookworm work) and Wickliffe Rose during the life of the antihookworm work in the U.S. South. As John Ettling sums it up, Stiles preferred basic sanitary measures such as the building of pit privies, and felt that strong authority and even coercion were necessary to force people to stamp out the disease; Rose "understood the long-range importance of attacking the disease at its source — soil contaminated by people with unsanitary habits . . . but he felt it more important for the time being for the Commission to demonstrate convincingly that hookworm sufferers could be cured." Stiles was put out to pasture in 1914; Rose was given charge of the new international machinery.[37] In his unfortunate demise, Jiménez was at least in good scientific company.

The first Rockefeller local director, Carter, soon moved on to another post, and his place was taken by Louis Schapiro, whose constancy as mission chief for the next six years had a great deal to do with the success and evolving shape of the office's public health work. He collaborated in the adaptation of the foundation's goals to an initiative of local making, transforming the narrow antihookworm focus of the imperial plan by combining it with the creation of a school health department. Schapiro warrants a short biographical assessment, as does Solón Núñez, the Costa Rican physician who became his most crucial ally in realizing the newly redefined mission.

In some ways, Schapiro was a classic Rockefeller recruit. His background as a physician included service in the military and Coast Guard, and three years as a senior public health official in the occupied Philippines from 1910–1913. Other aspects of Schapiro's profile set him apart from the norm. He was Jewish, spoke Spanish quite well, and according to Victor Heiser, who had been his superior in the Philippines, had "demonstrated very unusual executive ability" and "unusual tact in getting along with all classes of people."[38] Prior to arriving in Costa Rica, he had worked for two years in the public health department of Milwaukee and as a specialist in hygiene and tropical medicine at Marquette University. Judith Leavitt has described the exceptional success of public health reformers in making Milwaukee known, by the second decade of the twentieth century, as "the healthiest city" in the United States. Schapiro's tenure there followed the brief socialist incumbency in the city council that had consolidated a model of broad community mobilization in public health. It was the product of a Left-liberal coalition designed to defeat traditional politicians who had preyed on the rapid growth of the city while impeding public health initiatives.[39]

Núñez was a young physician appointed by the government to be the assistant director of the School Health Department in early 1916. A year later, he was appointed by Schapiro the subdirector of the Department of Ancylostomiasis, while retaining his authority over the school health program. Núñez was the key Costa Rican in the seven-year direct Rockefeller involvement, and subsequently became undersecretary of public health in 1922 and then secretary of the new Ministry of Public Health and Social Protection in 1927. His background is worth some comment since it also brushes against the grain of the stereotypical local "collaborator" central to the assumptions of dependency theory and proponents of cultural imperialism.

Prior to 1913, when he departed to study medicine in Geneva, Núñez was a high-profile member of a group of embittered young dissident intellectuals who had dedicated themselves to the cause of antiimperialism and social justice.[40] Often teachers in the country's leading schools, and grouped around radical periodicals and cultural centers for workers, this loosely affiliated network included many of Costa

Rica's most inspired Left intellectuals, like Joaquín García Monge and Carmen Lyra. Núñez had been a teacher in two rural schools, a school inspector, and a professor of hygiene in the principal girls' secondary and normal school. He also established himself as a critic of dominant society by taking an active role in publications like *Aurora* (1908) and *Cultura* (1910). His 1911 essay in *Renovación*, "Jesús y Tostoi," is considered a classic expression of the romantic anarchist and social Christian vision that animated the project of this generation of *ácratas* (the bitter and disaffected ones).[41]

It is unlikely that Núñez had lost his anti-imperialist principles by the time he returned from his studies in Switzerland and his apprenticeship on the battlefields of France. Yet it was clear to him, and to many other progressives of the day, that there was a difference between, say, the Department of Ancylostomiasis and the building of a U.S. canal or the annexation of the country. Direct Rockefeller control was designed to phase itself out by 1921, whereupon the state would assume complete control over the operations. The basic Rockefeller public health plan was quite compatible with that proposed by Costa Rican reformers, particularly given Schapiro's willingness to integrate the mission with the school system.

In short, the project promised a way of circumventing the severe fiscal crisis as well as the obstacles thrown up by the retrograde elements of the medical and political establishments, and thus represented a possible shortcut to a centralized apparatus of public health that Núñez very much conceived of as a socialist advance over laissez-faire. For the Rockefeller plan involved a marked shift away from the de-centered regime (characteristic of the first antihookworm program) and toward a centralist and much more statist model of public health management. Ironically, it was the imperial institution from the United States that insisted on a statist model associated with socialism, while the Latin American system, traditionally associated with the statist stereotype, had actually evolved as a disaggregated system incorporating private initiative and practitioners.

Núñez caught his share of criticism for making this Faustian bargain. He never hesitated, however, and vociferously defended Schapiro on more than one occasion, insisting that he was a great Costa Rican patriot. Like many of his generation who had nourished themselves on the works of the great anarchists, Núñez's energies were now turned to imaginative leadership in expanding the role of the state. The trade-offs and compromises involved in this incorporation were similar to those faced by the intellectuals of the Progressive Era who were interpellated into state reformism in the United States at this time—proponents of social medicine like Louis Schapiro, for example.[42]

The Intensive Method

Lynn Marie Morgan, following the research of E. Richard Brown, proposes that the Rockefeller antihookworm campaign targeted coffee pickers and plantation workers in Costa Rica, and that they were coordinated with the United Fruit Company's medical apparatus and the coffee oligarchy.[43] In fact, there was no direct relationship between the evolution of the antihookworm program and the immediate needs of foreign or local agrarian capital. In the first year of operations, for example, from September 1914 through September 1915, campaigns were undertaken in extremely isolated peasant communities in Guanacaste and Puntarenas, and in the public schools in San José, as well as along the Pacific littoral and in the coffee-growing regions of the Central Valley.

At the end of this experimental period, Schapiro decided to institute his own version of the "intensive method": the country was broken down into a grid and systematically worked through, with the intention to test, and treat if necessary, every individual in the area. Neither the schedule nor the method were determined by the nature of agricultural production in the region. As for the United Fruit Company, when a hookworm team inaugurated its campaign in the province of Limón in June 1915, Schapiro complained to his superiors in New York that "the showing by the officials of the United Fruit Company was not that of cooperation." Schapiro only made headway in the area after meeting the Hispanic governor and principal officials, the Roman Catholic priest and the British consul to Costa Rica who called together and secured the cooperation of the "colored ministers."[44] The actual politics of the campaign were much more in the nature of this delicate negotiation with the multiple nodes of provincial power, and gaining such a consensus became increasingly necessary as Schapiro implemented a more intrusive method.

Carter had begun the Costa Rican work using the same dispensary

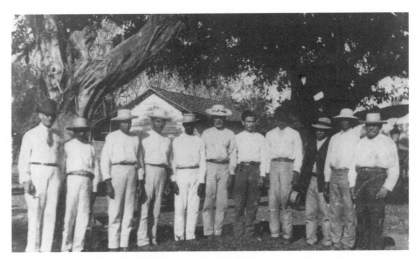

Fig. 4. Rockefeller Foundation agents in Guanacaste, 1917.
Archivo Nacional de Costa Rica.

method pioneered by Bailey Ashford in Puerto Rico and then adapted
in the U.S. South. A laboratory was established in the district with as
much fanfare as possible, and people were urged to come out en masse
for an informational session, followed by a physical and blood and fecal
exams after which, if they were found to be infected, they were given
medicines to take at home and a pamphlet explaining how to build a pit
privy. In November 1914, prior to taking up his Costa Rican assignment,
Schapiro had toured the hookworm programs in the U.S. South and he
may have learned of misgivings about the dispensary system from Sanitary Commission workers: while spectacular and exciting, it merely
passed over the surface of the area without achieving compliance or
long-term prophylaxis.[45]

Under the intensive method, the country was divided into "units" of
three to four thousand people, which usually corresponded to the established political jurisdiction of the canton. The distant and most
heavily infected areas were targeted for work during the dry season,
while areas close to the railroads were slated for work during the rainy
season.[46] At the height of the campaign, six teams were in operation in
six different areas at the same time. One microscopist and two hygiene
inspectors were assigned to work the unit, though Schapiro himself or
the Costa Rican assistant director would oversee the setup of the work
and the field director would monitor the activities.[47]

Prior to the beginning of the work, letters would be sent to the governor of the province, the jefe político of the area, the municipality, large landowners who employed many laborers, the president of the school board, and the district physician in whose jurisdiction the campaign was to operate. Aside from general information about the work, these letters stressed the important increase in agricultural productivity that could result from eradicating hookworm infection, the patriotic nature of the campaign, and the need for the authorities and influential citizens to set good hygiene examples.[48]

Local community leaders were then convoked: the clergy and those who, "due to the position they occupy in society, in teaching, farming, commerce, and the liberal arts, have the greatest influence on the people." They got a brief lecture on the hookworm, probably accompanied by magic lantern slides, charts, and handouts. The senior officer explained the campaign method, and asked for suggestions on a local person who knew the area well and could assist the team in its work. He also described the law on the mandatory construction of latrines and stressed that this was the major prophylactic task of the campaign. At this point, he would invite an exchange of ideas and try to get the municipality to commit some funds, or at least horses and lodging for the team, as well as agree to enforce the law on the construction of privies.[49]

The campaign would kick off with the official opening of the laboratory in the main village or town of the canton. When a new lab opened in Paraíso in September 1915, the public conference was attended by the president, minister of war, and governor of Cartago province. Sixty schoolteachers were marshaled for the event, and over five hundred "very enthusiastic" people attended.[50] At the opening of the laboratory in Liberia in May 1916, over eight hundred people attended and "the commander of the troops of this province sent the military band to liven up the meeting."[51]

In the U.S. South, the dispensaries had proven so successful because they were structurally similar to the evangelical tent revival meetings that were such a crucial part of the festive cycle in rural popular culture. Organizers began to self-consciously fashion the meetings as such, developing fiery oratorical skills, eliciting testimonials from the "cured," and so on.[52] In Costa Rica the model was the *fiesta cívica*, or *turno*—the carnivalesque celebrations coinciding with a town's patron saint.[53] As

Schapiro noted after the opening of labs in Pacaya, Juan Viñas, and Capellades in August 1917, "public enthusiasm" and the event were "in the nature of public feasts."[54]

Smaller places had less pomp and circumstance, but people inevitably attended the conference at the local church or school decked out in their best clothes, the entire family in tow. Even in places too small to have a marching band, people were convoked en masse "by ensuring their arrival at the meeting place with the exhibition of cinematographic views and projections of intestinal parasites, their life cycle, the damages they cause, and so forth."[55] The Costa Rican assistant director Núñez remarked in 1921 that in the public conferences, "the person who addresses the crowd cannot always adapt himself to the mental capacity of all those listening in the audience."[56] These were official ceremonies, their didactic effect at least matched by their function as signifiers of erudite and official knowledge that invested the subsequent work with power. This solemn and official modern mass was then followed by celebration.

Núñez was no doubt correct in saying that the more effective educational work was done in the subsequent house-to-house visits, "especially if the hygiene inspector is skillful, capable of insinuating himself into the soul of the simple people of the village."[57] Such a capability was likely given that they were "of the people," recruited from a lower social class than the microscopists, and because they came "accompanied by someone with intimate knowledge of the area," quite often a teacher.[58]

The inspectors effected a complete census of the area during these visits. Each house was assigned a number and its occupants registered. Talks on hookworm disease and its prevention were given at each home, along with general hygiene counsel, while at the same time the employees "put simple literature popularizing hygiene into the hands of the family" and copies of the law on latrine construction accompanied by instructions on how to build a sanitary privy.[59] José León Quijano, field director of the campaign in the canton of Nicoya, one of the most peripheral and poor of the country, wrote that "more than half of the residents know how to read and write, and they get great pleasure from reading our pamphlets" (in effect, according to the raw census data of 1927, 52 percent of the people of Nicoya were literate).[60]

They received pleasurable texts like the instructional pamphlet on latrine construction, a handsome six-page booklet that explained that hookworms were "dangerous worms whose poisons thin the blood, sap strength, bottle up the intelligence, and lead to misery and death." The reason for this contamination? There are no toilets, and those that do exist are improperly built. The toilet was a mark of civilization and the progress of the community. "From the time of the great legislator Moses, the urgent need to bury human excrement was understood, and from this came the idea of the toilet."[61] It is worth keeping in mind that these pamphlets and single sheets would have been among the few pieces of literature in the possession of peasant families who were none-theless increasingly literate.[62]

Once the preparatory work had been done, most of the inhabitants were given a blood test, the anemia quotient serving as a guide to calcu-late the amount of medicine needed. Finally, properly marked speci-men containers were left for each member of the family, and people were invited to present their fecal samples ("the size of a kernel of corn is enough") at the district dispensary on a certain day for examination. Those who tested positive were issued a summons, with a registration number and their name in printer's type, explaining the procedure and giving them an appointment at the dispensary. Initially, people were given medicines to take home with instructions for use, but this was soon discontinued because compliance was spotty, and people often saved up the drugs and purgatives (one family in Nicoya organized a constant flow of infected samples in order to get a commercial stock of purgatives).[63] As a result, doses of anthelmintic (and often purges as well) were given in the central office of the district field lab "as the only means by which to control the efficiency of the drugs."[64]

The sick were given a dose of magnesium sulphate (Epsom salts) to take on the evening prior to the treatment. Early the following morn-ing, usually a Sunday, they returned to the lab and were administered two equal doses of thymol or oil of chenopodium, one at six o'clock and another at eight. Finally, another saline purge was administered two hours after the last dose of anthelmintic.[65] During Elmendorf's 1915 visit to Miramar, a large crowd of all ages assembled on a Sunday morn-ing and the roll was called. The men stepped up "in answer to their name as in answer to a patriotic call to arms." The ability to withstand the stronger medicine of thymol was part of manhood in the country areas, and it was "preferred by the men."[66] The women "merely took the medicine" (which increasingly was oil of chenopodium instead of thymol), while terrified children were cajoled into taking their medicine by the adults.[67] For women and children, the oil of chenopodium was mixed with brown sugar to create a syrup, and then mixed again with coffee extract, "which eliminates the nausea and dizziness for the subsequent purge."[68] The medicine was given in the presence of the microscopists and sanitary inspectors, "and sometimes the sick have received the medicine from the very hands of the employees."[69]

The employees of the lab would allow the oil of chenopodium to be mixed with castor oil—brought along by the patients.[70] The fact that the treatment relied so heavily on a purge mirrored the important role of purgatives in popular medical approaches that were still governed by humoral principles, and this may have made it more comprehensible and convincing to sufferers. The logic of the specific treatment may also have sat more easily with popular medical practice in that, until the 1880s, the idea of such targeted treatment was much more common to popular medicine than to its learned counterpart, which saw "specifics" as the mark of quackery.[71]

Each infected person was required to take two treatments. The subsequent stool sample was tested two or three times; when these were negative, another test would be taken eight days later, and only then, if still negative, were people given "a diagnosis of 'cured.'"[72] Frequently, persons "pronounced cured were given a subsequent blood test for the purpose of determining the increase in hemoglobin resulting from treatment." This second examination was "of great value in pointing out the immediate physical benefits of treatment and thus enlisting permanent interest in the work."[73] Meanwhile, follow-up visits were made by hygiene inspectors to urge "delinquents" to present their specimens at the lab or, if they had failed to respond to the summons after positive results, to present themselves at the lab for treatment. The extent to which people were meeting their obligations to construct latrines was measured, and advice was given to those in the process of doing so. Those who had not complied were threatened with official action, and the municipality was encouraged to fulfill its policing function and provide the money for latrine construction for those really too indigent to afford the materials.[74]

Exceptions to this uncompromising regime were made only in the cities, larger towns, and most distant peripheries with scattered populaces. In the cantons of General, Buenos Aires, and Boruca (where leading residents petitioned for a Rockefeller Foundation mission since there had been no medical attention for years), an ambulatory dispensary was set up due to the extreme dispersal of the populace (most of them indigenous). The percentage of hookworm infection was high (94.9). The large percentage of cures obtained in the area (98.9) was "a clear indication of the interest which the people had in freeing themselves of infection, for many had to travel long distances for treatment."[75]

Exceptions were made in the urban areas on class grounds. In Alajuela city and the canton of La Unión, instead of getting people to come to the lab with their samples, "special employees" went from house to house to pick them up, and then later to deliver the diagnosis and purgative; subsequently medicines were distributed in the lab or directly to homes. "This system is necessary when the work is done in places whose elements belong to decent society, wealthy people, with their family physicians, who would never dream of going to the laboratory."[76]

San José was exempt from the intensive method. Schools served as focal points for examining and dosing children en masse, while adults could come to the dispensary on a voluntary basis.[77] Examination and treatment for hookworm also continued in the Hospital San Juan de Dios. The departmental offices in San José became an ongoing public health exhibition. The prominent merchant and philanthropist John M. Keith presented the office with glass models of the male and female ancylostoma, and an enlarged cross section of the head of a hookworm done in wax.[78] During the Christmas season of 1919, traditionally a time of festive outings corresponding to San José's saint day, a permanent display was opened, with graphs showing morbidity and mortality rates for the country, specimens of various types of intestinal parasites, charts depicting the progress of the antihookworm work, and models of sanitary latrines. Demonstrations with the microscope were "an important feature of the exhibition."[79]

When the Costa Rican government formally assumed full fiscal and administrative control over the antihookworm work, the tallies of seven years of the intensive method were impressive. Over three-quarters of the Costa Rican population had been tested (314,968 people) — 97 percent of those who had been registered in the health censuses. Just over half of these had been diagnosed with hookworm infection; roughly 90 percent of these had received at least one treatment, and 40 percent (about 65,000 people) had received treatment until they were pronounced cured. Over four hundred public conferences and almost a thousand school conferences had been held. The central office in San José had received over seventy thousand visits. One hundred thousand pamphlets had been distributed along with another hundred thousand flyers, and five hundred articles on hookworm disease and related hygiene issues had been published in local newspapers and journals. Of the more than forty thousand homes inspected, only 13 percent had had a latrine on the first visit; by the final inspection, 46 percent had some sort of privy.[80]

More important than these statistics was the mass experience of receiving a dose of strong medicine at the hands of inspectors and microscopists; viewing a pathogen through a microscope; feeling rapidly cured of a condition diagnosed scientifically; receiving an official and personalized summons with one's name typeset at the top; and having an agent of the state extract one's blood and examine one's feces. All this was done amid great patriotic celebration, and accompanied by literature, magic lantern displays, and films, which for some may have been their first cinematic experience.

Allies and Reactions

There is no evidence about a clash of medical worldviews between commoners and the treatment teams, though this was almost certainly a muted undercurrent. What is clear is that agricultural waged workers were made nervous by the campaign if it looked like the treatment might disrupt migrant labor schedules or require them to be absent from work because they feared (often with good reason) that employers would dock their pay or let them go.[81] Political allegiances also caused noncompliance, and it was virtually impossible to conduct the work effectively during the semiannual election period. At the outset of the campaign in 1914–1915, it was not uncommon to have to use "threats" to get people out to the laboratory, and "in various places . . . it was necessary to resort to violence to achieve the building of privies."[82] Unfortunately, no details exist of the many incidents in which the hookworm teams, along with the authorities, resorted to coercion to enforce compliance with the public health plan.[83]

The Rockefeller teams had two groups of key allies in the rural areas. They found that priests remained faithful to their role as learned medics and generally counseled cooperation with the hygiene work. Father Chinchilla of Escazú was typical in this regard. According to Guillermo Ortíz, a technical assistant who worked the area in 1917, "he recommended in his talks from the pulpit that the people look to be cured and called their attention to the benefits it would bring, and said that opportunities of this kind should not be missed, suggesting to them that in a healthy body there was a like soul."[84] The public schoolteachers were the most important allies. As Núñez put it in 1921, as "the intellectual part of the localities," teachers had always "viewed our work with fondness [and] continue to lend us their most enthusiastic support."[85] According to the report of one sanitary inspector, women schoolteachers were more enthusiastic than their male colleagues, and this may have been especially the case in schools where the teachers were graduates of the women's normal school (it was virtually impossible to find a graduate of the men's normal school in a rural teaching post); from 1900 onward, the students at the Colegio de Senoritas — among them, scholarship girls from the provinces — imbibed modern notions of hygiene and embraced an evangelical spirit of modernity.[86] Women teachers seem to have relished the idea of confronting the patriarchal provincial power structure, and the arrival of the hookworm teams invested with the most impeccable of civilizing credentials provided them a perfect vehicle. The fact that the hookworm office was also in charge of the School Health Department dovetailed nicely in this regard, not least because the office had the authority to provide written commendations for teachers, which would assist them in promotions.

The local power structures were dominated by the *gamonales,* or rural political bosses, who had acquired increased power after 1909 due to the introduction of the direct vote. Where before the vote had occurred in two stages, with a small number of electors holding the final and most powerful cards, now it was the locals who were capable of pulling the vote who had the power and were rewarded with appointment to local offices. If it was close to election time, they would not risk supplying ammunition to potential competitors by forcing people to spend money on privy construction. Núñez complained vociferously that the municipalities were made up of "simple folk who fail to meet their obligations" and whose fear of losing their positions showed them to be "deficient in moral authority."[87] Of course, they were also desperately short of funds, so that they were hard-pressed to ease the pain of forced privy construction by subsidizing it.[88] Besides the gamonales, some of the most serious resistance came from "foreign property owners" with large labor forces who "tyrannized" their workers if their participation in the antihookworm program looked to interfere with their work schedule.[89]

The law creating the School Health Department had placed all the town doctors under the control of the Rockefeller mission director. As a result, the resistance and indifference the district physicians displayed toward the antihookworm program is all the more notable. The only instance Schapiro mentioned explicitly was that they disliked the fact that the antihookworm units distributed medicine free to everyone (and not just to the indigent, as was the town doctors' charge) because it would further reduce their private business. Schapiro adopted the same strategy used by the Sanitary Commission in the U.S. South, arguing that a healthier populace would mean a wealthier one that would consult physicians with greater regularity.[90] But more telling is the absence of district physicians from the accounts of the hookworm work. As the Department of Ancylostomiasis had, in physicians' eyes, usurped a program that had formerly augmented their incomes, this is not too surprising. The resulting rift that opened up between the district physicians and the embryonic state public health apparatus was a long time in closing.

Irregular country doctors were also opposed to the Rockefeller teams for similar reasons. In Nicoya, the field director complained that there were "many curanderos," some of whom allege that once the campaign is over the government will charge people for the medicine "and other stupidities."[91] The stakes could be raised much higher. As Núñez explained, "The indifference of the people is often exacerbated by the curanderos, who find in the campaign against ancylostomiasis an obstacle to their commerce. They make war on the office, trying to malign its work by attributing to the drugs we use cases of death, whatever their origin."[92] Nevertheless, other curanderos may have welcomed the campaign, especially after it had gained some acceptance among sufferers. Christopher Abel reports a case from Cundinamarca in Colombia where three *teguas* (popular healers) selling "specifics" were arrested for claiming to represent the antihookworm office.[93] The campaign generated its own curanderos: in 1921, Núñez explained to a visiting Rockefeller dignitary that a number of those who had worked as inspectors and microscopists during the antihookworm campaigns had subsequently sold their services as curanderos in the rural areas.[94] Given that they had diagnosed illness using specialized instruments and administered often remarkably effective treatments for a debilitating condition, it is hardly startling that they were able to set themselves up as adept healers and that other popular healers might have been envious.

The Hygiene Catechism

On setting up operations in the country, the Rockefeller mission had dismissed Luis Jiménez, the director of the prior Costa Rican campaign, and proceeded without heeding his proposals about how the treatment of hookworm should evolve. Still, in a more important sense, the Rockefeller program was transformed by its hosts to embrace a more general, preexisting plan to piggyback a hygiene apparatus on the public education system. This agenda had been impeded by a lack of resources, itself the product of a political class not convinced of the need to push through the necessary budget appropriations. By mid-1915, despite an executive that was singularly disposed to effect this reform, the always precarious fiscal situation of the Costa Rican state was becoming ever more bleak with the onset of a deep recession induced by the European war.

Soon after his arrival, Schapiro was wooed by Minister of Education Luis Felipe González Flores (also, notably, the president's brother) to create a School Health Department under the auspices of the antihookworm program. He accepted the offer, thus committing the foundation to fill the fiscal and political void.[95] The Departamento de Sanidad Escolar was officially created in May 1915 as a subsection of the Rockefeller-controlled Departamento de Ankylostomiasis. One of Schapiro's first directives was issued to the country's Boards of Education urging that all schools have a toilet facility "and that the students should learn to use it."[96] The results were encouraging. In May 1916, Schapiro had the pleasure of visiting Acosta, where a holiday had been declared to celebrate the inauguration of a privy in the primary school.[97] A sanitary inspector in Escazú reported in 1917 that the central school had built a septic tank "as an experiment, and the results have been very good."[98]

Meanwhile, agents of the School Health Department or antihookworm units delivered almost one thousand school conferences between

1915 and 1921, where "every effort was made to inculcate in the minds of the children the principles of cleanliness, hygiene, and orderly habits of life."[99] Of the almost one hundred thousand pamphlets that were distributed during the same period, many were mass-produced titles in the "popular hygiene" series inherited from the state press that the department streamlined and expanded. The department's series editorship was inaugurated with a Schapiro pamphlet, *Mission of the Teacher in the Service of School Sanitary Inspection.* The pamphlet included a workbook in which teachers could take meticulous notes on each individual student: physical details such as the number of baths per week and the state of eyesight were to be tabulated in conjunction with "moral condition, extrascholarly work, family history," and grades.[100]

The workbook mirrored a system of sanitary cards introduced into the schools by the department in 1915 that also demanded that teachers register information concerning the physical and moral health of each student.[101] Other titles in the series, which stretched on into the 1930s and beyond, included Pupo Pérez's *Our Avoidable Diseases* and Núñez's *My Hygiene Catechism,* which combined the mantras of bourgeois manners (to thoroughly chew your food before swallowing, for example) with exhortations to regularly visit the Infants' Clinic and take fecal samples for testing to the public health lab. One of the commandments may be the origin of Costa Ricans' modern moral obsession with showering at least once a day: "Any day I go without bathing, even if I have good reason, I feel sad, in a bad mood, and without any desire to work."[102]

Because Costa Rica's schools of nursing were still not producing graduates with any regularity or quality, Schapiro secured the voluntary services of physicians to organize special classes in late 1915 where a select number of teachers were trained as nurses for the School Health Department. Four of these "sanitary assistants" were employed full-time by the Ministry of Education to work in the schools of the capital city; the number rose to eight by 1922 with one in each of the other three main towns and another staffing the capital's new Infants' Clinic. Four school physicians were also employed on a part-time basis, and they visited one school each morning. The principal task of the nurses was to visit the homes of students absent for more than three days or those pronounced "defective" by the physicians. These visits had the objective of gathering "systematic information on hygienic conditions" and to offer counsel to mothers. The program quickly achieved significant results: in 1919, 4,586 pupils received medical attention, and the school nurses effected 2,212 home visits. This ambitious network of child and maternal inspection was one of the earliest manifestations of professional social work in Costa Rica.[103]

In his 1921 summary of the Costa Rican program, Schapiro insisted that the organization and direction of the School Health Department "was the first step to centralize public health agencies towards the formation of the National Health Department."[104] The original scope of the Rockefeller mission had been radically altered. In 1921, at the end of the foundation's formal seven-year involvement, the budget for the School Health Department was greater than that devoted to hookworm relief.[105]

The Centralization of Public Health

The Costa Rican mission of the Rockefeller Foundation's International Health Commission was reshaped by its hosts almost as soon as it arrived. Within a year it had also become the School Health Department, assuming jurisdiction over the district physicians and implanting its public health project in the education system. The office benefited as well from the withering of the Faculty of Medicine, a product of generational exhaustion and the perceived collaboration of leading physicians with the Tinoco military dictatorship of 1917–1919 (a subject I will discuss in more detail in the following chapter). After the fall of the Tinocos, the new government of Julio Acosta began to invest greater jurisdiction over questions of public health in the antihookworm unit.

The hookworm teams were asked to treat malaria in the distant southeastern regions of the country in 1919 when an epidemic broke out, and government satisfaction with their work led to their enlistment in preparing the field for a smallpox vaccination campaign and subsequently carrying it out.[106] Then, in 1918–1919, the postwar influenza pandemic swept through the country, leaving some 2,300 people dead. Both the Faculty of Medicine and Department of Ancylostomiasis were asked to respond to the emergency, and only the latter provided any relief in an efficient manner.[107] In June 1920, the Ministry of the Interior chose to put a sanitary inspector dedicated to yellow fever control measures under the direction of the Department of Ancylostomiasis.[108]

The primacy of the foundation's office over public health matters was made more apparent in July 1920 when the government created Juntas Sanitarias Patrióticas in all cantons of the country, and declared that these local health councils were to follow the instructions of the Faculty of Medicine, Department of Ancylostomiasis, and School Health Department—the latter two, of course, were wings of the Rockefeller mission.[109]

After rejecting the Sanitary Code written by a physician who was a relative by marriage of the Tinocos, the new government asked Schapiro to prepare a replacement, which he did in 1920 (it was passed into law in 1923).[110] The new Infants' Clinic approved by Congress at the end of 1920 was also placed under the antihookworm department, and in June 1921, the control of malaria and all other epidemics was assigned to the office.[111] Schapiro ended his tenure as director of the Department of Ancylostomiasis in late 1921 when full fiscal and political jurisdiction reverted on schedule to the national government, and he was succeeded by his second-in-command, Núñez.

In June 1922, in a secret meeting between the Acosta cabinet with Núñez in attendance, Schapiro proposed that if the government gave the department undivided authority over matters of public health, the Rockefeller Foundation would be prepared to continue financial assistance in such areas as the creation of an advanced bacteriologic laboratory, fellowships for training Costa Rican sanitary personnel, and funding for sanitary engineering and other health-related pilot projects. Acosta noted that such a move would require "changing the laws of our country" in that the jurisdiction of the Faculty of Medicine over public health would be eliminated. Nevertheless, it was agreed that this fundamental shift would be pushed through by the government.[112] Acosta acted swiftly, and on 12 July 1922, he transformed the Department of Ancylostomiasis into the Subsecretariat of Hygiene and Public Health under the control of the Ministry of the Interior; it would be responsible for all questions of public hygiene in the country, the circuit of district physicians, and the provision of medical services in prisons and social assistance clinics. Núñez was appointed subsecretary.[113] The centralized, Rockefeller-inspired model of public health had won the day in Costa Rica in 1921–1922, and under Núñez's activist leadership the subsecretariat would achieve the stature of a full ministry in 1927. Costa Rica was one of the first countries in Latin America to raise public health to full ministerial status, preceded only by Cuba (1909), the Dominican Republic (1921), and Chile (1924).[114]

In 1915, when Schapiro offered to make massive quantities of hygiene literature available to the Ministry of Education, the minister responded by setting aside in the curriculum a half hour each week, "the day and the time to be uniform throughout the republic . . . for the instruction of pupils from the literature furnished." The image of this simultaneous instruction recalls Benedict Anderson's analysis of the nation as a group of people anonymous to one another, transformed into a political community through the simultaneous sharing of identical experiences. In the process, the distinction between physical and moral hygiene was blurred, and both were linked to national values, so that being a good Costa Rican became increasingly impossible unless one defecated in a latrine, bathed once a day, remained vigilant against invisible pathogens, and generally maintained good health.[115]

The combined local and Rockefeller Foundation antihookworm campaigns played a large role in developing a consciousness of preventive public health. In the process, they popularized the new laboratory-based medicine, and established in the popular mind the idea that official medicine, in its new scientific guise, could determine effective and specific cures for debilitating diseases. And yet these teachings were not necessarily accepted in orthodox fashion. Instead, they were recombined with existing ways of understanding illness and curing, and popular health culture grew more eclectic than ever.

8

The Magician versus the

Monopolists: The Popular Medical

Eclecticism of Professor Carbell

He arrived in Costa Rica toward the end of 1931, a magician and spiritist in a touring carnival called "Coney Island Park" that set up in the plaza in front of the Pacific Railway Station in one of the city's popular neighborhoods. Despite the biting economic crisis, perhaps based on a reputation won with the large crowds that visited the fair during the traditional year-end fiesta, no doubt with the aid of local fellow theosophists, the exotic foreigner had soon established an extraordinarily successful practice in the capital city—one ostensibly devoted to spiritism. His name was Carlos Carballo Romero, but he won fame under the pseudonym Professor Carlos Carbell, a healer who used supernatural powers, wondrous techniques, and special nostrums to cure diseases that official medical science was powerless to treat.[1]

Late one night in January 1932, in the heart of San José, Dr. Sotero Antillón, the capital city's chief of sanitation, crashed into Professor Carbell's apartment. In a scene worthy of comic opera, the young doctor forced the handsome magician from his bed at gunpoint and paraded him through the streets of the capital in his nightclothes. When they arrived at the offices of the municipality, Antillón tried to charge Carbell with the illegal practice of medicine. This vigilante action was unsuccessful, but soon after the Costa Rican Faculty of Medicine took up the case, and its counsel formally requested that the republic's principal police agent for public health and social protection lay charges against Carballo Romero.[2]

In his testimony before the public health police, Carbell declared that he was a Cuban national, thirty-two years of age, and that his "profession" was that of "occultist." According to his statement, he neither posed as a doctor or curandero, nor charged "honoraria" for healing services. The professor did not deny, however, that through the use of his "mediumistic faculties" he might well "exercise mental influences on the will of the individuals who consult me, obtaining in this way a moral improvement that would have its physical reflection, and thus an improvement in the state of these individuals and humanity in general."[3]

The Carbell dossier compiled by police provides a detailed glimpse of the inner workings of an urban curandero's practice, and offers a rare opportunity to explore common beliefs about medicine at a crucial moment in the relationship between popular and official medicine in the country. The incident occurred during a period of rapid increase in the number of physicians, and at a time when the maturing campaigns in state public health had nurtured the assumptions and techniques of biomedicine among the popular classes. The fact that the professor's eclectic healing included a deliberate mimicry of the poses, practices, and terminology of the medical profession suggests that a broad spectrum of Costa Ricans were more willing than ever to accept the authority of physicians. The scientific and professional guise had established itself as an indispensable element in the repertoire of healers and sufferers alike. Nonetheless, biomedicine and professionalism were simply the newest additions to constellations of popular medical beliefs and practices that remained heterodox and "extrascientific." The case of Carbell also indicates that these elements were imbibed in different ways according to the gender of the sufferers. Although the women interviewed by the police were not necessarily more averse than men to the scientific medicine embodied in a patriarchal profession, they were less satisfied that this approach alone could supply an ultimately satisfactory response to their health needs.

As might be supposed from the fury of the young Dr. Antillón, this episode is also a good one to explore relations between unlicensed healers and a resurgent medical profession making more aggressive attempts to enforce its monopoly on healing. Following a decade-long period of professional decadence and economic recession between 1914 and 1924—years in which new medical graduates slowed to a trickle while the medical elites began to show signs of age—the second half of the 1920s saw the influx of unprecedented numbers of young practitioners during a time of economic revival. Among them were some truly bright lights who would revitalize physicians' esprit de corps and challenge the ongoing proliferation of alternative healers in a medical marketplace that was soon constrained again by the Great Depression. This was the context for the confrontation between Carbell and the would-be monopolists of the medical profession.

A Modern Curandero and His Patients

Roy Porter has written that "the sick have always been ignored in histories of quackery, caricatured as gaping fools and mindless morons," whereas the more pertinent and revealing approach to flamboyant cases of irregular medicine should be to ask who consulted the quack, and what motives they might have had to seek out such an extraordinary doctor.[4] At one time or another, in various combinations according to circumstance, Carbell posed as a physician, psychotherapist, homeopath, physiotherapist, mesmerist, magician, and shaman as well as an apocalyptic visionary with a clear political message (he also had an office dispensary staffed by a chemist). The heterodoxy of his practice was inscribed on the diploma hung in his consulting room, conferred in 1927 by a Venezuelan office of professional titles, and certifying Carbell as a "Professor of Theosophy, Hypnotism, Magnetism, Astrology, Medical Chiromancy, Spiritism, and Biopsychology."[5] Indeed, this eclecticism is what made him such an exceptional figure—a veritable grand master of alternative healing. Yet in each case, the professor's alternative powers were complemented with orthodox connotations drawn from professional medicine and pharmacy.

The professor's offices mirrored those of any physician. He had a female receptionist, large waiting area, dispensary attended by a chemist, and consulting room where he displayed the eclectic diploma. The receptionist registered the arrival of the patients, took notes on their condition, and assigned them a seat. After the inevitable lengthy wait, Carbell would enter the waiting area to greet the patient and then see them individually in the consulting room. He would perform a diagnosis and prescribe drugs that had to be filled in his office dispensary. The professor's standard fee was five colones — a sum that slightly exceeded the cost of consulting a physician. The clearest composition in his carefully managed kaleidoscope of self-representation, then, was that of a physician in private practice. Nevertheless, the great majority of his patients knew that he was not merely a physician; indeed, they would not have come to consult him had they thought he was only that.[6]

The most detailed depiction of a consultation with Carbell was provided by a secret agent, Heriberto Araya, an artisan in the employ of the municipality. On the instructions of his boss, Antillón, he presented himself at Carbell's office. It was extremely crowded, and he was given a number and made to wait. Finally, Araya was received by the charismatic professor. A reporter who met him described his presence as "imposing": his speech was "considered," his voice was "firm and sure," and his "long, curly head of hair and his Nazarene beard" gave him "a certain resemblance to Christ" (a resemblance that Carbell carefully cultivated).[7] On entering the consulting room, the patient was greeted by the following set: the darkened room was illuminated by electric lamps and candlelight; its walls and doorways were decorated with multicolored curtains along with a cypress crown in the form of a star. There were books on occultism by various authors, and a variety of traditional séance and magic artifacts.[8]

In this environment, before the imposing professor, Araya complained that he suffered from pain when urinating. "After that it seemed like he wanted to call up the spirits because he made signs that aren't those of a doctor but those that they talk about in the books on occultism and other stuff that everyone knows about. Once he'd done this, he gave me a prescription and charged me the sum of five colones, and told me that I suffered from chronic gonorrhea. The prescription was for the chemist that he has in the same apartment, . . . who told me that I needed some injections starting right away because my case is serious."[9] Araya's workmate Federico Paniagua, also on assignment, had a similar encounter moments later after complaining of an ache in his hand. He, too, was put on medication to be purchased at the office dispensary and told he would have to return for further treatment.

Of course, Carbell's magic and mind reading relied on tricks. María Angela Alarcón, the young woman who worked as his receptionist, testified to the police that Carbell had trained her to casually interrogate each patient on entry. With widowed women (who were frequent clients), she was to find out the name of the dead spouse and the circumstances of their death; with others, she was to elicit any information that might be useful. This written down, she would pass the little dossier through a secret door that linked her reception space to his inner office. By means of this classic technique, Carbell was able to deeply impress patients with his powers of divination. One woman, who had come to consult him from the town of Sarchí, on the rural periphery, was stunned when the professor confirmed exactly what she herself already suspected: "she had been bewitched by señora Adelia de Cespedes."[10]

Carbell's constantly prescribed patent medicine was a syrup with a potent, and not altogether pleasant, odor and taste. According to his servant, Clemencia Hidalgo Torres, who prepared the mixture in bulk, it was made of onions, honey, sugar, and camphor (for the authentic pharmaceutical odor). Carbell also sold special talismans at fifteen colones a piece, "for falling in love, all classes of luck, and many things more." Fifteen colones (three- to five-days work for an artisan of that time) got the customer a little black leather bag containing a capsule of gelatin hardened around some graphite and powder; the gelatin was wrapped in a piece of red cloth decorated with silver paint, paraffin, and tinfoil (not a bad talisman, really, though perhaps on the expensive side).[11]

The testimonies in the Carbell dossier make it clear that he enjoyed a truly massive clientele, with reports of lines stretching into the street in front of the office.[12] His servant testified that a majority of clients were women, and that widows were well represented among the ranks. Most of the patients were from the capital city, but others came from the towns and villages surrounding San José, and some from the rural periphery. They were of all social classes, but it was more likely that a woman of middling or plentiful means would consult Carbell than would a man of similar standing. It is telling in this regard that Antillón asked two artisans in the municipality's employ to act as undercover agents rather than, say, a clerk or another physician.

Not all of Carbell's patients were specifically seeking his supernatural treatments. Some were simply shopping in the medical marketplace for a cure, and given his great reputation, the Cuban empiric seemed as good a bet as any officially sanctioned doctor. Rafael Solano, a young carpenter from San José who could only describe his illness as "really bad eye sickness," went to see Carbell after hearing that the Cuban was "very skillful at curing." Carbell told him that it was not serious, and charged him five and a half colones for the visit and some medicine. The medicine, however, had no effect, and the pain worsened. Fearing he was on the verge of losing his eyesight, Solano went to the hospital for treatment, "and it was there that they were able to cure me after doing various exams of my mouth, [my] blood, and my whole body to see if they could find the cause of my illness." He depicted the triumph of medical science in the following fashion: "After one month of being in the hospital, and when my relatives thought I was going to lose my eyesight, I left the hospital miraculously cured."[13] Whether or not the hospital stay had involved some calculated and successful treatment, Solano imagined his cure as a miracle that was nevertheless somehow associated with expert healers.

Others sought out Carbell when medical science had given up on them. A moving example of this was the petition by Regina Salazar that the professor visit her husband, seriously ill with fever. Carbell's enthusiasm dissipated abruptly at the man's bedside: faced with the mask of death, he opted for telling the young woman that he was unable to treat her husband due to the latter's imminent demise. It should be recalled that treating the husband would have called the attention of the authorities to Carbell at the moment of their inquiries into the cause of death. Furthermore, the professor probably followed a strategy that had been standard for doctors in the ancient and medieval world: in order to maintain and expand one's reputation, it was necessary to treat as far as possible only those diseases that were self-limiting and to avoid all association with death.[14]

The case of the dowager Isolina Castro viuda de Bustamante reveals a patient wealthy enough to consult a variety of healers concerning her heart condition. According to her daughter, these specialists included "foreign and Costa Rican physicians" who had demonstrated that the widow suffered from a "chronic heart condition," a diagnosis apparently supported by an X-ray plate. Carbell did not dispute the expert opinion in this case but did prescribe Isolina his special syrup as well as some injections of a substance called "Cardiotone." It is possible that her interest in the professor was heightened by a desire to make supernatural contact with her late husband in the great beyond; in any event, she soon joined him by natural means.[15]

In other instances, it is clear that the search for medicines was combined with the purchase of talismans and spiritist sessions. This was so in the case of the bewitched woman of Sarchí, who took medicines back home with her along, no doubt, with secret knowledge on how to break the spell. Other women came for a mixture of medicinal and spiritist comfort, to treat their physical ailments, communicate with the dead, and garner information about the future all in one session. One of Carbell's patients was a paralytic who came for therapeutic massages with Bay Rum.[16] All sought something more than a mere medical diagnosis and treatment based on scientific techniques and knowledge, though the majority wanted this as well. Ironically, although the witnesses who testified in the Carbell investigation were chosen by the Faculty of Medicine, four of the seven who offered an opinion on the matter were satisfied with the treatment they had received from the professor (two of those who did not register their feelings were dead, though apparently neither as a result of Carbell's treatment).

The array of spiritual and medical services offered by Carbell resonated loudly with historical trends in the alternative medicine of Latin America. His Cuban roots allowed him to trade on the connection between the images of the island and African healing mysteries, which had been reintroduced to Costa Ricans in a new form after 1880 by the Jamaican practitioners of Obeah and Myalist medicine. He combined herbal cures and magic in a way that recalls the practice of brujos, sorcerers, and wisewomen in Costa Rica and elsewhere. Indeed, in many respects Carbell can be understood in terms of the classic repertoire of the shamanic healer, with his counseling, fortune-telling, attempt to unify the natural and supernatural worlds, carefully orchestrated performances, and reliance on the belief of the patients in his special powers.[17] Carbell's "resemblance to Christ," dark gowns, and posturing recalled the traditional healing vocation of priests and monks (and the great healer, Christ himself). His professorial title emphasized the kind of learned erudition that had made all *bachilleres* potential healers during the colonial era. Like so many of the alternative healers of Western history, Carbell was itinerant, traveling about and combining his panacean offerings with carnivalesque performance. He picked up on a tradition of spectacular foreign healers like Esteban Courtí whose exotic erudition and miraculous healing powers had enthralled Latin Americans since the late eighteenth century. The professor accentuated his foreign mystique through the "internationalized" Franco-Anglo overtones of "Carbell" — also, of course, an essential part of a magician's stage mystique and one that echoed the most famous magician of all, Kardec, the reference point for much of Latin America's medical spiritism from the second half of the nineteenth century onward.

Carbell's success testified to the strengthening grip on the popular imagination of modern medicine, in both its regular and irregular guises. On a local scale, he was able to trade on the reputation of the Cuban country doctors of the turn of the nineteenth century who had spanned the divide between alternative and regular medicine. And Carbell combined many of the main unorthodox medical specialties — animal magnetism, psychology, spiritism, massage therapy, and homeopathy — with a straight mimicry of physicians in private practice and the provision of pharmaceutical services. Virtually all of the continent's well-traveled roads between official and unofficial medicine intersected in his impressive person.

In a recent analysis of the rise of the urban curandero in Latin America, James Dow distinguishes this figure from practitioners of the traditional "indigenous" style of curanderismo on the basis of his or her "synthesis of practices and beliefs" — elements that can be taken from almost any religion or healing theory.[18] But what is most interesting about Carbell's practice is his lack of concern with synthesizing the different elements from this expansive repertoire. At its heart was the simultaneous performance of each pole of the medical universe: the spiritual healer (*el médico de la bolita*) and conventional physician; the shaman and biomedical professional. This was nicely captured in the report of the artisan spy Araya, who remarked on the abrupt shift in Carbell's diagnostic performance from occultist gestures and utterances to the physician's certain diagnosis of syphilis and his writing of a prescription. These two poles sat on either side of an outlandish eclecticism that ranged from homeopathy to physiotherapy to psychological counseling to love magic. In this sense, Carbell was a herald of the more formally pluralistic medical configuration characteristic of Latin America in the second half of the twentieth century. Such medical pluralism is sometimes imagined as a patient-driven phenomenon, with sufferers appealing to different healing traditions. But Carbell shows that popular practitioners themselves promoted the idea that all of these medical approaches could work together. This posed a particular problem for a new generation of medical doctors for, though it almost goes without saying, the professor certainly did not live up to the anthropological stereotype of the curandero practicing outside the cash nexus.[19]

The Fall and Rise of the Medical Profession

The coherence, power, and jurisdiction that physicians of Durán and Ulloa's generation built up during the golden age of their professional association was almost crowned under the Tinoco dictatorship of 1917–1919, only to dissipate rapidly with the collapse of the regime itself. The physician old guard had close links with the Tinoco brothers, and sought to use these connections to further entrench the political power of the profession. Durán, like every former living president but one, expressed public support for the dictatorship in its early days (he was, in fact, one of the first to pay Federico Tinoco an official visit), while José María Soto Alfaro was a personal friend and physician to Federico Tinoco, and the head of the Faculty of Medicine, Emilio Echeverría, was a close relative by marriage.[20] In 1918, the Tinocos created a Superior Council of Health, with a permanent and powerful role for the Faculty of Medicine.[21] They also charged the faculty with overseeing the creation of a new Sanitary Code. Both were designed as the foundations for a national department of health in which the Faculty of Medicine would have been in a dominant position.

These plans were suspended when the regime was overthrown in 1919 and the medical elite was perceived to have collaborated with the dictatorship—an appearance that Soto did nothing to dispel by running as a presidential candidate in the elections of 1919 against the triumphant hero of the antidictatorial resistance, Julio Acosta.[22] As a result, the medical establishment suffered a marked decline in political influence. On top of this, the great patriarchs of Costa Rican medicine, the generation of the 1880s, were now in the twilight of their careers, and in the case of Durán, their lives (he died in 1922). Symbolic of the exhaustion of the second wave's energies, the *Gaceta Médica* ceased publication in January 1918, probably for reasons of an acute economic crisis and a drastic reduction in public expenditures (the state had subsidized its publication), and was not revived. Moreover, the profession had little capacity for generational succession. The latter third of the nineteenth century had been characterized by a rapid increase in the number of new physicians incorporating in the country, with a steep increase in the 1890s (see figure 5). The arrival of new practitioners slowed drastically over the first fourteen years of the twentieth century, and then all but came to a halt, with the appearance of a new professional a rare event during the years of the European war and its aftermath. It was in this context of a debilitated and discredited profession that the new government of Acosta was able to transfer jurisdiction over national medicine and public health to the Rockefeller-backed nucleus headed by Núñez.

Then, especially after 1924, there began a vertiginous ascent in young men (and a few young women) seeking incorporation into the Faculty of Medicine, almost all of them Costa Ricans returning from studies in the United States and Western Europe. The total number of physicians practicing in the country rose by almost 70 percent over the course of the decade. It soon outstripped the turn-of-the-century ratio of physicians per capita, considered a disaster of saturation at the time. From a physician for every 2,850 inhabitants in 1900, the proportion had changed by 1921 in favor of the profession to roughly 1 to 4,000 as the number of new practitioners declined; by 1932, at the worst moment of the depression, the ratio reached 1 physician for every 2,700 Costa Ricans.[23] That ratio, however, was at the national level, and the growing tendency of physicians to crowd into the capital city put more market pressure than ever on the bulk of official providers of medical care. In 1904, 29 of the country's 100 medical doctors lived in San José; in 1935, 67 of 140 (48 percent) lived there, making the physician to resident ratio about 1 to 1,000, meaning that half the doctors were concentrated among 10 percent of the populace.[24]

Though it put market pressure on physicians, the infusion of new blood after 1924 brought the medical patriarchy back to fighting shape. In that year, Antonio Peña Chavarría returned to practice and research, and by the end of the decade he was joined by Rafael Angel Calderón Guardia, Ricardo Moreno Cañas, and Mario Luján. All would play key roles in the country's professional and political life, and Peña Chavarría and Moreno Cañas had strong research interests. The scientific horizons also improved with the return in 1923 of the brilliant young serologist Clodomiro Picado after a research fellowship at the Pasteur Institute to resume his directorship of the laboratory at the Hospital San Juan de Dios.[25]

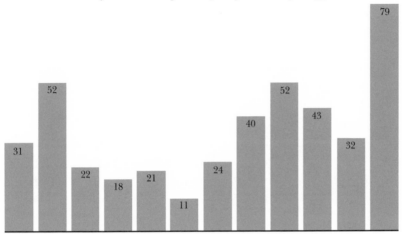

Fig. 5. Number of physicians incorporating into Costa Rica's Faculty of Medicine per five-year period, 1890–1950.

This self-conscious spirit of renovation was in evidence in Peña Chavarría's 1927 proposal to the faculty for a Día del Médico Costarricense (National Day of the Costa Rican Doctor) as well as the celebration of periodic assemblies in the country's major towns to present work on "national pathology and hygiene."[26] Efforts to revive a medical journal resulted in the annual publication of the *Anales de la Facultad de Medicina* between 1927–1929. Then, after sixteen years without a medical journal that would satisfy professional and scientific needs, two young medical researchers founded the bimonthly *Revista Médica* in October 1933. A year later, San José played host to the Second Central American Medical Congress, which produced a number of monographs based on papers read at the gathering. National publications devoted to medicine and hygiene, which numbered in the dozens prior to 1910, would be counted by the hundreds between 1927 and 1940.[27]

No steps were taken toward creating a medical school, however. Young Costa Rican medical students altered their preferences for countries of study after 1910. The period coincided with the creation of a new model of research-oriented medical instruction in the United States, following the impact of the Flexner report on North American medical education. Still, despite the aggressive push made by the United States — including the Rockefeller Foundation — for increased influence over medical instruction, the United States did not supplant

Magician versus Monopolists

Europe as a desirable academic destination. The United States retained its allure up until 1925, and the Rockefeller Foundation gave eight prestigious public health fellowships to Costa Ricans during the 1930s (though some went to nurses, statisticians, and engineers). Yet the U.S. position as academic supplier to a plurality of young Costa Rican physicians collapsed in the second half of the 1920s.[28] Indeed, the choice of medical education in the United States appears to have grown as a kind of surrogate in the context of the increased difficulty of studying in the more prestigious German schools. There were almost no Costa Rican graduates of German universities between 1910 and 1925; with travel to Europe again possible and a massive currency devaluation in Germany after 1919, 20 percent of those who incorporated in the final five years of the decade were returning from studies in the Weimar Republic.[29]

Specialization and New Offerings

One way that physicians met the challenge of increased professional competition was specialization. As distinct from the era of the great generalists like Durán, those who made the greatest mark for themselves in the profession in the new century were often specialists. Emilio Echeverría, who had graduated in general medicine from Columbia University in 1889, returned to study at the London School of Tropical Medicine in 1904 — a specialty that eventually earned him the direction of the United Fruit Company's Costa Rican Medical Department. The young surgeon Ricardo Jiménez Núñez quickly determined to devote himself exclusively to the practice and study of anesthetics after incorporating in 1902. Changes in hospital medicine also promoted this differentiation, and the country acquired its first specialist in orthopedic surgery, Ricardo Moreno Cañas, in 1919 and its first radiologist, Antonio Peña Chavarría, in 1924.[30]

With growing public confidence in the hospital, and the concerted effort of the medical community to represent the hospital as a disciplined and professional space of treatment and recovery, the Hospital San Juan de Dios rapidly lost its reputation as a place for the indigent and chronically ill. Between 1910 and 1916, the number of patients attended increased in great, steady leaps of about a thousand per annum, from 2,700 to 7,400.[31] The wealthy and respectable still were not entirely comfortable with the general hospital, and the 1910s and 1920s saw a vogue in the "little hospital"—the clinic. Emilio Roig de Leuch-senring has described the emergence of appendicitis as a "fashionable condition" among girls of good families in 1920s' Havana, with the melodrama of "recuperation in the clinic" becoming a kind of lifestyle consumer product. Certain doctors became *de moda,* and in order to be in vogue one had to submit oneself to these physicians' interventions. A market in aesthetic plastic surgery, breast reconstruction, and the re-duction of leg fat also took shape in the same decade.[32] Costa Rica had its own clinics, like the Clínica Victory-Pacheco with its art nouveau stylings and Mariano Figueres's electrotherapy clinic, both of which thrived in San José during the second half of the 1910s.[33]

Above all, the general public had become fascinated with injections, particularly of the famous "magic bullet," 606 or salvarsan. The chemi-cal compound, discovered in Germany in 1909, attacked the spirochete that caused syphilis, and as such was the first drug developed by labora-tory science capable of targeting a particular pathogen. According to the 1923 report of Teodoro Picado, director of the Public Assistance Service, it was nearly impossible to explain to people the real role of the antivenereal dispensaries he oversaw. He blamed "the mercantile pro-paganda that has been spread and the abuses of the curanderismo so in vogue for medicinal treatment by injection," which had "brought to the popular spirit the belief that at present all sicknesses must be cured through injections."[34]

This belief had combined with a belief associated with humoralism and apparently common to the popular classes throughout Latin Amer-ica: "the vague notion of illnesses of the blood, and the belief that all diseases derive from the poor state of the blood, [which has] sowed in the popular mind the idea that all ailments find their source there." Picado complained that a large number of people with rheumatism, malaria, varicose ulcers, tuberculosis, and other diseases, as well as those who had broken out in a rash—in short, anyone suffering from almost anything—came to the clinic "in the belief that the treatment estab-lished to combat venereal diseases, constitutes a universal panacea [*sic*]." Indeed, this idea was still present in 1932 in the mind of a young baker and sometime heroin addict, who explained to the public health police agent that the vice "must be cured with injections of Sal Varsan [*sic*], which they give me in the Clinic of Dr. Picado."[35]

Injections were certainly a staple of empirical practice, as we have seen in the case of Carbell. But the practice was propagated by physicians as well in an effort to live up to the expectations of their clients. In 1932, Dr. Pupo Pérez had concluded that in the domain of medicine and public health "chaos reins [*sic*]: drugs are handed out like blessed bread without examining the patient . . . ; money is spent in injecting very expensive and dangerous drugs that have no curative value."[36] Such willful attempts to win the popular classes over to the official agents of modern medicine were even promoted by the public health apparatus. In discussing the beginnings of the School Health Department's clinics, Núñez contended that "it was necessary to accustom the mothers to coming to the office, and this was only possible at first if they were sure they would return to their homes with pills, potions, and papers," while on the back cover of Núñez's 1923 pamphlet on whooping cough, the working classes of the capital were guaranteed that "in the Infants' Clinic and School Clinic poor children will be prescribed and provided drugs free of charge."[37]

Market Pressure from Other Healers

The professional rivalry between physicians and pharmacists was exacerbated by the influx of new doctors and continual graduation of cohorts from the College of Pharmacy. Each group now had better ammunition to throw at the other due to the greater legal precision in clauses relating to the professions in the 1923 Sanitary Code. After much lobbying by pharmacists, even physicians who were also titled pharmacists were prohibited from practicing both professions at once, and their office dispensaries had to be staffed by a licensed pharmacist, though in actuality many physicians continued to break this rule. Pharmacists, who complained that their profession was "not very prestigious," continued to diagnose customers' illnesses and prescribe a wide variety of medicines, many of them with narcotic bases that were prohibited by law.[38] This was quite common in the rural and semirural periphery, where pharmacists may have faced at least as much pressure as temptation to practice medicine. In 1929 Daniel Acuña, a pharmacist in the town of Pacayas, was denounced by a resident for dispensing his own concoction for the treatment of tuberculosis. Acuña claimed in his defense that he was constantly called on to prescribe medicines due to the absence of a physician in the area (though the fact that he promoted himself in this role is evidenced by the popular home medical manual he published in 1926, alleged to be "indispensable for families of the countryside").[39]

In the wonderful childhood memoir-cum-novel *Marcos Ramírez*, Carlos Luis Fallas recalls growing up in the hospital district of San José in the early 1910s. His mother constantly sent him round to the Botica La Victoria to make small purchases, and don Severo, the formidable pharmacist-proprietor, was forever engaged in "curing" children's ailments of one sort or another. Indeed, people of the working class could more reflexively turn to the barrio pharmacist than to a physician: after a nasty rock-throwing incident, Marcos and his friends automatically decide to leave an unconscious friend (thinking him dead) at the door of the pharmacist's house before running away.[40] In the census of 1927, there were 179 licensed pharmacists in the country (three of them women), and the small pharmacy had become a fixture of the barrios in the major towns and, especially, burgeoning popular neighborhoods of the capital.[41] The jurisdictional and market antagonisms between the two professions had become so acute by 1929 that they provoked a nasty propaganda war, with the Faculty of Medicine denouncing pharmacists for propagating heroin addiction among young, working-class artisans in San José — an accusation that prompted a general and pronounced moral panic.[42]

As table 3 suggests, physicians had cause to feel anxious about the general proliferation of allied health practitioners visible by the late 1920s, all of whom might offer their healing services in the tighter marketplace and many of whom had empiric counterparts who might also tread on the physicians' terrain. The Faculty of Medicine and Surgery had tried to maintain control over its junior surgical partner by creating a school of dentistry in 1906, but only one student enrolled and the effort was abandoned after a year. Legitimate dentistry remained a solidly capitalino affair, and in the hands of foreigners, although by 1914 there were practitioners in Alajuela, Heredia, and Limón to go along with the fourteen practicing in San José. In the 1920s, dentists created their own autonomous Faculty of Dental Surgery and battled petitions from the many dentist empirics — survivors of the ancient trade of the *sacamuelas*, or tooth puller — to have their status formalized by the government.[43] They were unsuccessful, despite support from the professional associations of pharmacists and physicians,

Table 3. All licensed health practitioners in Costa Rica, 1864–1950

	Pharmacists	Midwives	Nurses	Dentists	Physicians
1864	18[a]	24[b]	3	1	38[f]
1883	44[a]	—	0	7	35
1892	54[a]	—	0	6	42
1905	45[g]	14	—	11[e]	85
1914	75[g]	25[g]	—	19	106
1927	176	86	204	89[f]	145
1950	310	425[c]	425[d]	146	265

a. includes unschooled holders of retail patent to sell drugs in area without licensed pharmacist
b. unlicensed comadronas
c. includes nurses
d. includes midwives
e. 1898 figures
f. includes licensed empirics
g. estimated

Sources: GMCR 8, no. 5 (1904): 75; GMCR 11, no. 3 (1906): 46; República de Costa Rica, *Censo general de la República de Costa Rica (27 de noviembre de 1864* (San José: Imprenta Nacional, 1868), 86–95; República de Costa Rica, *Censo de la República de Costa Rica* [1883] (n.p., n.d.), 72–85; República de Costa Rica, *Censo general de la República de Costa Rica (1892)* (San José: Tipografía Nacional, 1893), lxxxviii–ci; *Directorio comercial de San José, 1898* (San José: Imprenta Greñas, 1898), 1; RFA, record group 5, series 51, box 7, folder 103; Mario Samper, ed., *El censo de la población de 1927: creación de una base nominal computarizada* (San José: Oficina de Publicaciones de la Universidad de Costa Rica, 1991), 82; and República de Costa Rica, *Censo de la República de Costa Rica, 22 de mayo de 1950,* 2d ed. (San José, 1975), 312.

and the national legislature passed a law in 1932 granting license to practice to "empirics in dental surgery."[44]

The state's efforts to expand the network of public health personnel inevitably caused trepidation among physicians. In 1929, the Ministry of Health created a School of Sanitary Inspectors. In answer to criticism that the school would simply create more curanderos, Minister Solón Núñez told Congress that "we are not trying to train curanderos, but even if that is the outcome at least they practice an educated curanderismo [*curanderismo culto*] that will prejudice the trade of the numerous Chinese, black, and other curanderos who practice their trade in full view of tolerant authorities."[45] Again, the medical profession might have felt its monopoly being ridiculed by a state satisfied to see the spread of licensed empirics.

When in 1926 the Subsecretariat of Hygiene received funding for an agency of public health policing, the profession's elites, practitioners in the capital city, demanded that it increase the pressure on empirics and curanderos, particularly those practicing in or around San José. The agency did its best to comply, in the first full year of operation investigating forty-eight cases concerning the illegal practice of medicine referred to it by the Faculty of Medicine and three cases against unlicensed midwifery.[46] But unlicensed empiricism and the challenge of rival medical sects continued apace, with the appearance of osteopaths, and a new wave of homeopath salespersons and practitioners crisscrossing the countryside, often with titles from schools of homeopathic medicine.[47] One empiric, Antonio Bayer Jaramillo, was convicted of seriously harming and even helping to kill a woman suffering from typhoid, yet he got off with a relatively small fine of one hundred colones and dared to wage a dispute with physicians in the national press over the way they had treated the patient prior to her death.[48] As for the continued popularity of the folk and religious healer, a violent mob of thousands gathered on the outskirts of the capital city in 1931 to intervene against the authorities after a town doctor orchestrated the arrest of don Roque, an elderly parish activist who had begun to practice faith healing. Such a tumultuous and spontaneous public reaction in this relatively domesticated and institutionalized political environment is a testament to the continued virulence of popular feelings against the persecution of irregular healers, especially those who emanated from the community.[49]

In 1923, the country's new Public Health Code consolidated the tendency toward strict medical ethics. Physicians were prohibited from offering to the public, "through newspapers, posters, or handbills, the cure of special diseases based on claims to have secret or unique means, knowledge, operations, or remedies for the objective that is proposed, or panaceas."[50] The strictures were reinforced in the 1932 *Code of Medical Ethics* adopted by the Faculty of Medicine, perhaps in the face of liberties taken by members to attract clientele in a context of economic depression.[51] One of the main goals of these measures was to raise the status of the medical profession by more clearly separating the empiric, and particularly the charlatan, from the physician. Yet it meant that

Magician versus Monopolists

those practitioners who wanted to enjoy the potential benefits of being a member of the official club had to swear off the advantages enjoyed by irregular practitioners. Meanwhile, empirics like Carbell were able to attract a massive clientele by combining a scientific discourse of medicine with others relating to secret, magical, and panacean powers that physicians were no longer allowed to profess. Only the alternative doctor was able to satisfy a broader spectrum of demands in a medical marketplace in which consumers showed a clear interest in this type of "mix-and-match" medicine. If physicians were no longer allowed to be quacks, then quacks should not be allowed to assume the poses of scientific medical practitioners.

Such was the outlook, at least, of anxious young physicians like Sotero Antillón, San José's chief of municipal sanitation and self-styled persecutor of offensive charlatans. Though not it would seem one of their brighter lights, Antillón was very much a representative of the new wave of physicians. He had graduated from medical studies in Germany and incorporated into the Costa Rican faculty in 1929.[52] His anxiety over the failure of the authorities to enforce the laws on the books was also exemplary of young physicians confronting the economic crisis, and he had stated to the press late in 1931 that Costa Rica was "a country where things can only be achieved through the use of force."[53] Carbell's ability to attract a huge clientele and practice medicine in the heart of San José with apparent impunity was too much for him, although the manner in which he chose to use force to solve this menace to professional and public health also had an explicit gender dimension, and revealed a lingering sense of impotence among the resurgent medical community.

The Medical Profession as Cuckolded Patriarchs

It was Carbell's sexual charisma that finally provoked Antillón to action. Among the professor's clients asked to testify by the public health police in the aftermath of the vigilante arrest was Irene Acuña, a thirty-nine-year-old schoolteacher from the capital who apparently sought no medical opinion at all from Carbell. Daniel Fernández, a small merchant and husband of the woman in question, complained to the health police agent that his wife visited Carbell at different times of the day, and that even at night he saw "many people" going in to see him. The worst thing about all this, worse even than Carbell's cures, was that "he gets into giving advice about private matters that are in every way off-limits to him." Fernández had also been horrified to hear from an acquaintance that his wife was paying for the therapy sessions by hocking her jewels in the state-owned pawnshop. Francisco Frutos, a neighbor of the unhappy couple, testified that he had overheard Acuña talking in the street with another woman. She referred to Carbell and then, in the same breath, spoke of her husband "in harsh terms."[54]

Acuña herself admitted to the health police agent that she had gone to see Carbell, but only once, and not for her health. "I simply went because he is a person of a certain erudition and I like that." She added, rather provocatively, that were she not "an extremely busy person, I would go to see him frequently because, well, I don't see the danger in it." Her noncompliant posture finds echo in the refusal of Teresa Infante, who was separated from her husband, to implicate Carbell in the sale of drugs that he had prescribed her. She consulted him only because "they told me that he could guess the present, past, and future"; further badgering from the police agent brought the curt reply, "Don't ask me any more questions than the ones I've already answered."[55]

Both may have been assuming an infinitely more compliant posture with Carbell. His servant Clemencia Hidalgo claimed that "behind a curtain adjacent to the consulting room, he has a bed where he takes advantage of the women who come." She never actually saw this going on because he closed the interior door, "but you could hear everything — what's more, he used to joke that he had to use like eight women a day."[56] Hidalgo's testimony should be taken with a grain of salt because she was a disgruntled ex-employee. Nevertheless, it jibes with Carbell's style and the concern of the husband who may have heard gossip about the professor's "therapy sessions."[57]

This dimension of his practice also offers a further clue to understanding Antillón's violent intrusion on Carbell as well as his expression of outrage in moral terms. He was voicing a professional censure that nonetheless was an authentic representation of the larger patriarchal community. That sympathies tended to align according to gender is not that surprising given the constitution of professional and scientific medicine as a domain of patriarchal authority. In England and the United States, the growing popularity of occultism in the late nineteenth century was clearly associated with the fact that it opened spaces for women that while "public," were claimed through the enactment of enclosed and private spectacles. Sessions of spiritism, with their trance states and summoning of other identities to speak through the participants, resonated with the symbolic liberation of female sexuality along with the possibility for women to assume masculine voices. Spiritists constantly offended the dignity of the leaders of the medical and scientific communities. These latter declared spiritism a disease, and associated it with "feminine conditions," from madness of uterine origin to paralysis in males. They likewise denounced practitioners as effeminate frauds and their (mostly female) followers as neurotic or mentally unstable. Not coincidentally, these attacks occurred simultaneous to the medical profession's growing role in the creation of psychology and psychiatry as specialized disciplines.[58]

Carbell's own booklet stressed that those most predisposed to project "the capabilities that science designates as psychic" had delicate nerves or showed signs of neurosis and hysteria. This implicit superiority of females as vehicles for supernatural powers was confirmed by the fact that Carbell had allegedly carried out the scientific experiments that were the basis of his book with "a female medium [*una medium*], G. M." In both instances, it might be noted that he assigned women a privileged role in a domain of inquiry and experiment whose scientific status he was championing against an exclusively male medical monopoly.[59]

Women like schoolteacher Irene Acuña embraced the encounters with the impressive and erudite professor as stimulating experiences that enriched their lives and served psychotherapeutic purposes. Together with a general dissatisfaction with their marriages, these women (and the other patients, male and female, for that matter) might have consulted Carbell as a product and an expression of their disappointment with the new species of scientific and professional physicians, and with a type of reason and progress that seemed only to strip away the spiritual dimensions of life without compensating for the loss. They accepted that medicine was a materialist science, but they wanted it to be something more than that. Whether the intercourse between Carbell and his patients was sexual as well as medical, occultist as well as intellectual, will never be known for certain (though it is worth noting that Carbell's book detailed his mastery of therapeutic "rotary digital impositions," "looks," and "blowing on the affected areas," which like all mesmerist techniques are charged with erotic promise).[60]

Popular Medicine to Medical Populism

Were the meetings between Carbell and women like Acuña really a cuckolding of the positivist system? Antillón saw them as such. The behavior of this public medical official offers an especially clear example of the parallels between professional, political, and gender transgressions. Antillón insisted that it was his responsibility as a physician in a public post to take the action, in order to "fulfill my duty and, above all else, to watch over the moral laws of the country." Moreover, he explained, "I did not prohibit the man from putting his clothes on; quite the contrary, I repeatedly asked him to dress but he didn't want to, and preferred to go outdoors in pajamas, and this is proven by the fact that his own male friend [*el propio compañero de él*] did dress in order to come with us."[61]

The commentary conjures the spectacle of a peculiar type of "rough music." Not only did Antillón noisily intrude on Carbell's privacy, apparently entering his very bedroom to make an aggressive arrest; he paraded him through the streets in his nightclothes along with a male companion. The transparent innuendo in Antillón's remarks to the press offered a second public suggestion that the occultist was a depraved homosexual. The patriarchs had to emasculate their rival in public to discredit not only a man who had had illicit "relations" with the women of the city but one who, in the words of Antillón, was "a charlatan who has attempted to ridicule all of us in the medical profession [*reirse de nosotros los médicos*]." Academic discussions of this type of ritualized charivari often invest it with a purely popular, communitarian character; as cultural form, however, it is plainly able to simultaneously express the threatened honor of professionals who identified their interests and public duty with nothing less than upholding the "moral laws of the country."[62]

This first part of Carbell's story demonstrates that by the beginning of the 1930s, after two decades of state hygiene campaigns, a significant number of Costa Ricans had embraced the authority of physicians and a scientific discourse on health. Nevertheless, in choosing to consult Carbell, a great many of these indicated that they wished to supplement that authority with the marvelous "specialties" he offered, from a touch of the shaman to homeopathy to psychotherapy and beyond. Popular beliefs about curing, far from being in a process of lineal transition toward an acceptance of official medicine and hygienism, were an outlandish stock constantly being reheated, added to, and stirred.

Magician versus Monopolists

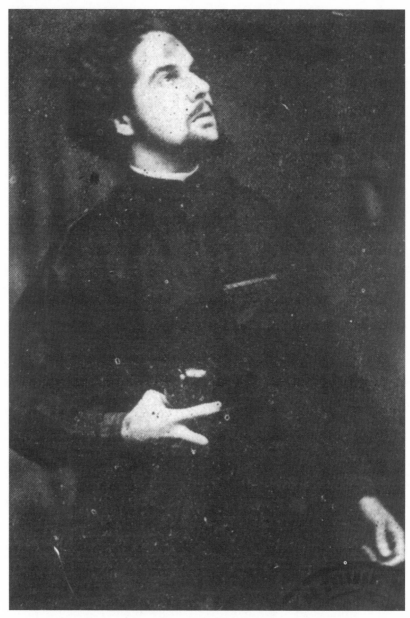

Fig. 6. Carlos Carballo Romero, alias Professor Carlos Carbell.
Biblioteca Nacional de Costa Rica.

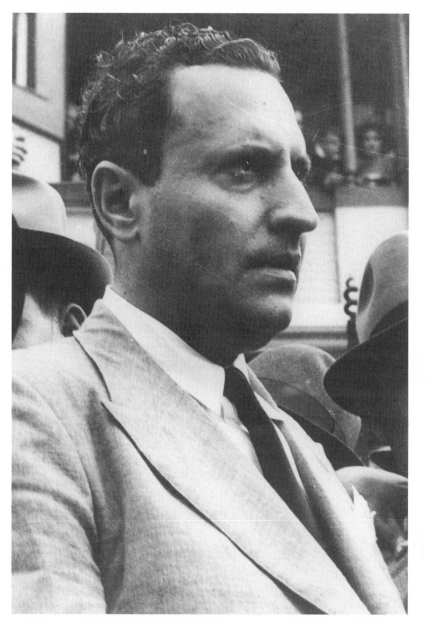

Fig. 7. Dr. Rafael Angel Calderón Guardia. Archivo Nacional de Costa Rica.

Typically, following his investigation by the public health police, Carbell received just a slap on the wrist, and only had to sign a document swearing that he would refrain from practicing medicine or face prosecution under the Law of Public Health and the Penal Code. He then proceeded to do exactly the opposite, making ever more audacious attacks on the medical profession, most conspicuously in a book he published in late April 1932 titled *The Other Side: A Brief Study of Today's and Tomorrow's Medicine in Relation to the Occult Forces of Nature*. With a serious national political crisis as backdrop, the Faculty of Medicine made fresh accusations that the good professor was still practicing cures. The authorities, this time including the intelligence services, began more extensive investigations of the practice of this marvelous mountebank. As they tightened the net, Carbell, by then a public figure of some notoriety, took the extraordinary step of refashioning himself as a charismatic political leader, announcing over the radio and in print an imminent apocalypse and the dawn of a socialist golden age in Costa Rica. This is the second part to Carbell's tale — one that brings us to the concluding chapter of this book, and helps clarify the rise of Costa Rica's populist physician-president Rafael Angel Calderón Guardia and the medical reform he undertook in Costa Rica in the early 1940s.

9

Medical Populism:

Dr. Calderón Guardia and the

Foundations of Social Security

A great act of medical creation lies at the heart of Costa Rica's modern polity. In 1941, a popular physician serving as president of the republic introduced medical and maternity coverage as the basis of a new regime of social security. This was the centerpiece of Dr. Rafael Angel Calderón Guardia's ambitious program of social reform, which included the founding of the University of Costa Rica (1940), inclusion of social guarantees in the Constitution (1942), and passage of a labor code (1943). Calderón Guardia was a leading member of Costa Rica's second great wave of national physicians — one of the large number of young men who left for studies abroad following the lean economic times and travel restrictions of the First World War years. He graduated from Louvain and incorporated as a physician in Costa Rica in 1927, the very year the country created a Ministry of Health. Calderón Guardia came of age professionally and politically, then, as physicians experienced their highest-ever levels of professional saturation, and as the public health system consolidated the centralizing and statist tendencies that had begun with the creation of the Rockefeller antihookworm department in 1914.

Despite this context, scholars have so far seen Calderón Guardia's implementation of social security as a historical enigma, having determined that there were no concrete forces propelling him to take the ambitious step. Explanations for social security fall into two basic camps. A Left perspective argues that Calderón Guardia was trying to co-opt an urban working class leaning toward a dynamic new Communist Party (even though neither party nor workers had articulated any demand for such a program).[1] A more social democratic school best represented by Mark Rosenberg, the only scholar to have studied the creation of Costa Rican Social Security in detail, determines that Calderón Guardia simply took it on himself to push through social reforms out of a Catholic philanthropism, and because the implementation of a program like Social Security in Costa Rica was inevitable given the historically reformist tenor of the country's politics and an accumulation of failed proposals to address the social question during the 1920s and 1930s.[2]

Both explanations are typical of the dominant schools of thought on the creation of social security programs in Latin America that began in the southern cone in the 1920s. Incipient industrialization and the rise of a pesky urban working class with a radical political face exacted social security programs from middle-class reformist parties and populist demagogues. As Patricio Marquez and Daniel Joly sum it up, with a slightly more leftward tint than might be found in the work of Carmelo Mesa-Lago or James Malloy, "The rise of the medical programs of social security institutions was . . . a response to the social demands of workers during the period of industrialization and served as an important mechanism of social control."[3] The context of industrialization and urban labor radicalism was obviously key to the timing of government programs to ameliorate workers' suffering and offer them some social guarantees. Nevertheless, as this chapter tries to show, the implementation of social security in Latin America can also be told as a medical history. And Costa Rica is an excellent country to tell this story in a compelling fashion, for industrialization was minimal and the working class was not formulating any such urgent demands, whereas the institutions of medicine and public health were ripe for such a program, and physicians and allied health workers had grown in number to the point where they could actually staff such a system.

But the introduction of medical social security also required a charismatic leader with great political will, for there were a number of serious obstacles to be overcome in order to implement the system. Chief among them was the resistance of the medical profession itself — a profession that had cohered again by the 1930s, encountered a strong new leadership cadre, expanded considerably in number, and worked out a new modus vivendi with the state public health apparatus centered on the development of rural health clinics. Over the medium term, physicians would learn that as long as it was implemented in a restricted fashion, social security could be a source of prosperity for the medical profession, increasing employment for its burgeoning lower ranks and expanding practitioners' share of the low-income market for medical attention without them having to abandon their existing private clientele. Yet at the outset, the grand ambitions Calderón Guardia harbored for the program's coverage made the profession balk.

It was Calderón Guardia's populist appeal that allowed him to overcome these obstacles—a populist appeal that was peculiarly medical in nature. Calderón Guardia's rhetoric resonated with the spiritual, antimaterialist, and antimonopolist strains of popular medical culture, even while it expressed a long-standing popular desire to benefit from official medical knowledge and practice. Calderón Guardia's stature as a revered physician had been won by his work among the popular sectors of the capital city—a long labor explicitly guided by Catholic devotion that recapitulated his father's professional journey. Populism eludes theory; it is also, by nature, more intangible than most political phenomena and so difficult to re-create historically.[4] The sources of Calderón Guardia's medical populism can perhaps best be grasped by returning to the saga of Professor Carbell. Though its last chapter was written some eight years prior to the rise of Calderón Guardia, Carbell's struggle against the medical monopolists reveals the limitations of professionalized biomedicine and the insistence at the heart of popular medical culture that, ultimately, healing can only be legitimately situated as a fundamental dimension of political community.

The Radiant Will of Professor Carbell

Carbell's confrontation with the medical profession took place at a critical juncture in Costa Rica, Latin America, and indeed throughout the West. Many of the countries of the continent, and all the other polities of Central America, fell to military dictatorships in the early 1930s. Though in the end Costa Rica was one of the few countries in the region to see its democratic institutions survive, it, too, had its brush with political unrest—an attempted coup d'état in February 1932 by a disgruntled political clique that had lost that year's presidential elections and wished to seize control before the new president, Ricardo Jiménez, was officially sworn in on the traditional May Day transfer of power. Although the coup failed, the mood in the capital was tense as the day of investiture approached. Under Costa Rican electoral law, Jiménez's victory would not be finally secured until the outgoing deputies in the Congress ratified the legitimacy of the electoral returns, and the pro-Jiménez deputies whose vote was required for ratification were put under armed guard.[5]

Given this explosive context, the Costa Rican secret police and the proregime politicians no doubt raised their eyebrows when Carbell's book, *The Other Side,* hit the stands at the end of April. Aside from its inflammatory assault on members of the Costa Rican elite, the book carried an endorsement from General Jorge Volio.[6] Volio was a charismatic political demagogue with an ardent following among elements of both the urban and rural popular classes. He was leader of a political party, the Reformists, which in the mid 1920s had been the first to introduce elements of a social democratic agenda into the electoral arena. He was also a theosophist and an anti-imperialist crusader (his military rank was granted by the Costa Rican Congress in 1912 after he had gone to fight with the Nicaraguan patriots against the U.S. occupying forces). While sitting as a deputy in the opposition camp of the Costa Rican Congress in 1932, he had been one of the leaders of the February putsch attempt. The failed rebels received amnesty from outgoing President Cleto González Víquez. As the first Costa Rican readers of Carbell's booklet, which could be bought for a modest one and a half colones, opened the cover to a prologue by General Volio assuring them that the pages contained "delicate honey collected from the esoteric gardens of humanity," Volio himself was poised to take his seat as deputy for San José in the tense May Day session of the legislature.[7]

The principal objective of Carbell's "rigorously scientific" work, the first installment of a larger project titled *The Radiant Will,* was to describe the psychic and "supranormal" manifestations of those occult forces that remain latent in human nature, "in particular the manifestations or exteriorizations of neuric [*sic*] fluid, or radiant will; that is, the sixth sense that Adam possessed and that he lost at the moment of abandoning Paradise." Carbell was on the verge of scientifically isolating nothing less than the qualities that had made humans magic and

Popular Medicine to Medical Populism

immortal before their alienation from God. These were the occult forces that could be applied "in the cure of illnesses that official science has declared itself impotent to treat."[8] Readers could find at the core of Carbell's book the powerful, erotic images of animal magnetism, virtually unchanged since the age of Franz Anton Mesmer himself: the body of the female sufferer ecstatically transfixed by the gazes, rubbings, blowings, and frenzied manipulations of the operator, whose magnetic fluids exerted a stimulus on the patient that resulted in the exteriorization of the radiant will, an ectoplasm, or opalescent aura generated by the "neuric" fluid in the spinal column and emanating from the eyes, nose, mouth, and fingers to unify the individual with the superior intelligence of the world. This was the incarnation of universal love, the sixth sense.[9]

The connecting thread of *The Other Side,* however, was political: an insistent claim that the book proved "to a certain group of professional mediocrities, obstacles to all progressive evolution in these parts, that OCCULTISM is not, as they affirm, a useless and harmful pastime but rather a positive science." Carbell was the oracle of the next phase in the dialectic evolution of the social sciences. Surgery, radiology, and bacteriology, though praiseworthy, were nothing but "the last glimmers of a dying bonfire." Their great failure lay in an exclusive reliance on an ultramaterialist understanding of humanity. It was the subconscious tendency in humans toward materialism that had resulted in the progressive erosion of the capacity to use the sixth sense. The next era would be one in which a scientifically understood and regulated ectoplasm would mediate between the worlds of matter and spirit.[10]

Inside Congress, to the surprise of many, the May Day transition of power went smoothly. The opposition deputies, most like Volio representing the interests of the *golpistas* (putschists), limited themselves to casting a protest vote. Significantly, the candidate they proposed for the presidency, a fellow deputy, was Dr. Ricardo Moreno Cañas, the young, Swiss-trained orthopedic surgeon who had garnered mass popularity as head of surgery at the Hospital San Juan de Diós. Although like most private practitioners Moreno Cañas set aside time each week to treat the poor free of charge, his popularity was probably more attributable to the way he deftly managed publicity surrounding a series of "miraculous" surgical interventions: the dramatic extraction of a bullet touching on a man's heart and the reconstruction of the leg of a poor young man suffering a monstrous deformity. Moreno Cañas had even produced a silent movie documenting the latter orthopedic case, complete with gruesome shots of the actual surgical procedure, that was played in the country's cinemas before the main features in the early 1930s.[11]

Ricardo Jiménez, the new president, took office without incident, but there was clearly some plotting going on behind the scenes, and Carbell was involved. On 12 May, Carbell made his play for political demagoguery with a one-and-a-half-hour conference broadcast on the capital's most popular radio station as part of its "gala" Thursday evening lineup, and advertised in advance in the papers. His talk was titled "Costa Rica and Its Prophecy."[12] With his firm, considered, and sure voice, Carbell dramatically announced that the end was nigh: "A monstrous wave of burning anxiety is sweeping across the world," he alleged. His rapid *tour du monde* indicted the Communist Soviets, decadent Chinese, and continued troubles between France and Germany, among other disturbing questions of the day. They were responsible for the "unbalance that precedes all liquidations of value systems." Astrological signs were also clear, in particular the effect that Mars was having on the earth. Eastern religions were invoked to support the prophecy. Everything pointed to the year 1935 as the moment of apocalyptic reckoning, the fulfillment of the "visions of Christ the mystic and of Daniel."

In that fateful year, a natural cataclysm would provoke the dawn of a new age. The Pacific Ocean would engulf virtually all of South America, except for the Andean cordillera. A similar fate would befall North America. The isthmus of Panama would also disappear under the tidal rise. Through some sort of dramatic tectonic shift, Cuba, Florida, and the Yucatán would unite with Central America to form a single continent without American rivals. "Over the course of four centuries, Central America shall be the center of world activities, especially in the arts, sciences, legislation, etc., representing in history the same role as Greece, Egypt, and Persia, because she shall be the cradle of a new civilization."[13]

Costa Rica was destined to be the ultimate seat "of the new civilization, of the new doctrine" (the new Messiah, according to Carbell, would come in the form of a doctrine). Over these four centuries, a spiritual communism, imposed by a "superior will," would eliminate from the face of the earth all that is inharmonious and useless, all that stands in its way, through a "five-year plan and persecution of all the churches." Carbell's talk was a call "to the chosen who must present themselves in the ranks of the select to wage the final battle." He was careful to ask for cooperation with the Jiménez government, "which today is beginning its labors, under the presidency of a wise and just man." Nevertheless, in the very act of doing so, he suggested that the government was anything but secure, noting "the intense, delicate, and very difficult task [it faces] in this hour of commotion." As *The Other Side* had come out two weeks earlier with an endorsement from Volio, among Jiménez's most conspicuous and dangerous opponents, listeners would have known how to read the professor's words.[14]

Carbell's message itself was quite ingeniously constructed: it played to and inverted some of the central motifs of a chauvinistic Costa Rican nationalism that had been drummed into the heads of citizens since their first years in primary school. In liquidating the United States from its northern homeland and also Panama (and by extension, Nicaragua as well), it met the desires of the anti-imperialist consensus of the era. Better yet, in drowning Mexico and the South American giants, Costa Rica was left with the run of the imperial terrain. The speech also touched on Spenglerian themes popular among, and made popular by, Latin American intellectuals during the 1920s. The decline of former imperial civilizations signaled the hour for Latin American civilizations to achieve their glory.[15]

The vision discarded Soviet communism, while preserving the idea of a spiritual communism that was implicit in the evolution of Costa Rican values and qualities. On the other hand, it eliminated institutionalized religion. At least in the mind of Carbell, this vision had the most possibility of capturing people's political imagination in that moment. It is worth reflecting seriously on at least this part of his judgment since the professor had proven himself a rather astute gauge of popular preferences in other camps. If he was right about this, then the political desires of the Costa Rican popular classes at that critical conjuncture were made up of what might be labeled patriotic socialism mixed with secular spiritualism.[16]

Carbell's "third wave" philosophy was part of a broad cultural current of the time, its spiritualist overtones and general vision of history in many ways close to the discourse of Haya de la Torre of the Alianza Popular Revolucionaria Americana (APRA) (who had only recently passed through Costa Rica, causing a minor political tumult). A few years earlier, in 1928, Haya de la Torre's mentor José Vasconcelos had likely won the Mexican presidential elections with a mystical message that promised redemption for a cosmic race (only to lose the presidency through fraud and be forced into exile, two months of which were taken up by a controversial stay in Costa Rica, in April and May of 1930). Vasconcelos inverted the materialist teleology of Auguste Comte's "law of the three stages" in favor of another tripartite philosophy of history that would culminate in an aesthetic and spiritual phase.[17]

Of most importance to the context in which Carbell spoke, only a few hundred kilometers to the north another theosophist, the General of Free Men Augusto César Sandino, had inspired a nation (and much of world opinion) against Yankee imperialism with a messianic guerrilla war of national redemption equally based on a vague spiritual communism. In his "Light and Truth Manifesto" of February 1931, Sandino had spoken of "the great will" that had filled the universe prior to creation. This was the preamble to a portrait of his struggle in apocalyptic terms. "The final judgment of the world must be understood as the destruction of injustice on earth, and the beginning of the reign of the spirit of light and truth, the spirit of love."[18]

The general flight toward a new mass politics of Left and Right throughout the West was inevitably borne along by just such desires for a glamorous spirituality — a radiant will — that would be generated through the charismatic leader's manipulation of the body politic. The Great Depression had to be read as proof of the spectacular failure of positivist materialism. How good it would be to capture a radiant will, one capable of soaring above those walls of history that trapped people in the grinding materiality of their little worlds and thus making them whole once more. Here, too, on the periphery, the intelligibility of Carbell's appeal must be seen as a world historical manifestation of the end of the age of positivism, in the manner in which Robert Darnton has understood the relationship between mesmerism and the Enlightenment, as one way in which the common man and woman lived these great ideological transformations.[19]

How delusional was the professor? Carbell had carried out a systematic and apparently successful attack on the "intellectual monopolists" of the medical profession, in the process explicitly flirting with a radical political tradition in alternative healing that encompassed a revolutionary strain in mesmerism and a plebeian spiritualist movement within late-nineteenth-century Owenite socialism.[20] The repression of alternative healers was a delicate affair and could spark popular tumult. As recently as 1930, riots had broken out in an outlying barrio of San José when the local district physician tried to bring charges against a respected local man who was performing miracle cures, illustrating that alternative healers with a mass following could be trouble for the elites.[21]

In Latin America, of course, much more than in most parts of the West, the leading physicians who came under attack by Carbell as monopolists were also among the most important members of the liberal oligarchy. His medical crusade could not help but be an explicitly political one. It is probably a testament to the political wisdom and maturity of San José's laboring classes that they did not respond to the professor's call to rise up against the cabal of doctor-politicians, just as they had stayed out of the coup attempt at the Bellavista barracks earlier in the year (surprising the leaders of the putsch, who had expected at least demonstrations of popular support). That is, no popular unrest is recorded in San José and its environs in the wake of the radio conference. Nevertheless, the Ministry of Public Security had begun investigating Carbell in April. The secret police can hardly have been amused by his radio performance and may have urged him to move along at this point.[22]

As the new regime consolidated itself, the professor was forced to pack his bags and leave the country via Puntarenas. Carbell arrived in the Pacific port "in the company of the most beautiful of little women, with an hourglass figure, as white as snow, and as graceful as a palm tree," according to the *Prensa Libre* correspondent sent along to cover the event. ("The duties she is fulfilling in the company of the doctor are unknown to us.")[23] The masses may not have rallied to his political message, but Carbell was more than ever now an object of truly national fascination. A large number of people sought him out at the Hotel Imperial, yet the professor refrained from offering any consultations, insisting that he was too tired. When Carbell paid a courtesy call to the offices of the local newspaper, "an infinite number of people from all social classes" squeezed in to greet him and listen to his chat with the staff.[24]

The comic opera closed on 30 June with one final incident on board the steamer that was to take him to El Salvador. He apparently informed his companion at the last moment that he was unable to take her along, which resulted in the summoning of a lawyer and threats of legal action that would keep him in the country. As the *Prensa Libre* correspondent reported, Carbell was saved through the intervention of "a kind woman traveler, as attractive and graceful as the first," who contracted a lawyer and guaranteed him representation should charges be brought. With that cleared up, Carbell finally left the shores of Costa Rica and, as readers devoured the salacious details of his colorful departure, was on the high seas, perhaps "enjoying a glass of fine wine in the company of his lovely savior."[25]

In *The Other Side,* sounding rather like a modern French philosopher, Carbell wrote that among "medicine's strange particularities" was its heartless, unregenerative materialism. "As far as it is concerned, the human body — man — is merely a compound of nerves, tubes, muscles, and bones that function subject to the rule of mechanical, chemical, physical, and biological forces. In this way, and on that concept, it constitutes its medico-therapeutic postulates. Does it know, per chance, what life is? What is its function? Its object?"[26] Carbell made himself popular by proposing to go beyond scientific medicine — by promising to subsume and surpass it by means of a "scientific," but fundamentally human and spiritual medicine. He was a learned wizard who promised restoration, body and soul, to a state of collective bliss, but only if the monopolists who were blocking the road to spiritual fulfillment were first pushed out of the way. The professor perhaps made his wager from too far on "the other side" for it to be accepted by those at the table. It was the medical profession itself that would throw up a series of leaders who proposed a social and spiritual transformation of the body politic from "this side," a melding of material and spiritual concerns, and the dawn of a new communitarian age.

The Luminous Guide of Dr. Calderón Guardia

To some degree, it was inevitable that a Costa Rican physician would achieve mass political appeal. Between 1920 and 1948, an extraordinary 39 percent of legislative deputies in Costa Rica were physicians.[27] Dr. Aniceto Montero — the first to speak publicly about the Bolshevik revolution in 1919, founder of the country's first socialist party, and leader of the anti-imperialist Civic League of the late 1920s — was the Costa Rican equivalent to the Argentine socialist physicians Octavio

Bunge, José Ingenieros, Alejandro Korn, and Juan Bautista Justo who shook up the politics of the southern cone nations in the 1910s and 1920s.[28] More significant in terms of the development of Costa Rican medical populism was Dr. Francisco Vargas Vargas. After returning from studying in France in 1935, Vargas developed a vocal following as head of the Confraternidad Guanacasteca, the political force of the country's underdeveloped and ethnically distinct northwestern pampa. This was a populist coalition whose nationalist, separatist threat was only just kept in check in the late 1930s.[29]

The key prefiguring of Calderón Guardia, however, was Ricardo Moreno Cañas. With Moreno Cañas's popular reputation and political star ever on the rise, by 1938 he was considered the leading candidate for the presidency in 1940, but was assassinated in his home by a disgruntled patient whose unhappiness with a surgical outcome triggered a killing spree that also claimed the life of another member of the elite.[30] Soon after he was murdered, Moreno Cañas became the object of a popular urban medical cult that is one of the more notorious of contemporary Latin America. Anthropologists have pointed to this cult, along with others like that of Dr. José Gregorio Hernández of Venezuela, as examples of modern alternative healing traditions that have reclaimed religious faith and the supernatural — as symbols of the demedicalizing impulse of the Latin American popular classes. Certainly, the religious quality of the Moreno Cañas cult is evident enough, as is its mystical nature (after his death, Moreno Cañas quickly became among the favorite spirits contacted by Costa Rican mediums).[31] Yet both Hernández and Moreno Cañas were exemplary proponents of the "new medicine" represented by bacteriology and surgery, and leading members of their national professional bodies. The obvious counterthesis might rather be considered: that Hernández and Moreno Cañas are figures of the medicalization of healing cults; that their transformation into popular saints involved the apotheosis of biomedicine, the hospital system, and the very power of physicians.[32]

Although he was physically eliminated from the political scene in 1938, the martyrdom of Moreno Cañas played into the overwhelming victory in the 1940 presidential elections of another popular San José physician, Calderón Guardia. The son of an influential patrician doctor who had been one of the first presidents of the Faculty of Medicine, Calderón Guardia studied medicine at the progressive Belgian Catholic

University of Louvain in the 1920s. Biomedical discourse might have become ever more positivist and materialist, but Calderón Guardia offers excellent proof that leading doctors did not necessarily lose their vitalist beliefs and spiritual mission. He would write that "as the son of a physician, I felt at an early stage in my life the pain and misery that surrounds us. My father knew how to inspire in me the apostolic sense of his profession."[33]

While in Belgium, Calderón Guardia also attended the seminary in Malines, where his stay coincided with the new social doctrine of the church initiated in the *Rerum Novarum* of 1893 (later reinforced in the *Quadragesimo Anno* of 1931) and the heyday of the reformist theology of Cardinal D. J. Desiré Joseph Mercier.[34] Part of Mercier's vast neo-Thomist project of intellectual renovation for a modern church was the founding of a Catholic psychology and sociology, a "synthesis of the growing results of the sciences of observation," but superior to "positivist empiricism and classical spiritualism in its ability to explain the matrix of facts established experimentally and testified to by consciousness."[35] Profoundly influenced by the papal critique of the excesses of liberalism and materialism, and by Mercier's search for a social and spiritual synthesis, Calderón Guardia returned to establish a private practice in San José at the outset of the depression, and was moved by the poverty of the sufferers he attended.[36]

The progressive Catholic influences remained his guiding light. In his 1940 inaugural address, Calderón Guardia boldly asserted that his new administration "supports, in political terms, the doctrines of social Christianism, as they are explained in the admirable encyclicals of León XIII and Pius XI, and as they are blended in Cardinal Mercier's 'Sketch of a Social Synthesis.' " Calderón Guardia made a great deal of the need for modern people to find the "principle, impulse, and will of justice lacking in a materialist world," and declared that the social code of Malines was his "sure and luminous guide" in formulating the social reform — Calderón Guardia's radiant will.[37] Like Carbell, Calderón Guardia the devout physician also proposed that national alienation would be overcome, and a transcendant experience encountered, at the point where politics met the human physiological and spiritual condition.

It is worth stressing that the medical populist was not a phenomenon confined to Costa Rica, and its Latin American pantheon includes some rather well-known figures. Salvador Allende Gossens had begun identifying with the poor and studying marxism in the late 1920s while living in the slums of Santiago with other medical students from the provinces. In 1933, he became one of the youngest founders of the Partido Socialista.[38] Allende Gossens built his reputation as a medical reformer, editing the journal *Medicina Social* and publishing a book while minister of health (1939–1942) titled *La realidad médico-social chilena* (1940), an examination of health conditions among the working classes.[39] Panama's most important populist leader during the 1930s and 1940s was the Harvard-educated physician Arnulfo Arias, one of a formidable pair of brothers who led the "generation of '31" and, as a cabinet minister and director of the country's Sanitation Bureau, effected the reform of Panamanian public health.[40] In Cuba, Ramón Grau San Martín owed his ascent in the anti-Machado rebellion of 1933 to his principled career as a professor in the medical faculty of the university, where he forged close links with the student federation, and his political participation in the Cuban Medical Federation, which was an active player in the popular mobilizations against the regime.[41] Juscelino Kubitschek's medical career in Belo Horizonte underlay his rise in politics and influenced his vision of social transformation.[42] His ascent was prefigured by Pedro Ernesto, one of the brightest stars in the Brazilian populist constellation. The mayor of Rio was not only a well-known physician; his political campaigning of the 1930s was built on a platform of medical and public health reform.[43]

It might be said that the professional occupation of these men was incidental, that they could easily have been populists who happened to be lawyers like Jorge Eliécer Gaitán or (more commonly) military officers. Yet a medical strain saturated the new mass politics of Latin America — it was a central part of capturing the political imagination of the popular sectors, and in many countries it also sustained a real expansion of health services. One need only consider the most famous case of all. The Peróns led their own dramatic manipulation of the body politic with *justicialismo*, a quasi-spiritual social philosophy that sought to create an organized community living in harmony through the development of a "third position" beyond capitalism and communism. The dream was to be realized by the union of the masculine Perón — "the conductor" (think mesmerism) — with the feminine Evita — Argentina's first minister of health — the medium in Perón's contact with the *descamisados* (destitute) and semisecular patron saint of *justicialista* beneficence.

Five days after the death of Eva Perón, a young medical student returned to Buenos Aires to complete his degree after a long journey of discovery. He did so successfully, becoming Dr. Ernesto Guevara de la Serna in April 1953, and then embarking on a real tour of revolutionary social and spiritual transformation that reached one glorious culmination five and a half years later in the Havana streets still traversed by Carbell.[44] Had they met, the by then middle-aged professor of all forms of irregular medicine and the dashing young guerrilla physician might well have sat down together to discuss the possible connections between the radiant will and the new man.

Completing the Centralized Model of Public Health

By the late 1920s, the Ministry of Public Health and Social Protection had achieved primary jurisdiction over all matters of public health and medical regulation but one. From the moment he became a full member of the cabinet, Solón Núñez's efforts were absorbed by two battles: achieving effective power to police the system and gaining control over the Juntas of Charity, especially that of San José. Between 1922 and 1936, Núñez had marginal luck on the fiscal front, succeeding in raising the share of state expenditures on public health from 2 to 3.5 percent of the budget.[45] He was unable to crack the bastion of oligarchic philanthropy and banking power that was the Junta of Charity of San José. From his very first address as minister in 1927, he railed eloquently though impatiently against the "absurd" fact that the central institutions of medicine and public health were being run as though they were charity balls: "It is illogical that hospitals, sanatoriums, and asylums had been under the immediate control of the secretary of foreign relations [and beneficence]. . . . [I]n the same way that the public schools are not managed by committees of ladies, neither should any of these institutions be led by organisms independent of the state."[46]

In 1936, the new government of León Cortés finally ended Núñez's extraordinary fifteen-year tenure as the country's chief public health official (twenty years if his subdirection of the antihookworm department is included), appointing Antonio Peña Chavarría to the position. Peña Chavarría was a strong choice, named just as he was reaching the apogee of power within the medical profession. Returning from medical studies in Colombia in 1924, he had quickly emerged as the country's most important medical scientist after Clodomiro Picado, maintaining a constant stream of publications aimed at establishing a treatable national nosology. He was named head of medicine in 1935 at the Hospital San Juan de Diós and president of the Faculty of Medicine in 1936, followed in short order by an appointment to the ministry.[47]

Núñez had never cultivated a power base from within the community of physicians. Although he had achieved an entente cordiale, he was a formidable outsider, a consummate bureaucrat, but ultimately not "one of the club." Peña Chavarría was the elect of the Junta of Charity and the Faculty of Medicine, and was able to bring finally this behemoth of beneficence at least formally within the ambit of the institutions of state medicine. A good deal of autonomy, however, was maintained due to the creation of a mediating National Council of Health, Public Beneficence, and Social Protection. Gone were the archbishop and ladies committee, but the council of ten was still to be made up of the elites of civil society (including two physicians from the faculty) rather than technocrats under the direction of the ministry. The first ministry budget to include operating revenues from the Juntas of Health, that of 1936, confirmed Núñez's estimates of the enormous funds that had once been controlled by the Juntas of Charity: the government appropriation totaled only 45 percent of the whole, while the funds coming from the juntas accounted for 55 percent.[48]

Peña Chavarría had some notable successes. He gained a substantial increase in the government appropriation for public health right off the bat and then pushed the portion of the state budget devoted to public health over the 6 percent mark by 1940.[49] His first political triumph, and part of a great centralization that occurred in public health during the Cortés years, was to bring the modern hospital "into the common machinery of national health" by bringing the juntas under the jurisdiction of the ministry—a move that it was hoped would allow the coordination of services and programs.[50] The second achievement in this centralizing thrust was getting the major municipalities to agree to allow their public health offices to be absorbed into the ministry, which took over control of budgets, personnel, facilities, and policy.[51]

The building of an impressive new headquarters for the ministry symbolically hammered home the centralizing process, while also making its logistics easier. In this Peña Chavarría made good use of the new

Cortés government's attempt to alleviate unemployment and reduce social tension through massive public works (a policy that led to its nickname, "the government of cement and iron"). The vast new central edifice (still in use today) was designed to house the offices of the Ministry of Public Health and Social Protection along with its dependencies like the School Health Department, offices of the Rockefeller Foundation, department of epidemiology and sanitary engineering, bacteriology lab, national office of the public health police, Red Cross, Child Welfare Board and all its dependencies, dispensaries for tuberculosis and venereal disease control, municipal hygiene offices, and Infant Meal and Drop of Milk centers. It was built right beside the bastion of San José's Junta of Social Protection, the Hospital San Juan de Diós.[52]

In the late 1930s, Costa Rica enjoyed a marked decline in infant mortality. An erratic tendency in this direction had been visible since the early teens of the century, and it is likely that the mass rural hygiene education campaigns of the local and Rockefeller antihookworm teams had immediate effects on improving infant mortality. Certainly, dramatic increases in other basic health indicators like mortality rates and life expectancy at birth are visible starting in the early 1920s. The apparent improvement in public health that coincided with the first phase of mass hygiene campaigns is occluded by the fact that except for the years 1923 through 1928, virtually the entire stretch from 1910 to 1935 was marked by periods of severe economic duress, political turmoil, and epidemic disaster, all of which took a toll on mortality: the economic recession of World War I, Tinoco mass conscription campaign of 1916–1917, influenza pandemic of 1919, and worst years of the slump, 1929–1932, are reflected in the country's basic health indicators.[53]

In tandem with the expansion of the public health apparatus, infant mortality declined from an average of 232 to an average of 132 per thousand live births between 1925 and 1940. A sizable portion of the ministry's increased resources was invested in expanding the rural health units. Begun in 1928 in Turrialba, and based on the County Health Units promoted by the Rockefellers in the rural United States, by 1936 this model was superseding the old institution of the town doctor. Whether or not the criticisms were valid, health bureaucrats had never had much good to say about the district physicians; once they were marginalized in the institutional web of antihookworm work, they went into a marked decline, salaries stagnated, and the posts ceased to attract promising young men of science (reinforcing the dynamic, at the same time, between 1914 and 1925, spaces for physicians in San José began to open up again). The plan to replace the town doctors with more comprehensive nuclei of public health action came to fruition rapidly under Peña Chavarría. Again, good use was made of the expansion of state public works spending to build the rural posts and subsidize basic sanitary engineering projects. In 1936, there were experimental Health Units in Turrialba, Orotina, Grecia, and Santa Cruz; a year later there were six more, and the nineteen remaining town doctor posts were upgraded to include a nurse-midwife.[54]

The Health Units were integrated medical and public health facilities with a small laboratory and staff covering the range of health functions. A full-time physician was in command, and his staff included a part-time dentist, nurse, midwife, microscopist, sanitary inspector, secretary, and squad of workers.[55] Aside from the purely curative medical treatment meted out by the doctors (22,699 *enfermos pobres* (destitute sufferers), 8,000 malaria sufferers, and 27,000 cases of hookworm and other intestinal parasites were treated in 1937) and ongoing preventive work (4,719 immunizations for diphtheria, smallpox, and typhoid, along with over 8,000 home visits by hygiene inspectors), the Health Units brought into the rural cantonal centers the model developed by the School Health Department in the major towns.[56] A corps of fifty nurse-midwives was employed by the ministry for work with the Health Units and district physicians — the Health Units having one dedicated purely to obstetrics and another to home visiting. Between August 1936 and March 1937 alone, these health- and maternity-oriented social workers made 16,573 home visits.[57]

In the coffee-growing area of La Unión, the ministry even experimented with three day care centers during the harvest period in an effort to improve the health of the children of the large female contingent of agricultural laborers. The people of the area enjoyed a startling decline in infant mortality rates: from 1932 to 1936, the rate was 152.2 per thousand live births; from 1937 through 1942 it dropped to 99.4.[58] These are perhaps the most eloquent data to support the ministry's triumphal declaration that the decline was a direct result of the expansion of public health infrastructure and, in particular, the widening of the rural Health Units' radius of action after 1936.[59]

The days when the vast majority of Costa Ricans went an entire lifetime without being attended by a physician were quickly coming to a close, even if the attention was the very last they received. The trend toward doctors performing medical last rites rose dramatically as the public health infrastructure matured: in 1927, 40 percent of deaths were "attended by a physician" (that is, the death certificate was authorized by a licensed practitioner), rising slowly to 47 percent in 1936 and then jumping abruptly to 55 percent in 1937.[60] That was largely because, as the minister of health explained in his annual report, the "official medical posts, and especially the Health Units, have extended and intensified their free medical services, making them available in particular to the rural population."[61] These "free medical services" and others like them familiarized the population with the care of certified health workers, but also led them to expect the state to foot the bill for such care. As a result, they were at the heart of an antagonistic but symbiotic relationship between the increasingly powerful state public health apparatus and the country's body of physicians — one that would soon come to a head over the limits of state-subsidized medicine.

Professional Growth

The number of physicians incorporating into the Costa Rican Faculty of Medicine grew rapidly in the 1930s and 1940s, though this hardly put the country among the Western leaders of physicians per capita. The growth took place despite the fact that the country remained without a medical school of its own until the 1960s. The economic and international political uncertainties of the era promoted an eclectic shift in preferred countries of study among young people. Two trends were notable in the training of Costa Rican physicians. The first was the continued appeal of continental Europe and diminishing attraction of the United States (the destination of a mere 6 to 8 percent of Costa Ricans during these two decades). Despite the best efforts of the Rockefeller Foundation to combat what it saw as the pernicious influence of the French clinical model of medical instruction, U.S. hegemony over styles of medical instruction in Latin America was a phenomenon of the 1950s and after.[62]

The other was the meteoric rise of Mexico as a destination for medical studies after 1939. From the place of study of 9 percent of those returning to practice between 1935 and 1939, Mexican medical academies accounted for the training of 16 percent during the war years, and then trained 54 percent of Costa Rica's physicians during the first five years of the postwar period.[63] The dramatic shift to Mexico was again brought about by the closing of European destinations during the war as well as restrictions on maritime travel that made it difficult to study in the United States. Mexico was inexpensive, government scholarships were made available for study there, and students could travel overland — an arduous journey, to be sure, but feasible. As for the training, it was a "typical French system," according to Manuel Aguilar Bonilla, who sweated on a bus for almost a week in order to arrive in Mexico City in time for his first year of studies in 1937. The quality of instruction was high, but the complex of teaching institutions was not technically sophisticated or up-to-date.[64] One of the main effects of this Mexican pole of medical instruction was to expose Costa Rican students to the revolutionary fervor of Mexican state medicine, which demanded a rural tour of duty from graduates prior to their full incorporation into the profession. This experience dovetailed with the expansion of Costa Rican state medicine during the same period.

Although physicians were now present in a greater number of locales throughout the country, almost all of those who practiced outside the six major towns still relied on state postings as town doctors or heads of Health Units. The most extensive web of physicians was in Alajuela province. In 1935, less than half of the seventeen physicians practicing in the province lived in the city of Alajuela, with ten distributed in seven other secondary towns. Surprisingly, Guanacaste also had a fair distribution, with eleven doctors scattered in seven centers, even though this was the area with the poorest infrastructure and strongest traditional medicine. The city of Cartago was home to thirteen of the nineteen physicians practicing in the province in 1935, and all eight of the doctors of Heredia lived in the city center (Heredia was the closest of the three major centers to San José, and its medical community was the smallest of the four main urban centers as a result of this market overlap).

The towns of Puntarenas (seven of nine) and Limón (six of seven) likewise were host to almost all the physicians in their area. These latter two were the areas that enjoyed the greatest growth in resident physicians between 1935 and 1950, with Puntarenas almost tripling its number of practitioners to twenty-one. The expansion reflects the major

Medical Populism

growth of the populace due to in-migration as the United Fruit Company shifted its operations to the Pacific coast; Limón, the loser in this boom-bust cycle, nevertheless almost doubled its number of physicians to twelve during the same period.[65]

The most basic professional fact was that through the 1930s and 1940s, with only 10 percent of the national populace, San José was home to at least half of the country's physicians, and the tendency was toward an increasingly encephalitic concentration in the capital city. In 1935, 67 of Costa Rica's 140 physicians (48 percent) lived in the capital city, making the physician to resident ratio about 1 to 1,000; by 1950, 150 of 265 practitioners (57 percent) resided in San José, each one corresponding to 700 residents.[66] With economic conditions oscillating between desperate and weak throughout these decades, these greater numbers of physicians had to maximize their urban working- and middle-class clientele in order to prosper. These were precisely the social groups targeted by Calderón Guardia for medical coverage in his first social security proposal, which was designed to consolidate a constituency among this small but politically crucial stratum of the populace.[67]

Social Security

Given the populist vector in Costa Rican healing culture, institutional development and extension of state medicine, and profile of the growing medical community, the scholarly assumption that Calderón Guardia's social reforms, and particularly social security, were mandated ex nihilo begins to seem strange indeed. Though more research would be required to establish the exact figure, it is clear that the rapid expansion of rural health clinics during the 1930s had already brought a range of state-subsidized medical services, including obstetric care, to a large proportion of the semirural population. Analogous clinics existed in the cities, again including lying-in hospitals and obstetric services for birthing women of the laboring classes. To some degree, Calderón Guardia's social security program simply formalized and normalized a regime that was already in place, and one that many laboring Costa Ricans had come to expect.

In support of his argument that Calderón Guardia's social reform initiatives of 1940–1941 were purely voluntarist and did not respond to the evolution of institutional or social forces, Mark Rosenberg shows that they came about after Calderón Guardia consulted with a "close inner circle" made up of his father, Dr. Rafael Calderón Muñoz; his minister of health, Dr. Mario Luján; Guillermo Padilla Castro, a lawyer who was director of the National Child Welfare Board (PANI); and Dr. Solón Núñez, who had been minister of health up until 1936 and was invited back to resume the reins in 1943.[68] Considering the cast of characters, it seems reasonable to propose that some of the deepest roots of the Costa Rican welfare state are to be found in the country's nexus of medical and public health institutions.

Aside from the preponderance of physicians in this inner circle, all five were exemplary representatives of the most important private, state, and political medical currents in the country. Calderón Guardia embodied a new breed of populist practitioner. His father, Calderón Muñoz, had served as president of the Faculty of Medicine as well as chief of medicine and superintendent of the Hospital San Juan de Diós, and his political career had included stints as a deputy, senator (under the Tinoco reign), and first designate to the presidency.[69] Núñez, of course, had been the prime Costa Rican mover in the rise of a strong Ministry of Public Health almost since its earliest incarnation as the Rockefeller-sponsored Department of Ancylostomiasis.

Luján was a young firebrand pediatrician who had led urban hygiene and housing reform from the seats of the municipality and Parliament since graduating in medicine in France in 1928, and had been one of the first heads of the children's medicine section of the hospital prior to becoming Calderón Guardia's minister of health. And though Padilla Castro, the lawyer, may initially seem the odd man out in this mix, the PANI's origins are to be found in the School Health Department that had so broadened the mandate of the Department of Ancylostomiasis, and in the obsession of the turn-of-the-century medical community and state hygiene reformers with maternal and child protection. Indeed, it was no accident that Luis Felipe González Flores, who as minister of education had initiated the School Health Department in 1914, would resurface as the country's foremost expert on "paedofilaxis," and the great promoter and first president of the PANI from the late 1920s through the 1930s.[70]

But Calderón Guardia did introduce social security without consulting the Faculty of Medicine, and this would cause enormous problems with the implementation of the system. Soon after Calderón Guardia was sworn in, Padilla Castro had been quietly dispatched to Chile to study that country's pioneering social security program and develop blueprints for Costa Rica. He returned with an enthusiastic scheme to begin social security with medical coverage, confident in the public medical infrastructure of the country (planning for a social security hospital in the capital quickly got underway, and it was inaugurated in 1943). He also hoped to rapidly extend coverage to most urban workers in Costa Rica, including white-collar employees in most cities — precisely the popular base of most private physicians' practices.[71]

It is likely that the extraordinary amount of physicians in Congress, numbering close to 40 percent of the deputies, was responsible for reducing the percentage of middle-salaried workers who would be eligible for the plan when the legislation was modified by a parliamentary commission. Nevertheless, within two years of the institution's creation, and following an alliance between the regime and Communist Party along with an improvement in Calderón Guardia's parliamentary fortunes after the midterm election of deputies, the government dramatically increased the number of workers eligible for medical coverage under social security. By 1943, 20 percent of economically active Costa Ricans enjoyed medical coverage under this centralized state insurance program.[72]

The Faculty of Medicine responded by forming the National Medical Union and threatening a physicians' strike. Peña Chavarría emerged as one of the principal foes of the social security plan as well as the regime of Calderón Guardia itself. Calderón Guardia left the presidency in 1944, but remained a powerful influence over the successor government that, with Padilla Castro still in the direction of the Social Security Institute, moved ahead with plans to universalize the system. In 1946, the National Medical Union struck, and compromise was only reached after a bitter labor dispute between the state and physicians. The conflict further polarized the country during the period of marked instability that preceded the Civil War of 1948, one whose immediate cause was Calderón Guardia's hugely controversial attempt to win reelection on a progressive ticket.[73]

Calderón Guardia's populist style and his social reform were at the center of Costa Rica's great democratic breach in 1948. His attempt to have himself reelected became complicated by ideological disputes, fears that he was a potential dictator and a standoff over accusations of electoral fraud. The opposition leader who emerged victorious from the Civil War, however, was not part of the political old guard. José "Pepe" Figueres proved himself the greatest populist in Costa Rican history. As one of the prime movers of the country's hegemonic Party of National Liberation, Figueres would ensure that the welfare state begun by his despised predecessor expanded dramatically between 1950 and 1980, and that medical coverage of the populace under social security approached universality. It is worth noting that he, too, was the son of a physician, Mariano Figueres, who had immigrated from Spain in 1906 and worked as a town doctor on the periphery of the Central Valley, participating actively in the initial antihookworm campaign before opening a successful clinic in San José in 1917. In a further curious echo of the strains of mesmerist medical populism, the specialty of the Figueres clinic was electrotherapy.[74]

Conclusion

This book has argued that the history of healers in modern Costa Rica — and by extension, modern Latin America — is best comprehended by dispensing with the idea of a fundamental opposition between authentic forms of folk medicine or ethno-medicine, on the one hand, and a colonizing and suspect biomedicine, on the other. I have stressed instead the complex interchange among a broad range of practitioners, and the role of the state in mediating this exchange. Costa Rica's was a heterodox healing culture — one in which different types of practitioners borrowed liberally from one another to refashion medical identities and practices. Over time, and particularly by the beginning of the twentieth century, the heterodoxy of Costa Rican medicine was reined in under the hegemony of professional medical practitioners and agents of state medicine who ostensibly promoted a rigorous biomedical agenda. Yet they did not homogenize medical practice, nor did they implement an effective monopoly for schooled and titled practitioners. It might be said that the new official medical apparatus succeeded in sublimating rather than suppressing key strata of popular medical practice. The traditional partera was transformed into the obstetric midwife, the barrio herbalist was transformed into the barrio pharmacist, the foreign empiric was transformed into the town doctor on the agricultural frontier, while the village curandero was interpellated into official medicine through the preparation of death certificates for the modern secular state or reincarnated in the technical cadre of the new public health apparatus. Meanwhile, a still-thriving variety of unorthodox and alternative healers continued to operate, as physicians so often complained, "*a vista y paciencia de las autoridades*" (in full view and with the sympathy of the authorities).

A fairly standard Western biomedical apparatus achieved strategic command of the healing universe in Costa Rica by the 1940s. Nevertheless, this was not won through state, professional, or international efforts to suppress popular medicine. It is true that healing tended toward a hegemony of conventional medical styles and practices. This was in part due to the general dynamic of Western modernity as it came home to roost in Costa Rica as well as to the steady expansion of an influential community of physicians and public health experts. It was also due, however, to the tendency of popular healers of all stripes to incorporate central elements of conventional medicine, including clinical procedures, into their own practices. Even before the arrival of titled medical practitioners, popular healers engaged learned medical culture through the consultation of books and manuals. Secular approaches to healing gained greater space in popular medicine over the course of the nineteenth century, and many popular healers — "irregular" mostly by virtue of not having an official title — introduced conventional medical beliefs, styles, and practices into common medical culture. They were encouraged to do so by the persistent attempts of the Costa Rican public power to train or reward empirics who would execute a basic range of conventional medical and public health procedures.

This study has identified three notable phases in the creation of a community of physicians in Costa Rica, each one corresponding to a different type of medical association and public health administration. Between 1820 and 1860, foreigners made up a large majority of the country's original community of certified medical practitioners. They also shaped the first government effort to institutionalize state power over medical practice and the public health, thereby ensuring that the postcolonial model of the Protomedicato was adopted. This was a halfway point on the road to modern medical monopoly and state jurisdiction over public health, but it recognized the role of irregular healers outside the major towns and legitimized medical pluralism.

During the last third of the nineteenth century, a wave of native patrician lads returning from medical studies in the United States and Europe formed a grassroots movement that modernized professional association, identity, and practice. This book has identified an interesting paradox in the relationship between the medical profession and state — one that bears further exploration. The elite among these physicians were significant members of the political class that consolidated the liberal state. The application of bacteriology in public health made "scientific medicine" the apparent incarnation of the truths of positivist ideology and magnified the physicians' warnings that barbaric healing customs endangered the body politic. Yet in the cities, where physicians cried foul most often due to a question of market competition complementing their ideological concerns, government officials might fail to enforce the laws against the unlicensed practice of medicine out of sympathy for individual healers — or for alternative medicine more generally. In the cities, towns, and country, political bosses and police officials might resist enforcement from a practical sense that it was futile or a political intuition that such crackdowns would provoke extreme popular reactions. Not only were earnestly "civilizing" liberal regimes reluctant to suppress unconventional practitioners but the exigencies of state formation continued to demand their recruitment into the tenuous web of public power, and the old system of officially licensed empirics was not so easily suppressed.

So the modernizing state played a double game in regulating the domain of healing — a game that simultaneously augmented and attenuated the political and ideological power of the medical profession. Physicians were assigned (and being of the oligarchy, the medical elite assigned themselves) a privileged place at the apex of public power; they were given missions of great national importance, and their professional association was granted a portion of state jurisdiction over health and healing. Despite this, the formal monopoly that they enjoyed was never effectively enforced by the policing wing of that public power. From the earliest stages of Costa Rican state formation, official efforts were made to promote empiricism in medicine and surgery. As a result, the state never really endorsed the legitimacy of the medical profession's right to monopoly, and an ethos of tolerance toward uncertified medical practitioners was widespread among the authorities throughout my period of study. Such an ethos had its own pragmatic logic while also reflecting common sentiments.

Latin American medical elites of the late nineteenth century have been portrayed as agents of alien and colonizing discourses and practices. This book has presented the obverse side of the coin, emphasizing that in Costa Rica, the creation of a medical community with scientific and professional ambitions is best understood as a nationalist and, in some sense, decolonizing movement whereby a largely foreign body of licensed practitioners was replaced and a regulatory system that referred back to Spanish colonialism was substituted for a modern model. This allowed even a distant periphery like Costa Rica to generate a nucleus of medical scientists with a national research agenda that might even precede the giants of imperial public health in the discovery and design of a treatment strategy, and to transform subsequent imperial public health programs according to local priorities. The model of colonizing biomedicine presumes the lineal transmission of knowledge and practice from a Euro-American center to a Latin American periphery, and such a model cannot be sustained in the face of facts coming from many different countries in the region.

A third, and larger, wave of physicians led by some notable members of the country's political class renewed the domains of medicine and public health during the interwar period. This group laid the foundations for Costa Rica's contemporary medical system, one based on overlapping jurisdictions for private medicine, state public health, and the important new addition of social security. The dominant school of thought on the origin of social security in Latin America is that beginning in the southern cone in the 1920s, incipient industrialization and the rise of an urban working class with a radical political perspective exacted such benefits from middle-class reformist and populist demagogues. Yet this book has tried to show — and the case of nonindustrialized Costa Rica strongly suggests — that the history of social security needs also to be told as a medical story. Moreover, this was not only a positivist tale of ministries, professional bodies, and other institutions. A fundamentally political dimension of popular medical culture was involved in the advent of Costa Rican social security, encompassing the antimonopolistic and heterodox ethic of popular medical practitioners along with the social and indeed spiritual vision of a generation of physicians who one might otherwise be tempted to lump under the rubric of biomedical ideologues.

I have tried, with limited evidence, to explore the relationship between gender and medical practice. What emerges here challenges both the stereotypical image of women healers as practitioners of an herb- and a faith-based medicine that was radically distinct from conventional medicine, and the idea that they were subject to systematic persecution by the liberal state. It is true that, in the eyes of professionals and the state, women occupied the lowest level of the medical hierarchy in the nineteenth century, and were rarely included in the network of curanderos and empirics mobilized informally by the state for pragmatic reasons. But they could command the respect of the populace as well as sympathy of the authorities, and their expertise might be recognized in legal medicine. Although the tracks of unlicensed women healers rather disappear from the Costa Rican records in the twentieth century, it is suggestive that the realm of popular medical practice represented so powerfully by Professor Carbell—one that challenged the monopoly of the self-styled patriarchs of professional medicine and sought to exceed the limited, material claims of orthodox biomedicine—was cast in fundamentally feminine terms by friends and foes alike.

Midwives were a special case of the woman healer. Scorned for their superstition and ignorance, and cited as prime examples of the costs of such backwardness to the populace and nation, they were nevertheless widely tolerated by both the state and medical profession. Through a variety of formal and informal means, many a traditional Latin American partera modernized her approach to childbirth over the course of the nineteenth and twentieth centuries. In Costa Rica, the medical profession did not move to suppress women's dominion over labor; rather, physicians along with governments at the national and local levels sought to make it more effective and prestigious by transforming midwifery into a women's professional specialty that was at once patriotic and biomedical. The training of a cadre of midwives during the first twenty years of the twentieth century generated Costa Rica's first group of female scientists and certified medical practitioners. If it was a restricted domain of medicine that was entrusted to them—and conditional on the ultimate sanction of a patriarchal profession—it was also one considered to be of great national import and one in which they practiced with considerable autonomy. To simply dismiss obstetric midwives as agents of an alien and dehumanizing biomedicine is to miss the continuity—or perhaps rather the transposition—from popular medical to biomedical culture.

This book has also tried to reframe an understanding of the nature of the biomedicine that was promoted by the new apparatus of professional medicine and public health, and to move away from the idea that

Conclusion

it was the antithesis of the qualities associated with popular medicine. The hegemony of the biomedical model could only be negotiated by infusing its discourses and practices with analogous qualities. To deliver a child for the good of the republican nation is not the same thing as delivering it for the good of the lord and barrio, but neither is it necessarily incompatible, and both are acts of healing whose significance is located in terms of political community.

The same might be said for submitting oneself to treatment for hookworm disease, a ritual that as much as it might be portrayed as part of a systematic, transnational campaign to reproduce biomedical discourse and institutions throughout the globe, was enacted at the local level as a community ritual with marked ethnic, moral, and civic meanings. As for the religious or spiritual aspects of popular medicine, the strong Catholic strain in official medicine did not necessarily die out as the twentieth century progressed, as this study underlines: the devout and progressive Catholic Calderón Guardia justified the introduction of medical benefits under social security as the realization of a synthesis of the spiritual and material advocated by his great theological mentor, Cardinal Mercier.

To what extent is the history of Costa Rican medical practice relevant to understanding the Latin American experience? On the one hand, the emergence of a hegemonic social democratic order in the tiny Central American republic was a relatively rare outcome, and it might be proposed that the development of a biomedical hegemony with crucial popular influences is reflective of the larger picture and so equally anomalous. In some minor areas Costa Rica was relatively unique — in not having a medical school until the 1960s, for example. Perhaps of most significance, the Costa Rican liberal state was unusually early and ambitious in developing a rural health program, and this may ultimately be explicable only in terms of the precocious development of a hegemonic nationalism that denied ethnic difference, and mechanisms of political negotiation between the central state and municipal governments on the agricultural frontier.

Still, a vital medical pluralism operating rather openly within a framework of biomedical hegemony is characteristic of almost all Latin American countries. Like Costa Rica many countries began independence with few or no certified practitioners, and many countries preserved the colonial model of public health oversight well into the nineteenth century. In terms of the development of a complex of national medical institutions and a stratified community of professionals, Costa Rica's patterns also seem typical. In the late nineteenth and early twentieth centuries, many Latin American countries had a powerful positivist medical establishment that transformed the profession and medical institutions into vehicles for nationalist expression. They seem to have been equally ineffectual in enforcing professional monopoly. Indeed, the fact that medical pluralism thrived even in Costa Rica where social conflict was muted, where other ethno-medical traditions were relatively weak, and where even alternative medicines like homeopathy were not particularly imposing, indicates that one might have to look elsewhere than class resistance, ethnic otherness, and state impotence to find reasons for the vitality of popular medical currents. It may be that the colonial heritage of state pragmatism and recognition of medical heterodoxy combined with the exigencies of national state formation and the tendency of physicians to agglomerate in the cities to promote an official as well as semiofficial recognition of the legitimacy of medical pluralism. While it is true that professional organizations are clearly part of the modernizing positivist state — that is, professional formation *is* state formation in Latin America — that state also proved capable of acting beyond (or perhaps rather beneath) its professional component. In Costa Rica, medical pluralism did not just occur despite public power; it was also produced by it.

NOTES

Introduction

1 See, for example, the results of a study carried out in 1967 in the Pacific port town of Puntarenas: Miles Richardson and Barbara Bode, "Popular Medicine in Puntarenas, Costa Rica: Urban and Societal Features," in *Community Culture and National Change*, ed. Richard N. Adams et al. (New Orleans: Middle American Research Institute, 1972), 261–69. Another anthropologist found a similar eclecticism and familiarity with conventional medicine among mestizo sufferers in Peru and Chile in the early 1950s; see Ozzie G. Simmons, "Popular and Modern Medicine in Mestizo Communities of Coastal Peru and Chile," *Journal of American Folklore* 68, no. 267 (1955): 57–71.

2 The phrase is from Julyan G. Peard, "Tropical Disorders and the Forging of a Brazilian Medical Identity, 1860–1890," *Hispanic American Historical Review* 77, no. 1 (1997): 3. See also Julyan G. Peard, *Race, Place, and Medicine: The Idea of the Tropics in Nineteenth-Century Brazil* (Durham, N.C.: Duke University Press, 1999); Nancy Leys Stepan, *Beginnings of Brazilian Science: Oswaldo Cruz, Medical Research, and Policy, 1890–1920* (New York: Science History Publications, 1981); Nancy Leys Stepan, "The Interplay between Socio-economic Factors and Medical Science: Yellow Fever Research, Cuba, and the United States," *Social Studies of Science* 8 (1978): 397–424; Nancy Leys Stepan, *"The Hour of Eugenics": Race, Gender, and Nation in Latin America* (Ithaca, N.Y.: Cornell University Press, 1991); Marcos Cueto, *Excelencia científica en la periferia: Actividades científicas e investigación biomédica en el Perú, 1890–1950* (Lima: Tarea, 1989); Jaime L. Benchimol, *Dos micróbios aos mosquitos. Febre amarela e a revolução pasteuriana no Brasil* (Rio de Janeiro: Editorial Fiocruz, 1999). Jaime Benchimol, ed., *Manguinos do sonho à vida* (Rio de Janeiro: Fiocruz, 1990); and Jaime L. Benchimol, "Domingo José Freire e os primórdios da bacteriologia no Brasil," *Manguinhos: História, Ciência, Saúde* 2, no. 1 (1995): 67–98.

3 Among them, see Ricardo González Leandri's impressive *Curar, persuadir, gobernar: La construcción histórica de la profesión médica en Buenos Aires, 1852–1886*

(Madrid: Consejo Superior de Investigaciones Científicas-Centro de Estudios Históricos, 1999), and Edmundo Campos Coelho, *As profissões imperiais: medicina, engenharia e advocacia no Rio de Janeiro (1822–1930)* (Rio de Janeiro: Record, 1999). See also Ricardo Cruz-Coke, *Historia de la medicina chilena* (Santiago: Editorial Andres Bello, 1995); and Miranda Canal, Nestor, Emilio Quevedo Vélez, and Mario Hernández Alvarez. *Medicina (2): La institucionalización de la medicina en Colombia,* vol. 8 of *Historia social de la ciencia en Colombia.* Edited by Emilio Quevedo Vélez. (Bogotá: Instituto Colombiano para el Desarrollo de la Ciencia y la Tecnología Francisco José de Caldas, 1993).

4   Fascinating accounts of popular practitioners in conflict with the new medical authorities of the nineteenth century can be found in Sidney Chalhoub, *Cidade febril: Cortiços e epidemias na Corte imperial* (Rio de Janeiro: Companha das letras, 1996); and David Sowell, *The Tale of Healer Miguel Perdomo Neira: Medicine, Ideologies, and Power in the Nineteenth-Century Andes* (Wilmington, Del.: Scholarly Resources, 2001). Joseph W. Bastien's classic study of the Kallawaya includes a brief historical account: *Healers of the Andes: Kallawaya Herbalists and Their Medicinal Plants* (Salt Lake City: University of Utah Press, 1987), 21–24. Two other works that contain valuable accounts of popular healers past are Lycurgo de Castro Santos Filho, *História geral da medicina brasileira,* 2 vols. (São Paulo: Editora da Universidade de São Paulo, 1977–1991); and Luz María Hernández Sáenz, *Learning to Heal: The Medical Profession in Colonial Mexico, 1767–1831* (New York: Peter Lang, 1997), 227–63. Carlos Viesca Treviño, "Curanderismo in Mexico and Guatemala: Its Historical Evolution from the Sixteenth to the Nineteenth Century," in *Mesoamerican Healers,* eds. Brad R. Huber and Alan R. Sandstrom (Austin: University of Texas Press, 2001), 47–65, unfortunately does not live up to its billing, basing its discussion almost entirely on sixteenth-century sources and including a mere page of anecdotal material from the nineteenth century.

5   On the new agenda, see Judith Walzer Leavitt, "Medicine in Context: A Review Essay of the History of Medicine," *American Historical Review* 95, no. 5 (December 1990): 1471–84; and, for Latin America, Diego Armus, "Disease in the Historiography of Modern Latin America," in *Disease in the History of Modern Latin America: From Malaria to AIDS,* ed. Diego Armus (Duke University Press, 2003). Exceptional examples of new research on ethnicity, gender, social stature, and medical regulation are Marcos Cueto, "Indigenismo and Rural Medicine in Perú: The Indian Sanitary Brigade and Manuel Núñez Butrón," *Bulletin of the History of Medicine* 65 (1991): 22, 41; Ann Zulawski, "Hygiene and the 'Indian Problem': Ethnicity and Medicine in Bolivia, 1910–1920," *Latin American Research Review* 35, no. 2 (2000): 107–28; and Anne-Emanuelle Birn, "A Revolution in Rural Health? The Struggle over Local Health Units in Mexico, 1928–1940," *Journal of the History of Medicine* 53, no. 1 (January 1998): 43–76.

6   Important attempts to tackle the issue head-on are Willem de Blécourt and Cornelie Usborne, "Preface: Situating 'Alternative Medicine' in the Modern Period," *Medical History* 43 (1999): 283–85; Matthew Ramsey, "Alternative

Medicine in Modern France," *Medical History* 43 (1999): 286–322; Matthew Ramsey, *Professional and Popular Medicine in France, 1770–1830: The Social World of Medical Practice* (Cambridge: Cambridge University Press, 1988), 1–13; Norman Gevitz, "Three Perspectives on Unorthodox Medicine," in *Other Healers: Unorthodox Medicine in America*, ed. Norman Gevitz (Baltimore, Md.: Johns Hopkins University Press, 1988), 1–28; W. F. Bynum and Roy Porter, introduction to *Medical Fringe and Medical Orthodoxy, 1750–1850*, ed. W. F. Bynum and Roy Porter (London: Croom Helm, 1987), 1–4; and Irwin Press, "Problems in the Definition and Classification of Medical Systems," *Social Science and Medicine* 14B (1980): 45–57.

7 Irwin Press, "The Urban Curandero," *American Anthropologist* 73, no. 3 (1971): 741.

8 Lynn Marie Morgan, *Community Participation in Health: The Politics of Primary Care in Costa Rica* (New York: Cambridge University Press, 1993), 17, 18–19.

9 This binary opposition is central to the influential work of Michael Taussig, *Shamanism, Colonialism, and the Wild Man: A Study in Terror and Healing* (Chicago: University of Chicago Press, 1987); see, for example, 447–48.

10 Juan César García, *Pensamiento social en salud en América Latina* (Mexico City: Interamericana McGraw Hill/Organización Panamericana de Salud, 1994), 95–96. I might also mention in this vein the recent work of Ronn F. Pineo, which from a less polemical perspective frames the rise of scientific medicine in Guayaquil in the context of the late-nineteenth-century export boom and rapid urbanization; see Ronn F. Pineo, "Misery and Death in the Pearl of the Pacific: Health Care in Guayaquil, Ecuador, 1870–1925," *Hispanic American Historical Review* 70, no. 4 (1990): 609–37, and *Social and Economic Reform in Ecuador: Life and Work in Guayaquil* (Gainesville: University Press of Florida, 1996).

11 After the initial rush of enthusiasm that marked the study of medicine and empire in the 1980s, some second thoughts emerged about the degree to which Western medicine and Western imperialism were essentially as opposed to instrumentally related, and the extent to which biomedicine is intrinsically colonizing; see Shula Marks, "What Is Colonial about Colonial Medicine? And What Has Happened to Imperialism and Health?" *Social History of Medicine* 10, no. 2 (1997): 205–19. For a critical call to arms, see Warwick Anderson, "Where Is the Postcolonial History of Medicine?" *Bulletin of the History of Medicine* 72, no. 3 (1998): 522–30.

12 David Arnold's review essay on the subject begins with the historiography of medicine and colonization in Europe and North America in the nineteenth and twentieth centuries, and then explains that "the rest of the world has come increasingly under scrutiny as well," listing Africa, South and Southeast Asia, the Pacific region, and Australasia, but omitting Latin America ("Introduction: Disease, Medicine, and Empire," in *Imperial Medicine and Indigenous Societies*, ed. David Arnold [Manchester: Manchester University Press, 1988], 1). Though he does mention in passing some specific cases from Latin Amer-

ica, they do not warrant a categorical discussion, and the collection is without a Latin American case study. In a later review of medicine and colonialism, Arnold advances a typology that includes virtually every European colonizing configuration except those of Spain and Portugal; see David Arnold, "Medicine and Colonialism," in *Companion Encyclopedia of the History of Medicine*, ed. W. F. Bynum and Roy Porter (London: Routledge, 1993), 1:394–95. Studies of Latin America are also absent from another key collection on the subject: Milton Lewis and Roy Macleod, eds., *Disease, Medicine, and Empire: Perspectives on Western Medicine and the Experience of European Expansion* (New York: Routledge, 1988). The fact that the U.S. occupation of the Philippines receives attention in both the Arnold and the Lewis and Macleod anthology underlines the point. A Latin American case study is included in a more recent collection by Arnold, Julyan G. Peard, "Tropical Medicine in Nineteenth-Century Brazil: The Case of the 'Escola Tropicalista Bahiana,' 1860–1890," in *Warm Climates and Western Medicine: The Emergence of Tropical Medicine, 1500–1900*, ed. David Arnold (Amsterdam: Editions Rodopi, 1996), 108–32. As Warwick Anderson notes, however, Peard's contribution sits awkwardly within the editorial framework of the anthology; Anderson, "Where is the Postcolonial History of Medicine?" 525.

13   A collection of important examples of this scholarship can be found in Marcos Cueto, ed., *Missionaries of Science: The Rockefeller Foundation in Latin America* (Bloomington: Indiana University Press, 1994). See also the major contribution of Christopher Abel, "External Philanthropy and Domestic Change in Colombian Health Care: The Role of the Rockefeller Foundation, ca. 1920–1950," *Hispanic American Historical Review* 75, no. 3 (1995): 339–76; and Steven Palmer, "Central American Encounters with Rockefeller Public Health, 1914–1921," in *Close Encounters of Empire: Writing the Cultural History of U.S.–Latin American Relations*, ed. Gilbert M. Joseph, Catherine LeGrand, and Ricardo D. Salvatore (Durham, N.C.: Duke University Press, 1998), 311–32.

14   Chalhoub, *Cidade febril*, 97–150. See also Jeffrey Needell, "The *Revolta Contra Vacina* of 1904: The Revolt against 'Modernization' in Belle-Epoque Rio de Janeiro," *Hispanic American Historical Review* 67, no. 2 (1987): 233–69; Sidney Chalhoub, "The Politics of Disease Control: Yellow Fever and Race in Nineteenth-Century Rio de Janeiro," *Journal of Latin American Studies* 25, no. 3 (1993): 441–63; and Teresa A. Meade, *"Civilizing" Rio: Reform and Resistance in a Brazilian City, 1889–1930* (University Park: Pennsylvania State University Press, 1997), 87–120.

15   Though their work has been roundly and rightly criticized for its "presentist" validation of the inevitable triumph of Western medical science in their particular countries, these traditional works invariably contain a wealth of information, and sometimes document folk and popular medical practices, if only in the interests of jocular folklore. See Victor M. Ruiz Naufal and Arturo Gálvez Medrano, "La *Historia de la Medicina en México* dentro de la histo-

riografía médica mexicana." Ruiz and Medrano's piece is a preface to the reprint edition of Francisco de Asis Flores y Troncoso, *Historia de la Medicina en México desde la época de los indios hasta el presente*, 4 vols. (Mexico City: Instituto Mexicano de Seguro Social, 1982), 1:xix. Particularly useful works in the genre are Hermilio Valdizán and Angel Maldonado, *La medicina popular peruana: Contribución al "folk-lore" médico del Perú*, 2 vols. (Lima: Imprenta Torres Aguirre, 1922); Carlos Martínez Durán, *Las ciencias médicas en Guatemala: Orígen y evolución*, 3d ed. (Guatemala City: Editorial Universitaria, 1964); Vicente Láchner Sandoval, "Apuntes de higiene pública: Organismos, institutos y profesiones en relación con este ramo," in *Revista de Costa Rica en el siglo XIX* (San José: Imprenta Nacional, 1902), 189–222; Ricardo Archila, *Historia de la medicina en Venezuela* (Mérida, Mexico: Universidad de los Andes, 1966); Benjamín Vicuña Mackenna, *Médicos de antaño* (1877; reprint, Santiago: Editorial Francisco de Aguirre, 1974); Pedro Lantaro Ferrer, *Historia general de la medicina en Chile* (Talca, Chile: Imprenta Talca, 1904); Juan B. Lastres, *Historia de la medicina peruana*, 3 vols. (Lima: Imprenta Santa María, 1951); *Historia general de la medicina argentina*, 2 vols. (Córdoba: Universidad Nacional Autónoma de Córdoba, 1976–1980); Velarde Pérez Fontana, *Historia de la medicina en el Uruguay con especial referencia a las comarcas del Río de la Plata*, 2 vols. (Montevideo: Ministerio de Salud Pública, 1967); Edgar Cabezas Solera, *La medicina en Costa Rica hasta 1900* (San José: Editorial Nacional de Salud y Seguro Social, 1990); Carlos Eduardo González Pacheco, *Hospital San Juan de Dios: 150 años de historia* (San José: Editorial Nacional del Seguro Social, 1995), 192; Francisco Asturias, *Historia de la medicina en Guatemala*, 2d ed. (1902; reprint, Guatemala City: Editorial Universitaria, 1958); Emilio Roig de Leuchsenring, *Médicos y medicina en Cuba, Historia, biografía y costumbrismo* (Havana: Museo Histórico de las Ciencias Médicas "Carlos J. Finlay," 1965); and finally, the classic study of late-nineteenth-century Mexican medical historiography, Asis Flores, *Historia de la Medicina en México*.

16   There have been some notable attempts to apply Foucauldian method to the Latin American history of medicine. One good example is Pedro Barran's study of the deployment of a medical discourse for regulating the public body and private sexuality in his *Historia de la sensibilidad en el Uruguay*, 2 vols. (Montevideo: Ediciones de la Banda Oriental, 1990). Suggestive and beautifully written, the study's processing of European discourses without any attempt to assess their intersection with a specifically Uruguayan social configuration is a perfect instance of the problems with the simple passing of raw local data through the Foucauldian apparatus, which can only result in a new intellectual transmission perspective.

17   González Leandri, *Curar, persuadir, gobernar*, 51.

18   In 1995, James Dow offered a synthetic description of curanderos that although careful to distinguish between the "Amerindian" and the more eclectic "urban" curandero (following Press, "Urban Curandero"), nevertheless

maintained that the latter are defined by their claim to have special religious power and their synthesis of alternative medical beliefs, the varieties of which are too great to be analyzable; see James Dow, "Curandero/Curandeiro," in *Encyclopedia of Latin American History and Culture,* ed. Barbara Tenenbaum (New York: Charles Scribner's and Sons, 1995), 2:344.

19 Press, "Urban Curandero," 741.

20 Ramsey, "Alternative Medicine in Modern France," 289.

21 See, for example, the essays collected in Gilbert M. Joseph and Daniel Nugent, eds., *Everyday Forms of State Formation: Revolution and the Negotiation of Rule in Modern Mexico* (Durham, N.C.: Duke University Press, 1994).

22 See Aristides A. Moll, *Aesculapius in Latin America* (Philadelphia, Pa.: W. B. Saunders Company, 1944). This is particularly true of the work of John Tate Lanning and Francisco Guerra. See, for example, John Tate Lanning, *The Royal Protomedicato: The Regulation of the Professions in the Spanish Empire,* ed. John Jay TePaske (Durham, N.C.: Duke University Press, 1985); John Tate Lanning, *Academic Culture in the Spanish Colonies* (Folcroft, Pa.: Folcroft Press, Inc., 1949); Francisco Guerra, *Las medicinas marginales: Los sistemas de curar prohibidos a los médicos* (Madrid: Alianza Editorial, 1976); and Francisco Guerra, *El médico político: Su influencia en la historia de Hispano-América y las Filipinas* (Madrid: Afrodisio Aguado, 1975). Guerra's generation of medical historians is well represented in the 1971 conference collection of John Z. Bowers and Elizabeth F. Purcell, eds., *Aspects of the History of Medicine in Latin America* (New York: Josiah Macy Jr. Foundation, 1979).

23 For work that proves the exceptionalist proposition to be at the very least in need of a thorough overhaul, see on the colonial and early independence period: Claudia Quirós, *La era de la encomienda* (San José: Editorial Universidad de Costa Rica, 1990); Carolyn Hall, *El café y el desarrollo histórico-geográfico de Costa Rica,* 3d ed. (San José: Editorial Costa Rica, 1982); Lowell Gudmundson, *Costa Rica before Coffee: Society and Economy on the Eve of the Export Boom* (Baton Rouge: Lousiana State University Press, 1986); Mario Samper, "Generations of Settlers: A Study of Rural Households and Their Markets on the Costa Rican Frontier, 1850–1935" (Ph.D. diss., University of California at Berkeley, 1987); and Iván Molina Jiménez, *Costa Rica (1800–1850): El legado colonial y la génesis del capitalismo* (San José: Editorial de la Universidad de Costa Rica, 1991). On the politics of the modern state, see Mercedes Muñóz Guillén, *El Estado y la abolición del ejército en Costa Rica, 1914–1949* (San José: Editorial Porvenir, 1990); and Fabrice Lehoucq and Ivan Molina Jiménez, *Stuffing the Ballot Box: Fraud, Electoral Reform, and Democracy in Comparative Perspective* (New York: Cambridge University Press, 2002). For a revisionist cultural history of Costa Rica from 1750 to 1950, see Iván Molina Jiménez and Steven Palmer, eds., *Héroes al gusto y libros de moda: Sociedad y cambio cultural en Costa Rica (1750–1900)* (San José: Plumsock Mesoamerican Studies, 1992); and Iván Molina Jiménez and Steven Palmer, eds., *El paso del cometa: Estado, política social y culturas populares en Costa Rica (1800–1950)* (San José: Plumsock Mesoamerican Studies, 1994).

Notes to Introduction

An effort to incorporate the new historiography into a short, general history is Iván Molina Jiménez and Steven Palmer, *The History of Costa Rica: Brief, Up-to-date and Illustrated* (San José: Editorial de la Universidad de Costa Rica, 1998).

24 Hector Pérez Brignoli, "El crecimiento demográfico de América Latina en los siglos XIX y XX: Problemas, métodos y perspectivas," *Avances de Investigación* (Centro de Investigaciones Históricas, Universidad de Costa Rica) 48 (1989): 12–13.

25 On Costa Rica, see Láchner Sandoval, "Apuntes de higiene," 190–201. For a sample of deaths attributed to different diseases, see "Enfermedades que han causado la muerte en 1867," in *Censo general de la República de Costa Rica (27 de noviembre de 1864)*, República de Costa Rica (San José: Imprenta Nacional, 1868), 62–71. For Latin America, see Mary C. Karasch, "Disease Ecologies of South America," in *The Cambridge World History of Human Disease*, ed. Kenneth F. Kiple (Cambridge: Cambridge University Press, 1993), 535–46. See also Stephen J. Kunitz, "Disease and Mortality in the Americas since 1700," in *The Cambridge World History of Human Disease*, ed. Kenneth F. Kiple (Cambridge: Cambridge University Press, 1993), 328–33.

26 See Blécourt and Usborne, "Preface," 283–85; and Ramsey, "Alternative Medicine in Modern France," 286–89.

27 Archivos Nacionales de Costa Rica, Policía 4660, f. 2v.

Chapter 1. Healers before Doctors

1 John Tate Lanning, *The Royal Protomedicato: The Regulation of the Professions in the Spanish Empire,* ed. John Jay TePaske (Durham, N.C.: Duke University Press, 1985), 138–45; Aristides A. Moll, *Aesculapius in Latin America* (Philadelphia, Pa.: W. B. Saunders Company, 1944), 83; Julyan G. Peard, "Tropical Disorders and the Forging of a Brazilian Medical Identity, 1860–1890," *Hispanic American Historical Review* 77, no. 1 (1997): 6 n. 13; Lycurgo de Castro Santos Filho, "Medicine in Colonial Brazil: An Overview," in *Aspects of the History of Medicine,* ed. John Z. Bowers and Elizabeth F. Purcell (New York: Josiah Macy Jr. Foundation, 1979), 97–108; and Nancy Leys Stepan, *Beginnings of Brazilian Science: Oswaldo Cruz, Medical Research, and Policy, 1890–1920* (New York: Science History Publications, 1981), 49.

2 Lanning, *Royal Protomedicato,* 143.

3 Ronald L. Numbers, introduction to *Medicine without Doctors: Home Health Care in American History,* ed. Guenter B. Risse, Ronald L. Numbers, and Judith Walzer Leavitt (New York: Science History Publications, 1977), 1–4; and Roy Porter, "The Patient's View: Doing Medical History from Below," *Theory and Society* 14, no. 2 (1985): 182. The point has been made for Latin America in Emilio Quevedo and Amarillys Zaldúa, "Antecedentes de las reformas médicas del siglo XVIII y XIX en el Nuevo Reino de Granada: Una polémica entre médicos y cirujanos," *Quipu* 3, no. 3 (1986): 311–34.

4   Archivos Nacionales de Costa Rica (hereafter ANCR), Policía 5419, f. 1.

5   See Victor Campos and Alia Sarkis, *Curanderismo tradicional de Costa Rica* (San José: Editorial Costa Rica, 1978).

6   Lydia Cabrera, *La medicina popular de Cuba: Médicos de antaño, curanderos, santeros y paleros de hogaño* (Miami, 1984), 23–24. Santos Filho has conjured the analogous Brazilian pantheon: Santa Ágata for pulmonary ailments, Santa Luzia or Santa Odília in cases of ocular afflictions, São Benedito for snake bites, and so on; see Lycurgo de Castro Santos Filho, *História geral da medicina brasileira* (São Paulo: Editora de Universidade de São Paulo, 1977–1991), 1:354–55.

7   See Robert A. Voeks, *Sacred Leaves of Condomblé: African Magic, Medicine, and Religion in Brazil* (Austin: University of Texas Press, 1997), 132.

8   See José Daniel Gil Zúñiga, "Un mito en la sociedad costarricense: el culto a la Virgen de los Ángeles (1824–1935)," *Revista de Historia* (Costa Rica), no. 11 (January–June 1985): 47–129.

9   Wilhelm Marr, "Viajes a Centroamérica," in *Costa Rica en el siglo XIX: Antología de viajeros,* ed. Ricardo Fernández Guardia (1929; reprint, San José: Editorial Universitaria Centroamericana, 1985), 176. At roughly the same time, a U.S. traveler suffering the same affliction in Nicaragua reported that "the best surgeon is an Indian boy who always performs the operation skillfully." Ephraim George Squier, *Nicaragua: Its People, Scenery, Monuments, Resources, Condition, and Proposed Canal; with One Hundred Original Maps and Illustrations,* rev. ed. (New York: Harper and Brother Publishers, 1860), 45.

10 On Mexico, see Luz María Hernández Sáenz, *Learning to Heal: The Medical Profession in Colonial Mexico, 1767–1831* (New York: Peter Lang, 1997), 160–61; and on Costa Rica, Tulio von Bulow, "Apuntes para la historia de la medicina en Costa Rica durante la colonia," *Revista de los Archivos Nacionales* 9, nos. 1–2 (1945): 46–47. On the history of the Latin American trade, see Francisco Guerra, "Drugs from the Indies and the Political Economy of the Sixteenth Century," in *Analecta Médico-Historica: I Materia Médica in the Sixteenth Century* (London: Pergamon Press, 1966), 29–54. Risse notes the incorporation of copal, a medicinal used by the Aztecs, into the Spanish pharmacopoeia by Agustín Farfán in his famous *Tractado Brebe de Medicina* of 1592; see Guenter B. Risse, "Medicine in New Spain," in *Medicine in the New World,* ed. Ronald L. Numbers (Knoxville: University of Tennessee Press, 1987), 49.

11 See Numbers, introduction to *Medicine without Doctors,* 1; and George M. Foster, "On the Origin of Humoral Medicine in Latin America," *Medical Anthropology Quarterly* 1, no. 4 (December 1987): 364–66. On the use of such manuals in rural Brazil in the 1860s, see Dain Borges, *The Family in Bahia, Brazil, 1870–1945* (Stanford, Calif.: Stanford University Press, 1992), 92.

12 "Instrucción práctica y sencilla del modo cierto de curar las viruelas," *El Noticioso Universal,* 22 November 1833; cited in Patricia Fumero Vargas, ed., *Centenario de la Facultad de Farmacia* (San José: Editorial de la Universidad de

Costa Rica, 1997), 179, 165–82. Commonly mentioned medicinal ingredients at this time correspond to the classic continental repertoire outlined in Hernández Sáenz, *Learning to Heal*, 134–43; and Carmel Goldwater, "Traditional Medicine in Latin America," in *Traditional Medicine and Health Care Coverage: A Reader for Health Care Administrators and Practitioners*, ed. Robert H. Bannerman et al. (Geneva: World Health Organization, 1983), 37–49.

13   On contraband, see Iván Molina Jiménez, *Costa Rica (1800–1850): El legado colonial y la génesis del capitalismo* (San José: Editorial de la Universidad de Costa Rica, 1991), 128. On British patent medicines in North America, see James Harvey Young, "Patent Medicines and the Self-Help Syndrome," in *Medicine without Doctors: Home Health Care in American History*, ed. Guenter B. Risse, Ronald L. Numbers, and Judith Walzer Leavitt (New York: Science History Publications, 1977), 97–98. For Mexico, see Hernández Sáenz, *Learning to Heal*, 154.

14   See ANCR 4660, f. 1v.

15   *Crónica de Costa Rica*, 29 January 1859, 4.

16   See Iván Molina Jiménez, *"El que quiera divertirse": Libros y sociedad en Costa Rica, 1750–1914* (San José: Editorial de la Universidad de Costa Rica, 1995), 27, 57. On Buchan in Spain, see Enrique Perdiguero, "The Popularization of Medicine during the Spanish Enlightenment," in *The Popularization of Medicine, 1650–1850*, ed. Roy Porter (New York: Routledge, 1992), 176–77. On the popularity of Buchan's work in Cuba, see Cabrera, *Medicina popular de Cuba*, 95.

17   See Molina Jiménez, *"El que quiera divertirse,"* 57. The title of Graham's work is the Spanish translation of his *Sure Methods of Improving Health, and Prolonging Life: Or, a Treatise on the Art of Living Long and Comfortably* (London: Simpkin and Marshall, 1827), popular enough to see three English editions within a year of its initial publication.

18   See Santos Filho, *História geral*, 1:349–52. On the U.S. adaptations, see John B. Blake, "From Buchan to Fishbein: The Literature of Domestic Medicine," in *Medicine without Doctors: Home Health Care in American History*, ed. Guenter B. Risse, Ronald L. Numbers, and Judith Walzer Leavitt (New York: Science History Publications, 1977), 15.

19   Charles E. Rosenberg, "Medical Text and Social Context: Explaining William Buchan's Domestic Medicine," *Bulletin of the History of Medicine* 57 (1983): 27, 33. See also Roy Porter, *Health for Sale: Quackery in England, 1650–1850* (Manchester: Manchester University Press, 1989), 38–39.

20   See Paulina Malavassi, "Entre la marginalidad social y los orígenes de la salud pública: Leprosos, curanderos y facultativos en el valle Central de Costa Rica, 1784–1845," master's thesis, Universidad de Costa Rica, 1998, 181–82.

21   For the classic argument for the European derivation of all indigenous and popular medicine in Latin America, see Foster, "On the Origin of Humoral Medicine in Latin America," 355–93. Powerful counterarguments can be

found in Joseph W. Bastien, "Differences between Kallaway-Andean and Greek-European Humoral Theory," *Social Science and Medicine* 28, no. 1 (1989): 45–51. For Mesoamerica, see Bernardo Ortíz de Montellano, *Aztec Medicine, Health, and Nutrition* (New Brunswick, N.J.: Rutgers University Press, 1990). The adoption of humoral categories in Afro-Brazilian medicine is discussed in Voeks, *Sacred Leaves of Condomblé*, 131–33.

22 See Vivian Nutton, "Humoralism," in *Companion Encyclopedia of the History of Medicine*, ed. W. F. Bynum and Roy Porter (London: Routledge, 1993), 1:281–91; and Nancy G. Siraisi, *Medieval and Early Renaissance Medicine: An Introduction to Knowledge and Practice* (Chicago: University of Chicago Press, 1990), 104–6.

23 Arthur Kleinman, "What Is Specific to Western Medicine?" in *Companion Encyclopedia of the History of Medicine*, ed. W. F. Bynum and Roy Porter (London: Routledge, 1993), 1:18.

24 "Deseando auxiliar a la humanidad en la espantosa peste del cólera morbus asiático si por desgracia tocase entre nosotoros, insertamos la siguiente," *El Noticioso Universal*, 1 November 1833; cited in Patricia Fumero Vargas, *Centenario de la Facultad de Farmacia* (San José: Editorial de la Universidad de Costa Rica, 1997), 175.

25 See Charles E. Rosenberg, *The Cholera Years: The United States in 1832, 1849, and 1866* (Chicago: University of Chicago Press, 1962), 73–78; and Lilia V. Oliver, "El cólera y los barrios de Guadalajara en 1833 y en 1850," in *Salud, cultura y sociedad en América Latina*, ed. Marcos Cueto (Lima: Instituto de Estudios Peruanos, 1996), 96–100. On the strength of atmospheric interpretations in Guatemala during the 1837 outbreak, see Greg Grandin, *The Blood of Guatemala: A History of Race and Nation* (Durham, N.C.: Duke University Press, 2000), 86–88.

26 See Caroline Hannaway, "Environment and Miasmata," in *Companion Encyclopedia of the History of Medicine*, ed. W. F. Bynum and Roy Porter (London: Routledge, 1993), 1:292–308.

27 See Malavassi, "Entre la marginalidad social," 102; and Gladys Rojas Chaves, *Café, ambiente y sociedad en la cuenca del río Virilla, Costa Rica (1840–1955)* (San José: Editorial de la Universidad de Costa Rica, 2000), 69, 87–90.

28 "Instrucción práctica y sencilla del modo cierto de curar las viruelas," *El Noticioso Universal*, 22 November 1833; cited in Patricia Fumero Vargas, *Centenario de la Facultad de Farmacia* (San José: Editorial de la Universidad de Costa Rica, 1997), 179.

29 David Sowell, "Miguel Perdomo Neira: Healing, Culture, and Power in the Nineteenth-Century Andes," *Anuario Colombiano de Historia Social y de la Cultura* 24 (1997): 172.

30 Kleinman, "What Is Specific to Western Medicine?" 16–17.

31 For a fascinating example of such eclecticism in the case of a Mexican physician who practiced between 1835 and 1880, see Francisco Durán, ed., *Bitácora médica del Doctor Falcón: La medicina y la farmacia en el siglo XIX* (Mexico City:

Universidad La Salle, 2000). On Pasteur, see Matthew Ramsey, "Alternative Medicine in Modern France," *Medical History* 43 (1999): 288.

32 See Santos Filho, *História geral,* 1:335; and Francisco de Asis Flores y Troncoso, *Historia de la Medicina en México desde la época de los indios hasta el presente* (1886–1888; reprint, Mexico City: Instituto Mexicano de Seguro Social, 1982), 3:276.

33 Risse, "Medicine in New Spain," 14; Ross Danielson, *Cuban Medicine* (New Brunswick, N.J.: Transaction Books, 1979), 21; Sandra L. Orellana, *Indian Medicine in Highland Guatemala: The Pre-Hispanic and Colonial Periods* (Albuquerque: University of New Mexico Press, 1987), 63–76; Santos Filho, *História geral,* 1:349; and Flores y Troncoso, *Historia de la Medicina en México,* 3:23.

34 Matthew Ramsay, *Professional and Popular Medicine in France, 1770–1830: The Social World of Medical Practice* (Cambridge: Cambridge University Press, 1988), 132.

35 See ANCR, Gobernación 4177, ff. 30–30v; cited in Malavassi, "Entre la marginalidad social," 178. República de Costa Rica, *Censo general de la República de Costa Rica (27 noviembre de 1864)* (San José: Imprenta Nacional, 1868), 89. See also Lowell Gudmundson, *Costa Rica before Coffee: Society and Economy on the Eve of the Export Boom* (Baton Rouge: Louisiana State University Press, 1986), 133.

36 See Tânia Salgado Pimenta, "Barbeiros-sangradores e curandeiros no Brasil (1808–1828)," *Manguinhos: História, Ciencias, Saúde* 5, no. 2 (1998): 354.

37 See Irvine Loudon, "The Nature of Provincial Medical Practice in Eighteenth-Century England," *Medical History* 29 (1985): 1–32.

38 See Hernández Sáenz, *Learning to Heal,* 181; see also 179–203.

39 See Malavassi, "Entre la marginalidad social," 176.

40 See Hernández Sáenz, *Learning to Heal,* 310; and Santos Filho, *História geral,* 1:225.

41 See Vicente Láchner Sandoval, "Apuntes de higiene pública: Organismos, institutos y profesiones en relación con este ramo," in *Revista de Costa Rica en el siglo XIX* (San José: Imprenta Nacional, 1902), 222.

42 ANCR, Mortuales Independientes (Cartago), 590.

43 Santos Filho, *História geral,* 1:226–28.

44 ANCR, Mortuales Independientes (Cartago), 590. Though there is no evidence that they were used this way in Costa Rica, such medicinal properties were commonly ascribed to these materials in the eighteenth and nineteenth centuries in Mexico, North America, and England; see John K. Crellin and Jane Philpott, *Trying to Give Ease,* vol. 1 of *Herbal Medicine Past and Present* (Durham, N.C.: Duke University Press, 1990), 183; and John K. Crellin and Jane Philpott, *A Reference Guide to Medicinal Plants,* vol. 2 of *Herbal Medicine Past and Present* (Durham, N.C.: Duke University Press, 1990), 214, 410, 450. See also Hernández Sáenz, *Learning to Heal,* 134–43.

45 On domestic material culture and social stature in Cartago during this era, see Arnaldo Moya Gutiérrez, "Cultura material y vida cotidiana. El entorno doméstico de los vecinos principales de Cartago (1750–1820)," in *Héroes al gusto*

y libros de moda: Sociedad y cambio cultural en Costa Rica (1750–1900), ed. Iván Molina Jiménez and Steven Palmer (San José: Plumsock Mesoamerican Studies, 1992), 9–44; and Iván Molina Jiménez, "Vivienda y muebles: el marco material de la vida doméstica en el Valle Central de Costa Rica (1821–1824)," *Revista de Historia de América* no. 116 (July–December 1993): 60–91.

46 Mary C. Karasch, *Slave Life in Rio de Janeiro, 1808–1850* (Princeton, N.J.: Princeton University Press, 1987), 202.

47 Lanning, *Royal Protomedicato*, 143.

48 See Bulow, "Apuntes para la historia de la medicina," 46–47; Eugenia Incera Olivas, "El Hospital San Juan de Diós: Sus antecedentes y su evolución histórica, 1845–1900," Licenciatura thesis, University of Costa Rica, 1978, 2; Láchner Sandoval, "Apuntes de higiene," 193, 215; "Receta para curar fácilmente las mordeduras de toda clase de culebra," *El Noticioso Universal*, 20 December 1833 (cited in Patricia Fumero Vargas, *Centenario de la Facultad de Farmacia* [San José: Editorial de la Universidad de Costa Rica, 1997], 181); and Malavassi, "Entre la marginalidad social," 180.

49 See ANCR, Policía 4965, f. 7.

50 ANCR, Policía 4730, f. 6v; for the patient's testimony, see f. 3v. On ginger, see Crellin and Philpott, *A Reference Guide to Medicinal Plants*, 225.

51 For the 1839 decree, see "Reglamento de Curanderos," *Libro de sesiones celebradas por la Junta de Sanidad del Partido de Cartago*, ANCR, Salubridad Pública 182, f. 9. For 1845, see Malavassi, "Entre la marginalidad social," 177.

52 ANCR, Policía 5540, f. 39.

53 Juan B. Lastres, *Historia de la medicina peruana* (Lima: Imprenta Santa Maria, 1951), 3:154–55.

54 See Luz María Hernandez-Sáenz, *Learning to Heal: The Medical Profession in Colonial Mexico, 1767–1831*, Ph.D. diss., University of Arizona, 1993. 419–25.

55 During the first half of the nineteenth century, the schooled and titled French midwives at the Brazilian court practiced phlebotomy and vaccination, and treated medical conditions, "particularly discomforts of the uterus" (Santos Filho, *História geral*, 1:231, 2:329). Among the slaves on the British Caribbean plantations, "a woman doctor commonly combined the functions of midwife, gynecologist, pediatrician, general practitioner, as well as surgeon when the girls were circumcised" (Richard B. Sheridan, *Doctors and Slaves: A Medical and Demographic History of Slavery in the British West Indies, 1680–1834* [Cambridge: Cambridge University Press, 1985], 74).

56 On this subject in early twentieth-century New Mexico, see Babette Perone, H. Henrietta Stockel and Victoria Krueger, *Medicine Women, Curanderas, and Women Doctors* (Norman: University of Oklahoma Press, 1989), 89–90.

57 For example, Robert Voeks can muster but a thin page of historical background in his *Sacred Leaves of Condomblé* (43), while Sandra Orellana's portrait in *Indian Medicine* of Mayan medicine in "colonial" Guatemala typically interpolates throughout on the basis of the agreement or difference between the chronicles of the conquerors and modern anthropological fieldwork.

Notes to Chapter One

58 For a brief historical overview of the Kallawaya, see Joseph W. Bastien, *Healers of the Andes: Kallawaya Herbalists and Their Medicinal Plants* (Salt Lake City: University of Utah Press, 1987), 21–24. See also Sowell, "Miguel Perdomo Neira," 167–88.

59 On this distinction among highland Guatemalan indigenous groups, see Orellana, *Indian Medicine,* 63–76.

60 On the founding of the town, see "Relación de la visita hecha por fray Juan Nieto á los pueblos indios de Nuestra Señora del Pilar de Tres Ríos . . . años de 1753 y 1754," in *Colección de documentos para la historia de Costa Rica,* ed. León Fernández (San José: Imprenta Nacional, 1881–1907), 9:492–93. On the awa, see W. M. Gabb, "On the Indian Tribes and Languages of Costa Rica," *Proceedings of the American Philosophical Society* 14 (1875): 483–601.

61 See Bulow, "Apuntes para la historia de la medicina," 61; and Crellin and Philpott, *A Reference Guide to Medicinal Plants,* 454.

62 For examples of the work of the friars in ministering to the sick Indians in Tres Ríos, see "Relación de la visita hecha por fray Juan Nieto," 497. On the 1805 vaccination campaign, see Edgar Cabezas Solera, *La medicina en Costa Rica hasta 1900* (San José: Editorial Nacional de Salud y Seguro Social, 1990), 102–3.

63 See Karasch, *Slave Life,* 203.

64 A. J. R. Russell-Wood, *The Black Man in Slavery and Freedom in Colonial Brazil* (New York: St. Martin's Press, 1982), 56.

65 Simón de Ayanque, *Lima por dentro y por fuera* [1792]; cited in José Luis Romero, *Latinoamérica: Las ciudades y las ideas,* 3d ed. (Mexico City: Siglo XXI, 1976), 131.

66 Ricardo Archila, *Historia de la medicina en Venezuela* (Mérida, Venezuela: Universidad de los Andes, 1966), 75.

67 Lanning, *Royal Protomedicato,* 198, 305. It might also be noted that the preponderance of blacks and mulattoes in the healing trades of Latin American has a striking parallel with the medical history of Rome, where in the first century B.C.E the majority of practitioners in Roman western Europe were Greeks or of Greek ancestry, most of them slaves, freed slaves, or their descendants; see Ralph Jackson, *Doctors and Diseases in the Roman Empire* (Norman: University of Oklahoma Press, 1989), 56.

68 Lowell Gudmundson, "De 'Negro' a 'Blanco' en la Hispanoamérica del siglo XIX: La asimilación afroamericana en Argentina y Costa Rica," *Mesoamérica* 12 (no. 7) 1986: 309–29.

69 Lanning, *Royal Protomedicato,* 143.

70 Ibid., 153–74; and Hernández Sáenz, *Learning to Heal,* 54–63.

71 See Manuel Valladares, "La causa del Dr. Esteban Cortí, alias Curti," *Revista de los Archivos Nacionales* (Costa Rica) 3, nos. 3–4 (1939): 132–69. See also Archivo General de la Nación (Mexico) (AGNM), Grupo de Documentos Inquisición, 1381, 1390, 1340, 1350. For an example of Courtí's learned discourse in legal medicine, see Anastasio Alfaro, *Arqueología criminal americana* (San José: Imprenta de Avelino Alsina, 1906), 112–13.

72 See ANCR, Gobernación 13.234.

73 Cited in ANCR, Congreso 5147, f. 1.

74 John Lloyd Stephens, *Incidents of Travel in Central America, Chiapas, and Yucatan* (New York: Harper and Brothers, 1841), 1:343–44.

75 The phrase is from Benjamin Orlove, ed., *The Allure of the Foreign: Imported Goods in Postcolonial Latin America* (Ann Arbor: University of Michigan Press, 1997). In fact, one of the key weaknesses of this important book is that it fails to deal in its introduction or articles with the notion of the "foreign" during the colonial period — and the desirability of foreign "things," including physicians and medicines.

Chapter 2. First Doctors, Licensed Empirics, and the New Politics of Practice

1 Forty-nine "licensed medical doctors" are listed for this period in Luis Dobles Segreda, "Catálogo completo de médicos incorporados, y que han ejercido la profesión en Costa Rica," in *Medicina e higiene*, vol. 9 of *Indice bibliográfico de Costa Rica* (San José: Imprenta Lehmann, 1927–1936), 403–7. Other sources put the number higher or mention practitioners not listed by Dobles Segreda, in particular Edgar Cabezas Solera, *La medicina en Costa Rica hasta 1900* (San José: Editorial Nacional de Salud y Seguro Social, 1990), 132–35; and Gonzalo González González, "Algunos datos sobre historia de la farmacia y la medicina en Costa Rica," *Revista de la Universidad de Costa Rica* 1 (September 1945): 66. Nevertheless, none are perfectly reliable since they all list practitioners who my own archival research has revealed definitely did not have medical degrees or who were only licensed as empirics, though they later represented themselves successfully as legitimate medical doctors. Given the fluid nature of professional borders at this time, trying to determine the precise number who were actually titled physicians versus those who were really titled surgeons or apothecaries, or just empirics successful and influential enough to be taken for full doctors, is not an exercise of the greatest urgency.

2 See Tulio von Bulow, "Apuntes para la historia de la medicina en Costa Rica durante la colonia," *Revista de los Archivos Nacionales* (Costa Rica) 9, nos. 1–2 (1945): 44; and Vicente Láchner Sandoval, "Apuntes de higiene pública: Organismos, institutos y profesiones en relación con este ramo," in *Revista de Costa Rica en el siglo XIX* (San José: Imprenta Nacional, 1902), 194.

3 See Archivos Nacionales de Costa Rica (hereafter ANCR), "Actas Municipales de San José, 24 July 1820," 197; cited in Paulina Malavassi, "Entre la marginalidad social y los orígenes de la salud pública: Leprosos, curanderos y facultativos en el valle Central de Costa Rica, 1784–1845" (master's thesis, Universidad de Costa Rica, 1998), 176.

4 See Cabezas Solera, *La medicina en Costa Rica*, 132–33.

5 See John Tate Lanning, *The Royal Protomedicato: The Regulation of the Professions in the Spanish Empire*, ed. John Jay TePaske (Durham, N.C.: Duke University Press, 1985), 310–24; Bulow, "Apuntes para la historia de la medicina," 47;

Cabezas Solera, *La medicina en Costa Rica,* 132; and Carlos Martínez Durán, *Las ciencias médicas en Guatemala: Orígen y evolución,* 3d ed. (Guatemala City: Editorial Universitaria, 1964), 333–38.

6 A perceptive analysis of this process is Rodolfo Cerdas Cruz, *Formación del Estado en Costa Rica (1821–1842)* (San José: Editorial de la Universidad de Costa Rica, 1985). See also Steven Palmer, "Prolegómenos a toda futura historia de San José, Costa Rica," *Mesoamérica* 31 (1996): 181–213.

7 Alexander von Frantzius, "El antiguo convento de la misión de Orosi en Cartago," in *Viajes por la República de Costa Rica,* ed. Elías Zeledón Cartín (San José: Academia de Geografía e Historia, 1997), 2:31–32. On the colonial ruling caste, see Samuel Stone, *Dinastía de los conquistadores* (San José: Editorial Universitario Centroamericana [EDUCA], 1983).

8 See Carlos Meléndez Chaverri, *Dr. José María Montealegre* (San José: Academia de Geografía e Historia, 1968), 31–35. Once enshrined by Meléndez Chaverri as the first native Costa Rican to graduate as a physician, Montealegre has suffered somewhat of a demotion with the discovery that he was really a "mere" surgeon (of course, Edinburgh's surgical milieu was one of the best places to study medicine at the time), and that Pablo Alvarado Bonilla actually graduated as a physician in Guatemala in 1823, even though he returned to practice in Costa Rica only in 1842. See Cabezas Solera, *La medicina en Costa Rica,* 103–6, 118–19.

9 See Luis Felipe González Flores, *Historia de la influencia extranjera en el desenvolvimiento educacional y científico de Costa Rica* (San José: Editorial Costa Rica, 1976), 32–47. Integration, and work in the most senior public positions, was made easier because of Costa Rica's participation in the doomed effort to forge a Central American federal republic (1823–1838) and its subsequent maintenance of a special shared citizenship arrangement with immigrants from the other isthmian republics. See Iván Molina Jiménez, *Costa Rica (1800–1850): El legado colonial y la génesis del capitalismo* (San José: Editorial de la Universidad de Costa Rica, 1991), 136–39.

10 See González Flores, *Historia de la influencia extranjera,* 57; ANCR, Gobernación 27,885; Lanning, *Royal Protomedicato,* 223; and Cabezas Solera, *La medicina en Costa Rica,* 114.

11 See González Flores, *Historia de la influencia extranjera,* 58.

12 See Cabezas Solera, *La medicina en Costa Rica,* 113–15. Salmon's unlucky encounters with cholera are from ANCR, Policía 4965, f. 29.

13 See Ricardo Archila, "Médicos alemanes en Venezuela: Siglos XVIII y XIX," *Humboldt* 21, no. 73 (1980): 74–79.

14 See González Flores, *Historia de la influencia extranjera,* 85–87. Humboldt's letter is reproduced in Elías Zeledón Cartín, ed., *Viajes por la República de Costa Rica* (San José: Academia de Geografia e Historia, 1997), 2:17.

15 See Cabezas Solera, *La medicina en Costa Rica,* 114–15; and Carlos Hernández Rodríguez, "Herbolarios, empíricos y farmacéuticos: Contribución a la historia de la farmacia en Costa Rica," in *Centenario de la Facultad de Farmacia,*

Universidad de Costa Rica, 1897–1997, ed. Patricia Fumero (San José: Editorial de la Universidad de Costa Rica, 1998), 30. The French physicians may have operated in the orbit of the Carit pharmacy.

16 See Pedro Lantaro Ferrer, *Historia general de la medicina en Chile* (Talca, Chile: Imprenta Talca, 1904), 329–48; Ricardo Cruz-Coke, *Historia de la medicina chilena* (Santiago: Editorial Andres Bello, 1995), 303; Nancy Leys Stepan, *Beginnings of Brazilian Science: Oswaldo Cruz, Medical Research, and Policy, 1890–1920* (New York: Science History Publications, 1981), 50–51; Julyan G. Peard, "Tropical Disorders and the Forging of a Brazilian Medical Identity, 1860–1890," *Hispanic American Historical Review* 77, no. 1 (1997): 1–43; and Aristides A. Moll, *Aesculapius in Latin America* (Philadelphia, Pa.: W. B. Saunders Company, 1944), 245.

17 E. Bradford Burns, *Patriarch and Folk: The Emergence of Nicaragua, 1798–1858* (Cambridge: Harvard University Press, 1991), 97. See also Lantaro Ferrer, *Historia general de la medicina en Chile,* 356–57; Cruz-Coke, *Historia de la medicina chilena,* 301; Stepan, *Beginnings of Brazilian Science,* 50–51; and Marcos Cueto, *Excelencia científica en la periferia: Actividades científicas e investigación biomédica en el Perú, 1890–1950* (Lima: Torea, 1989), 49.

18 Ross Danielson, *Cuban Medicine* (New Brunswick, N.J.: Transaction Books, 1979), 60.

19 Luz María Hernández Sáenz, "Learning to Heal: The Medical Profession in Colonial Mexico, 1767–1831" (Ph.D. diss., University of Arizona, 1993), 32.

20 See ibid., 92–93.

21 González Flores, *Historia de la influencia extranjera,* 84–87.

22 For figures on coffee exports by Brealey as well as Espinach and Giralt, see Lowell Gudmundson, *Costa Rica before Coffee: Society and Economy on the Eve of the Export Boom* (Baton Rouge: Louisiana State University Press, 1986), 164–65. On the Espinach family, see Gonzalo Chacón Trejos, *Tradiciones costarricenses* (San José: Trejos Hermanos, 1956), 109–11.

23 Frantzius, "El antiguo convento de la misión de Orosi en Cartago," 31–32.

24 *Crónica de Costa Rica,* 13 April 1859, 4.

25 See *Recuerdo del cincuagésimo aniversario de la Botica Francesa (1869–1918)* (San José: Imprenta Alsina, 1918), 11.

26 According to the fee regime established by the Protomedicato in 1858, normal consultations were to be charged at the rate of one escudo if the patient visited "the house of the doctor," and half that for a house call within the city, with repeat visits on the same day being charged at lesser rates. Visits outside the city, but within a one-mile range, were charged at one escudo, and a nighttime house call inside the city was valued at four times that. See ANCR, Congreso 5147, f. 4. Lydia Cabrera cites an official 1835 fee schedule from Cuba with similar rates in *La medicina popular de Cuba: Médicos de antaño, curanderos, santeros y paleros de hogaño* (Miami, 1984), 73.

27 See Paulina Malavassi, "Entre la marginalidad social y los orígenes de la salud

público: Leprosos, curanderos y facultativos en el valle Central de Costa Rica, 1784–1845" (master's thesis, Universidad de Costa Rica, 1998), 176–77.

28 ANCR, Congreso 5147, f. 4.

29 Fee regulations published in Cuba in 1835 stipulated that "the miserably poor should be served free, while for those who maintain themselves through their own labor and who are without fincas the fees should be reduced according to circumstance" cited in Cabrera, *Medicina popular,* 73.

30 See ANCR, Policía 4899, ff. 3, 12; and ANCR, Policía 4885, f. 1.

31 See "Ministerio General del gobierno al Rector de la Casa de Santo Tomás, 8 April 1839, ANCR, Gobernación 8,200.

32 Mexico's first hospital for lepers, the Hospital de Tlaxpana, was founded by Hernán Cortés less than a decade after the conquest of Tenochtitlán, and even San Martín de Tours in Buenos Aires dated from 1635. See Gordon Schendel, *Medicine in Mexico: From Aztec Herbs to Betatrons* (Austin: University of Texas Press, 1968), 92–96; Carlos Andrés Escudé, "Health in Buenos Aires in the Second Half of the Nineteenth Century," in *Social Welfare, 1850–1950: Australia, Argentina, and Canada Compared* (London: Macmillan Publishers Ltd., 1989), 63; Danielson, *Cuban Medicine,* 26; and A. J. R. Russell-Wood, *Fidalgos and Philanthropists: The Santa Casa de Misericordia of Bahia, 1550–1755* (Berkeley: University of California Press, 1968), 278–80.

33 See Bienvenido Ortíz Cartín, *Copilación de leyes, decretos y circulares referents a medicina e hygiene del año 1821 hasta 1920* (San José: Imprenta Nacional, 1921), 141–42.

34 Ibid., 143.

35 Alexander von Frantzius was earning the former scale while he was the town doctor of Alajuela from 1854 through 1859; Lucas Alvarado earned the latter when he was appointed to oversee an epidemic of whooping cough in Cartago in 1853. See ANCR, Policía 4897, f. 1; ANCR, Policía 5540, f. 38.

36 Juan Echeverría, "Advertencia," *Crónica de Costa Rica,* 2 February 1859, 4; and ANCR, Policía 4918, ff. 1–2.

37 See ANCR, Policía 4897, f. 1; and Ortíz Cartín, *Copilación de leyes,* 141–42.

38 See Charles E. Rosenberg, *The Care of Strangers: The Rise of America's Hospital System* (New York: Basic Books, 1987), 82–91.

39 See Iván Molina Jiménez, "Los catálogos de libros como fuentes históricas," *Revista de Filosofía de la Universidad de Costa Rica* 30, no. 71 (1992): 108–11. The strands of protoscientific culture discussed in the following pages perhaps deserve to be considered alongside the pioneering argument of Marshall C. Eakin, "The Origins of Modern Science in Costa Rica: The Instituto Físico-Geográfico Nacional, 1887–1904," *Latin American Research Review* 34, no. 1 (1999): 123–50.

40 Ortíz Cartín, *Copilación de leyes,* 177. A Brazilian Medical Association was created as early as 1829, while the American Medical Association dates from 1845. See Stepan, *Beginnings of Brazilian Science,* 50; and Rosenberg, *The Care of Strangers,* 163.

Notes to Chapter Two

41 See ANCR, Policía 5847. On yellow fever and medical theory in the 1850s, see Sidney Chalhoub, "The Politics of Disease Control: Yellow Fever and Race in Nineteenth-Century Rio de Janeiro," *Journal of Latin American Studies* 25, no. 3 (1993): 443–44.

42 See Cabezas Solera, *La medicina en Costa Rica*, 116–17.

43 See Dobles Segreda, *Medicina e higiene*, 3–4.

44 See German Tjarks, et al., "La epidemia de cólera de 1856 en el Valle Central: Análisis y consecuencias demográficas," *Revista de Historia* (Costa Rica) 3 (1978): 81–127.

45 Charles E. Rosenberg, *The Cholera Years: The United States in 1832, 1849, and 1866* (Chicago: University of Chicago Press, 1962), 152; and Donald B. Cooper, "The New 'Black Death': Cholera in Brazil, 1855–1856," in *The African Exchange: Toward a Biological History of Black People*, ed. Kenneth F. Kiple (Durham, N.C.: Duke University Press, 1988), 244, 247.

46 See ANCR, Policía 4899, f. 3. Yucca was occasionally mentioned in European accounts of American materia medica, but it was not commonly used outside the region; see John K. Crellin and Jane Philpott, *Herbal Medicine Past and Present* (Durham, N.C.: Duke University Press, 1990), 2:467–68.

47 Dobles Segreda, *Medicina e higiene*, 3–4.

48 ANCR, Policía 4965, f. 29.

49 See Martínez Durán, *Las ciencias médicas en Guatemala*, 605; Juan B. Lastres, *Historia de la medicina peruana* (Lima: Imprenta Santa Maria, 1951), 3:193; and Lycurgo de Castro Santos Filho, *História geral da medicina brasileira* (São Paulo: HUCITEC and Editora de Universidade de São Paulo, 1977–1991), 3:331–42.

50 ANCR, Policía 5540, f. 15.

51 Peard, "Tropical Disorders," 7; and John Harley Warner, "The Idea of Southern Medical Distinctiveness: Medical Knowledge and Practice in the Old South," in *Sickness and Health in America: Readings in the History of Medicine and Public Health*, ed. Judith Walzer Leavitt and Ronald R. Numbers, 2d ed. (Madison: University of Wisconsin Press, 1985), 53–70.

52 See Zeledón Cartín, *Viajes por la República de Costa Rica*, 3:11–13.

53 Frantzius, "El antiguo convento de la misión de Orosi en Cartago," 32.

54 See Cabezas Solera, *La medicina en Costa Rica*, 113. On the decline of the Guatemalan faculty, see Martínez Durán, *Las ciéncias médicas en Guatemala*, 563–66.

55 "Establecer un Protomedicato," ANCR, Congreso 5147, ff. 1–1v.

56 See Lanning, *Royal Protomedicato*, 58–91. Despite the vagaries this might encompass in the colonial American setting, there was a risk that a student who had persevered through the arduous years of medical training would be turned down for a license on the basis of suspect birth, as the unlucky orphan José Mariano Martínez Prado found out in late colonial Mexico; see Hernández Sáenz, "Learning to Heal," 25. The institution was similar to the

French colonial system of the *medicin-de-roi*. See James E. McClellan, *Colonialism and Science: Saint Domingue in the Old Regime* (Baltimore, Md.: Johns Hopkins University Press, 1992).

57   See Luz María Hernández Sáenz, *Learning to Heal: The Medical Profession in Colonial Mexico, 1767–1831* (New York: Peter Lang, 1997), 85–94.

58   For a discussion of Bourbon public health reforms in a more significant periphery, see Suzanne Austin Alchon, *Native Society and Disease in Colonial Ecuador* (Cambridge: Cambridge University Press, 1991), 112.

59   See Malavassi, "Entre la marginalidad social," 57–65; and Láchner Sandoval, "Apuntes de higiene," 193–94.

60   See Archila, *Historia de la medicina en Venezuela*, 310; Schendel, *Medicine in Mexico*, 122, 149; Danielson, *Cuban Medicine*, 60; and Peard, "Tropical Disorders," 6–7. The Spanish Protomedicato was disbanded in 1804. In imperial Brazil (1820) and colonial Cuba (1834), Royal Governing Boards of Medicine and Surgery were created to institutionalize hospital instruction in clinical medicine as part of the continuing effort to reform scholastic university programs. See also Daniel M. Fox, "Medical Institutions and the State," in *Companion Encyclopedia of the History of Medicine*, ed. W. F. Bynum and Roy Porter (London: Routledge, 1993): 1210–18.

61   See Moll, *Aesculapius in Latin America*, 99–100; Mario Flores Mescal, "Historia de la Universidad en El Salvador," *Anuario de Estudios Centroamericanos* 1 (1976): 111; Cruz-Coke, *Historia de la medicina chilena*, 308; and Lastres, *Historia de la medicina peruana*, 3:151.

62   Barber-surgeons were still being licensed at the municipal level elsewhere in Latin America at midcentury. See Archila, *Historia de la medicina en Venezuela*, 207–15; and A. J. R. Russell-Wood, *The Black Man in Slavery and Freedom in Colonial Brazil* (New York: St. Martin's Press, 1982), 57.

63   See ANCR, Congreso 5147, f. 4v.

64   See República de Costa Rica, *Censo (de 1864)*, 86–95. Eighteen men were registered under the general term "druggists" (boticarios), though only twelve were titled and fully licensed "pharmacists."

65   Danielson, *Cuban Medicine*, 21.

66   Ortíz Cartín, *Copilación de leyes*, 177.

67   See ANCR, Congreso 5147, f. 5.

68   See República de Costa Rica, *Censo (de 1864)*, 88, 91, 94–5.

69   See Juan B. Lastres, *La cultura peruana y la obra de los médicos en la emancipación* (Lima: Editorial San Marcos, 1954), 327–37.

70   Archila, *Historia de la medicina en Venezuela*, 175. The most prominent Latin American trajectory of this kind was that of the Chilean Pedro Morán. Of humble origins, he began his career in the early nineteenth century as a sixteen-year-old phlebotomist in Santiago's Hospital San Juan de Dios. He then began touring the country as an ambulatory bleeder while pursuing secondary studies and reading medical literature, and his skills and knowledge

were noticed by the physicians and surgeons of the hospital, who furthered his apprenticeship. Morán then joined the forces of a patriot general as a military surgeon and served with distinction in the wars of independence. Afterward, his physician colleagues helped him gain a surgeon's title from the Protomedicato, even though the country still had no medical school. One of the members of the tribunal tried to bar Morán's petition on the grounds that he was of impure blood (showing that this criterion, too, might survive independence), but the attempt was overcome through influential intercession on the young surgeon's behalf, and by 1833 Morán was a member of the Chilean Protomedicato and the medical school. See Lantaro Ferrer, *Historia general de la medicina en Chile*, 389–91. For similar cases in Guatemala and Colombia, see Martínez Durán, *Las ciencias médicas en Guatemala*, 608–10; and David Sowell, "Miguel Perdomo Neira: Healing, Culture, and Power in the Nineteenth-Century Andes," *Anuario Colombiano de Historia Social de la Cultura* 24 (1997): 168.

71 At Rio de Janeiro's medical school, for example, of the two thousand students enrolled between 1833 and 1843, only one hundred became licensed physicians; see Stepan, *Beginnings of Brazilian Science*, 50.

72 Cited in ANCR, Gobernación 8,200.

73 See Molina Jiménez, "Catálogos de libros como fuente," 108–16.

74 ANCR, Policía 5539, ff. 1v, 2. The process was remarkably agile: his request was granted a mere eight days after it was made.

75 ANCR, Policía 5540, f. 63.

76 ANCR, Policía 4688, ff. 1–1v.

77 See ANCR, Policía 4960; and ANCR, Policía 4631.

78 See Matthew Ramsey, *Professional and Popular Medicine in France, 1770–1830: The Social World of Medical Practice* (Cambridge: Cambridge University Press, 1988), 84–87.

79 Lastres, *La cultura peruana*, 72. For Mexico, see Hernández Sáenz, *Learning to Heal*, 235–37. On Brazil, where a license as a curandero could be acquired up until 1828, with restrictions to use only "herbs of the country," see Tânia Salgado Pimenta, "Barbeiros-sangradores e curandeiros no Brasil (1808–1828)," *Manguinhos: História, Ciencias, Saúde* 5, no. 2 (1998): 364–65.

80 See Michael M. Smith, "The 'Real Expedición Marítima de la Vacuna' in New Spain and Guatemala," *Transactions of the American Philosophical Society* 64, no. 1 (1974): 51–54; and Láchner Sandoval, "Apuntes de higiene," 193–94. For other instances of the appointment of juntas of "practical medicasters" in the face of epidemics, see Malavassi, "Entre la marginalidad social," 170.

81 ANCR, Salubridad Pública 182, f. 9v.

82 Ortíz Cartín, *Copilación de leyes*, 141–42.

83 The strategy had been common in peripheral parts of the colonies like Venezuela where, in the absence of qualified practitioners, the Crown gave to "the colored curanderos" (*curanderos pardos*) who could demonstrate talent and good conduct licenses to practice medicine and surgery "*en condición de por*

ahora" — literally, "for the time being." See Yolanda Texera Arnal, "Médicos y cirujanos pardos 'en condición de por ahora' en la provincia de Venezuela, siglo XVIII," *Colonial Latin American History Review* 8, no. 3 (1999): 321.

84 ANCR, Policía 4885, f. 1.

85 See ANCR, Policía 4899.

86 Cited in Moll, *Aesculapius in Latin America*, 25. It also mirrored the case of France, where women were excluded from the officiers de santé system; see Ramsey, *Professional and Popular Medicine*, 86.

87 See ANCR, Policía 4885, f. 1.

88 See República de Costa Rica, *Censo general de la República de Costa Rica (27 de noviembre de 1864)* (San José: Imprenta Nacional, 1868), 88–95; and Arodys Robles Soto, "Patrones de población en Costa Rica, 1860–1930," *Avances de Investigación* (Centro de Investigaciones Históricas, Universidad de Costa Rica) 14 (1986): 44.

89 Lanning, *Royal Protomedicato*, 143.

90 See República de Costa Rica, *Censo (de 1864)*, 86–95.

91 ANCR, Policía 4620, f. 2.

92 ANCR, Policía 4730, f. 6v.

93 Wilhelm Marr, "Viajes a Centroamérica," in *Costa Rica en el siglo XIX: Antología de viajeros,* ed. Ricardo Fernández Guardia (1929; reprint, San José: Editorial Universitaria Centroamericana, 1985), 174–75.

94 Ibid., 187.

95 *Nueva Era,* 16 May 1861, 4; cited in Patricia Vega Jiménez, "From Benches to Sofas: Diversification of Patterns of Consumption in San José (1857–1861)," in *The Allure of the Foreign: Imported Goods in Postcolonial Latin America*, ed. Benjamin Orlove (Ann Arbor: University of Michigan Press, 1997), 75.

96 *Crónica de Costa Rica,* 28 April 1858, 4; cited in ibid., 73.

97 *Crónica de Costa Rica,* 9 October 1858, 4; cited in ibid., 74.

98 *Nueva Era,* 17 November 1860, 4; cited in ibid., 73.

99 See, for example, Thomas Kruggeler, "Changing Consumption Patterns and Everyday Life in Two Peruvian Regions: Food, Dress, and Housing in the Central and Southern Highlands (1820–1920)," in *The Allure of the Foreign: Imported Goods in Postcolonial Latin America*, ed. Benjamin Orlove (Ann Arbor: University of Michigan Press, 1997), 55; and Patricia Fumero Vargas, "La ciudad en la aldea: Actividades y diversiones urbanas en San José a mediados del siglo XIX," in *Héroes al gusto y libros de moda: Sociedad y cambio cultural en Costa Rica (1750–1900),* ed. Iván Molina Jiménez and Steven Palmer (San José: Plumsock Mesoamerican Studies 1992), 77–106.

100 ANCR, Policía 4660, f. 3.

101 *Album Semanal,* 22 June 1858; cited in Patricia Vega Jiménez, "From Benches to Sofas: Diversification of Patterns of Consumption in San José (1857–1861)," in *The Allure of the Foreign: Imported Goods in Postcolonial Latin America*, ed. Benjamin Orlove (Ann Arbor: University of Michigan Press, 1997), 75.

102   ANCR, Policía 4660, ff. 1v, cover.
103   ANCR, Congreso 6638, f. 3.

Chapter 3. The Formation of a Biomedical Vanguard

1   The best treatment of this intellectual transformation is Charles A. Hale, "Political and Social Ideas in Latin America, 1870–1930," in vol. 4 of *The Cambridge History of Latin America*, ed. Leslie Bethell (Cambridge: Cambridge University Press, 1984–1996), 367–441.

2   On the relationship of Comte's thought to the life sciences, and particularly to the propositions of the early-nineteenth-century French physician F. J. V. Broussais, see Georges Canguilhem, *On the Normal and the Pathological* (London: D. Reidel Publishing Co., 1978), 17–28. On Barreda, see Charles A. Hale, *The Transformation of Liberalism in Late-Nineteenth-Century Mexico* (Princeton, N.J.: Princeton University Press, 1989), 140–47. On the Mexican society that included Francisco de Asís Flores y Troncoso and Porfirio Parra, see Victor M. Ruiz Naufal and Arturo Gálvez Medrano, "La *Historia de la Medicina en México* dentro de la historiografía médica mexicana," in vol. 1 of Francisco de Asis Flores y Troncoso, *Historia de la Medicina en México desde la época de los indios hasta el presente* (Mexico City: Instituto Mexicano de Seguro Social, 1982), xxviii.

3   See Roy Porter, *The Greatest Benefit to Mankind: A Medical History of Humanity from Antiquity to the Present* (London: Harper Collins, 1997), 330–33; and Francisco Guerra, *El médico político: Su influencia en la historia de Hispano-América y Filipinas* (Madrid: Afrodisio Aguado, 1975), 135–53.

4   The liberal physician head-of-state was a phenomenon peculiar to Central America. The brief tenure of Carlos Durán is eclipsed by the crucial reformist presidencies of Rafael Zaldívar in El Salvador (1876–1884) along with the positivist conservatives Adán Cárdenas and Roberto Sacasa in Nicaragua (1883–1893). More significant than all of them — and a man in dire need of a good biographer — was the Honduran Marco Aurelio Soto, who in 1871 went from medical studies at San Carlos to right-hand man and minister of everything during the formidable early reign of Guatemala's "liberal Napoleon," Justo Rufino Barrios, and then became the liberal reformist president of Honduras in the late 1870s. See Guerra, *El médico político*, 207–9.

5   Mauricio Tenorio-Trillo, *Mexico at the World's Fairs: Crafting a Modern Nation* (Berkeley: University of California Press, 1996), 151, 153.

6   Ricardo Cruz-Coke, *Historia de la medicina chilena* (Santiago: Editorial Andres Bello, 1995), 463–67.

7   Of the major Western democracies at this time, only French parliaments had a medical face, with physicians making up 10 to 12 percent of each legislature between 1870 and 1914. In Germany, Austria, Hungary, England, and the United States, their presence was miniscule, although the doctor-politician was more common in Italy, Spain, and Portugal. The reformist political strain

of medicine in Latin America has some similarities to the *zemstvo* medicine that emerged as a nationalist force for social reform in Russia at this time. See Jack D. Ellis, *The Physician-Legislators of France: Medicine and Politics in the Early Third Republic, 1870–1914* (Cambridge: Cambridge University Press, 1990), 4–6.

8 See Guerra, *El médico político*, 140–44; Cruz-Coke, *Historia de la medicina chilena*, 465; and Eduardo A. Zimmerman, *Los liberales reformistas: La cuestión social en la Argentina, 1890–1916* (Buenos Aires: Editorial Sudamericana, 1995), 102. In Mexico, Barreda made his mark as the great reformer of education, as did Rafael Villavicencio under the reformist Venezuelan dictatorship of Guzmán Blanco (himself a former medical student), while Puga Borne occupied the Chilean Ministry of Foreign Relations on three occasions.

9 See Donna J. Guy, *Sex and Danger in Buenos Aires: Prostitution, Family, and Nation in Argentina* (Lincoln: University of Nebraska Press, 1990), 77–104; Diego Armus, "Enfermedad, ambiente urbano e higiene social: Rosario entre fines del siglo XIX y comienzos del XX," in *Sectores populares y vida urbana*, ed. Diego Armus (Buenos Aires: CLACSO, 1984), 40–43; Juan César García, *Pensamiento social en salud en América Latina* (Mexico City: Interamericana McGraw Hill/ Organización Panamericana de Salud, 1994), 102–8; Zimmerman, *Los Liberales reformistas*, 101–25; and Teresa A. Meade, *"Civilizing" Rio: Reform and Resistance in a Brazilian City, 1889–1930* (University Park: Pennsylvania State University Press, 1997), 75–101.

10 On Cruz, see Nancy Leys Stepan, *Beginnings of Brazilian Science: Oswaldo Cruz, Medical Research, and Policy, 1890–1920* (New York: Science Publications, 1981). On Finlay, see Nancy Leys Stepan, "The Interplay Between Socio-economic Factors and Medical Science: Yellow Fever Research, Cuba, and the United States," *Social Studies of Science* 8 (1978): 397–424; Ross Danielson, *Cuban Medicine* (New Brunswick, N.J.: Transaction Books, 1979), 80–84; and François Delaporte, *The History of Yellow Fever: An Essay on the Birth of Tropical Medicine* (Cambridge, Mass.: MIT Press, 1991). On Freire, see Jaime Larry Benchimol, *Dos micróbios aos mosquitos: Febre amarela e a revoluçao pasteuriana no Brasil* (São Paulo: Editorial Fiocruz, 1999), 19–167.

11 See Iván Molina Jiménez and Fabrice Lehoucq, *Urnas de lo inesperado: Fraude electoral y lucha política en Costa Rica (1901–1948)* (San José: Editorial de la Universidad de Costa Rica, 1999), 148. In Peru, by comparison, 13 percent of the deputies were physicians between 1895 and 1918; see Marcos Cueto, *Excelencia científica en la periferia: Actividades científicas e investigación biomédica en la Perú, 1890–1950* (Lima: Tarea, 1989), 62.

12 Five were Cuban, five came from Central America and Colombia, three from Canada, and one or two from England, Germany, France, the United States, Spain, Ecuador, and Poland (the country's first woman physician, Jadwisa de Picado). Unfortunately, the complete list of physicians who incorporated to practice in Costa Rica during these years — contained in Luis Dobles Segreda, *Medicina e higiene*, vol. 9 of *Indice bibliográfico de Costa Rica* (San José: Imprenta

Lehmann, 1927–1936), 407–16 — gives the country of study but not of origin. The information on national origins has been pieced together from Luis Felipe González Flores, *Historia de la influencia extranjera en el desenvolvimiento educacional y científico de Costa Rica* (San José: Editorial Costa Rica, 1976); Edgar Cabezas Solera, *La medicina en Costa Rica hasta 1900* (San José: Editorial Nacional de Salud y Seguro Social, 1990); the San José municipal census of 1904, and obituaries from the *Gaceta Médica de Costa Rica* (hereafter GMCR).

13 The data on the country of study of all 195 practitioners presents a similar picture: 37 percent were graduates of European universities, 35 percent graduates of academies in the United States and Canada, and only 28 percent trained in Latin American universities. Over half of these latter had studied in Central America, but only 11 of them at San Carlos, while 15 were products of the new medical programs of San Salvador and Granada, or the older school of León.

14 The main difference between the two series is that only two of the thirty-four Costa Rican physicians had degrees from Latin America. This squares with the impressionistic evidence, but it should be kept in mind that they may be underrepresented by the simple fact that those who studied in Central America were not likely to occupy leading positions in the profession on their return, and so would have left fewer marks on the historical record.

15 Two Canadians, two Guatemalans, a Nicaraguan, a Colombian, two Frenchmen, and a Spaniard.

16 See "El Censo Municipal de San José, 1904," Centro de Investigaciones Históricas de América Central; and Dobles Segreda, *Medicina e higiene*, 407–16. The place of study of one physician is not listed.

17 See "Censo, 1904." Unfortunately, there is no good social history of the cafetalero caste of late-nineteenth-century Costa Rica. For an innovative social history of the cafetalero oligarchs of the late nineteenth and early twentieth centuries, see Florencia Quesada Avendaño, *En el Barrio Amón: Arquitectura, familia y sociabilidad del primer residencial de la elite urbana de San José, 1900–1935* (San José: Editorial de la Universidad de Costa Rica, 2001). On Mauro Fernández, see Astrid Fischel, *Consenso y represión: Una interpretación socio-política de la educación costarricense* (San José: Editorial Costa Rica, 1987), 115–33.

18 For brief biographies of Durán, see Carlos Pupo Pérez, *Nuestros males: Principios sanitarios que nadie debe ignorar*, 2d ed. (San José: Tipografía Nacional, 1936), 145–66; and Cabezas Solera, *La medicina en Costa Rica*, 121. For the surgical context, see Ulrich Tröhler, "Surgery (Modern)," in *Companion Encyclopedia of the History of Medicine*, ed. W. F. Bynum and Roy Porter (London: Routledge, 1993), 2:988–90. On Howse's influence at Guy's in the early 1870s, see H. C. Cameron, *Mr. Guy's Hospital* (London: Longman, 1954), 197, 250.

19 On Nightingale's influence on hospital reform and the general debate over antisepsis, see Guenter B. Risse, *Mending Bodies, Saving Souls: A History of Hospitals* (New York: Oxford University Press, 1999), 366–78. See also Porter, *Greatest Benefit*, 375.

20 Pupo Pérez, *Nuestros males,* 149; and Carlos Eduardo González Pacheco, *Hospital San Juan de Dios: 150 años de historia* (San José: Editorial Nacional del Seguro Social, 1995), 67. González Pacheco has Andres Sáenz as the attending surgeon, and the story may be an urban physician's legend that evolved to dramatize the surgical "dark ages" that Durán heroically fought; as pointed out in chapter 2, anesthesia was commonly used in Latin America soon after its first use in 1846.

21 Vicente Láchner Sandoval, "Apuntes de higiene pública: Organismos' institutos y profesiones en relación con este ramo," *Revista de Costa Rica en el Siglo XIX* (San José: Imprenta Nacional, 1902), 205. On Johns Hopkins, see Risse, *Mending Bodies,* 403–4.

22 See Cabezas Solera, *La medicina en Costa Rica,* 187; González Pacheco, *Hospital San Juan de Dios,* 66–67; and Tröhler, "Surgery," 993.

23 For example, in Guatemala, it is Juan J. Ortega, who returned from medical training in Paris 1882 to complete a thorough reform of hospital surgery. In Chile, Manuel Barros Borgoño is the Durán figure, studying in France in the mid-1870s under disciples of Lister, then returning to introduce antisepsis and modern hospital methods. See Carlos Martínez Durán, *Las ciencias médicas en Guatemala: Orígen y evolución,* 3d ed. (Guatemala City: Editorial Universitaria, 1964), 649–55; and Cruz-Coke, *Historia de la medicina chilena,* 467–69.

24 On the Olympian reformers of the 1880s and their confrontation with a Church-backed opposition, see Patricia Badilla Gómez, "Ideología y derecho: El espíritu mesiánico de la reforma jurídica costarricense (1882–1888)," *Revista de Historia* (Costa Rica), no. 18 (January–June, 1988): 187–202; Claudio Antonio Vargas Arias, *El liberalismo, la Iglesia y el Estado en Costa Rica* (San José: Guayacán, 1991); and Steven Palmer, "A Liberal Discipline: Inventing Nations in Costa Rica and Guatemala, 1870–1900," Ph.D. diss., Columbia University, 1990.

25 See Paulino Villalobos González, *La Universidad de Santo Tomás* (San José: Editorial de la Universidad de Costa Rica, 1989), 90; Dobles Segreda, *Medicina e higiene,* 400; and González Pacheco, *Hospital San Juan de Dios,* 68.

26 See Manuel Aguilar Bonilla, "Centenario de la primera revista médica de Costa Rica," *Acta Médica Costarricense,* special issue (1982): 27–38. González, *Universidad de Santo Tomás,* 90; and GMCR 1, no. 1 (1896): 4.

27 See GMCR 1, no. 3 (1896): 91; GMCR 5, no. 5 (1900): 116; and Norman Howard Jones, *The Pan-American Health Organization: Origins and Evolution* (Geneva: World Health Organization, 1981), 8–13.

28 See Gerardo Jiménez and Enrique Jiménez, *Higiene de las habitaciones y del agua en Costa Rica* (San José: Tipografía Nacional, 1902); and Benjamín de Cespedes, *Higiene de la infancia* (San José: Tipografía Nacional, 1900).

29 The Ley de Profilaxis Venérea is reprinted in Bienvenido Ortíz Cartín, *Copilación de leyes, decretos y circulaires referentes a medicina e higiene del año 1821 hasta 1920* (San José: Tipografía Nacional, 1924), 174–76.

30 See ibid., 143–47. Juan José Marín Hernández, "Prostitución y pecado en la

bella y próspera ciudad de San José," *El paso del cometa: Estado, política social y culturas populares en Costa Rica (1870–1950)*, ed. Iván Molina Jiménez and Steven Palmer (San José: Plumsock Mesoamerican Studies, 1994), 69–71. On the increasingly dense grid of public power projected over the country between 1880 to 1910, see José Daniel Gil Zúñiga, "Delito y control social en la provincia de Heredia, 1885–1941" (paper presented at the symposium Las sociedades centroamericanas siglos XIX y XX, San José, 1990.

31 *GMCR* 1, no. 1 (21 October 1880): 2; and Anguilar Bonilla, "Centenario de la primera revista médica de Costa Rica," 27–38.

32 On the number of practicing physicians at this time, see República de Costa Rica, *Censo de la República de Costa Rica* [1883] (n.p., n.d.), 85.

33 According to P. W. J. Bartrip, Lister's interventions in the *British Medical Journal* in 1879–1880 made these "decisive years in the history of Listerism" (*Mirror of Medicine: A History of the British Medical Journal* (Oxford: British Medical Journal and Clarendon Press, 1990), 134; and on Lister's important association with the *Journal* during this period more generally, 125–36. The translated article appeared as Joseph Lister, "Observaciones sobre los micro-organismos y sus relaciones con las enfermedades," *La Gaceta Médica* I (2) 31 May 1881, 32–36. Lister's original appeared in the *British Medical Journal* on 4 September 1880.

34 An excellent, but not complete list of journals can be found in Aristides A. Moll, *Aesculapius in Latin America* (Philadelphia, Pa.: W. B. Saunders Company, 1944), 404–5. See also Nancy Leys Stepan, *Beginnings of Brazilian Society: Oswaldo Cruz, Medical Research, and Policy, 1890–1920* (New York: Science History Publications, 1981), 51; Julyan G. Peard, "Tropical Disorders and the Forging of a Brazilian Medical Identity, 1860–1890," *Hispanic American Historical Review* 77, no. 1 (1997): 10; and Ross Danielson, *Cuban Medicine* (New Brunswick, N.J.: Transaction Books, 1979), 72.

35 See "Solicitud del cuerpo médico de la República para que se reforme el Reglamento del Protomedicato," Archivos Nacionales de Costa Rica, Congreso 3374.

36 The critique is from Vicente Láchner Sandoval, "Apuntes de higiene pública: Organismos, institutos y profesiones en relación con este ramo," in *Revista de Costa Rica en el siglo XIX* (San José: Imprenta Nacional, 1902), 217.

37 See *GMCR* 14, no. 5 (1910): 80.

38 See *GMCR* 4, no. 1 (1899): 13–14.

39 See *GMCR*, 1, no. 5 (1896): 141.

40 On this issue, see González Villalobos, *La Universidad de Santo Tomás*, 212–37; Fischel, *Consenso y repression*, 155–83; and Astrid Fischel, *El uso ingenioso de la ideología en Costa Rica* (San José: Editorial Universidad Estatal a Distancia, 1992), 61–64.

41 Marcos Cueto, "Nacionalismo y ciencias médicas: Los inicios de la investigación biomédica en el Perú, 1900–1950," *Quipu* 4, no. 3 (1987): 328. See also Zimmerman, *Los liberales reformistas*, 101; Moll, *Aesculapius in Latin America*, 245–47; and Ronn F. Pineo, "Misery and Death in the Pearl of the Pacific:

Health Care in Guayaquil Ecuador, 1870–1925," *Hispanic American Historical Review* 70, no. 4 (1990): 621.

42   See Moll, *Aesculapius in Latin America,* 102.

43   See Ronn F. Pineo, *Social and Economic Reform in Ecuador: Life and Work in Guayaquil* (Gainesville: University Press of Florida, 1996), 112; Danielson, *Cuban Medicine,* 70.

44   Gilberto Freyre, *Order and Progress: Brazil from Monarchy to Republic* (Berkeley: University of California Press, 1986), 124; cited in Peard, "Tropical Disorders," 8.

45   Dain Borges, *The Family in Bahia, Brazil, 1870–1945* (Stanford, Calif.: Stanford University Press, 1992), 87, 88.

46   Cueto, "Nacionalismo y ciencias médicas," 328.

47   See Miguel J. C. de Asua, "Influencia de la Facultad de Medicina de París sobre la de Buenos Aires," *Quipu* 3, no. 1 (1986): 79–89.

48   See Pineo, *Social and Economic Reform,* 112; and Asua, "Influencia de la Facultad de Medicina de París," 81.

49   See Jaime Benchinol, ed., *Marguinos do sonho à vida* (Rio de Janeiro: Fiocruz, 1990); and Stepan, *Beginnings of Brazilian Science.*

50   See Stepan, *Beginnings of Brazilian Science,* 85–91; Fabián de Jesús Díaz, *Vida e historia de la medicina en la provincia* (Valencia, Venezuela: Secretaría de Educación y Cultura, 1966), 31; and Cueto, "Nacionalismo y ciencias médicas," 328–31.

51   See Pineo, "Misery and Death," 621; República de Costa Rica, *Censo general de la República de Costa Rica (27 de noviembre de 1864)* (San José: Imprenta Nacional, 1868), 91, 94–95 (the total number of "doctors" in the 1864 census is thirty-eight, but the figure almost certainly includes some licensed empirics). The 1914 figures come from the Rockefeller Foundation Archives, record group 5, Series 1, Box 7, Folder 103.

52   See Cueto, *Excelencia científica,* 49, 64.

53   Julyan G. Peard, *Race, Place, and Medicine: The Idea of the Tropics in Nineteenth-Century Brazil* (Durham, N.C.: Duke University Press, 1999), 169–70. See also Stepan, *Beginnings of Brazilian Science,* 50–51.

54   See Guy, *Sex and Danger,* 94; GMCR 7, no. 4 (1903): 98; and Borges, *The Family in Bahia,* 92.

55   Peard, "Tropical Disorders," 8.

56   GMCR 3, no. 9 (1899): 136; and GMCR 3, no. 12 (1899): 194–202. On the academy effort, see GMCR 3, no. 12 (1899): 187–89.

57   On the total number of publications, which is probably not complete, see Dobles Segreda, *Medicina e higiene,* 8–91.

58   GMCR 3, no. 12 (1899): 194–202.

59   Cueto, "Nacionalismo y ciencias médicas": 334.

60   "Breves datos históricos sobre los análisis clínicos en Costa Rica," *Revista Médica* (Costa Rica) 1, no. 67 (1934): 139.

61   The story has been pieced together from three sources, which although conflicting on minor points, add up to this portrait of the discovery: Gerardo

Jiménez Nuñez, "El cansancio: Notas para contribuir al estudio de esa enfermedad en Costa Rica," GMCR 5, no. 8 (1901): 206–7; Pupo Pérez, *Nuestros males*, 154–57; and Solón Núñez, "La Ankylostomiasis," *Boletín de la Subsecretaría de Higiene y Salud Pública* 1, no. 1 (May 1923): 11–15.

62 On Perroncito's discovery, see John Ettling, *The Germ of Laziness: Rockefeller Philanthropy and Public Health in the New South* (Cambridge: Harvard University Press, 1981), 25–26.

63 See Núñez, "La Ankylostomiasis," 12; and Peard, "Tropical Disorders," 18.

64 Ettling, *Germ of Laziness*, 24–25.

65 See Ettling, *Germ of Laziness*, 31–33.

66 Peard, "Tropical Disorders," 10.

*Chapter 4. Conventional Practice: New Science,
Old Art, and Persistent Heterogeneity*

1 Carlos Durán, "Algunas observaciones sobre la difteria y su tratamiento por la antitoxina," *Gaceta Médica de Costa Rica* (hereafter GMCR) 2, no. 4 (1897): 57.

2 Debórah Dwork, "Childhood," in *Companion Encyclopedia of the History of Medicine*, ed. W. F. Bynum and Roy Porter (London: Routledge, 1993), 1082–83; and Ross Danielson, *Cuban Medicine* (New Brunswick, N.J.: Transaction Books, 1979), 72.

3 See Luis Dobles Segreda, *Medicina e higiene*, vol. 9 of *Indice bibliográfico de Costa Rica* (San José: Imprenta Lehmann, 1927–1936), 411–15.

4 Vicente Láchner Sandoval, "Apuntes de higiene pública: Organismos, institutos y profesiones en relación con este ramo," in *Revista de Costa Rica en el siglo XIX* (San José: Imprenta Nacional, 1902), 217. One of Costa Rica's first novels has among its principal characters the Cuban "physician" Oscar González. Originally from a rural part of Havana province, González is named to a district physician post on the frontiers of the Central Valley in 1897. He is portrayed as a cheat, liar, charlatan, and an all-around cad who soaks the townspeople, deflowers the town's most precious young virgin, and then abandons the girl and the area to settle into a comfortable life in San José. See Joaquín García Monge, *Abnegación* (San José: Imprenta de Padrón Pujol, 1902), esp. 27, 71–72.

5 See Arodys Robles Soto, "Patrones de población en Costa Rica, 1860–1930," *Avances de Investigación* (Centro de Investigaciones Históricas, Universidad de Costa Rica) 14 (1986): 44.

6 Borges, *The Family in Bahia, Brazil, 1870–1945* (Stanford, Calif.: Stanford University Press, 1992), 87; Peard, "Tropical Disorders," 8.

7 Dain Borges, *The Family in Bahia, Brazil, 1870–1945*, 88; and Julyan G. Peard, "Tropical Disorders and the Forging of a Brazilian Medical Identity, 1860–1890," *Hispanic American Historical Review* 77, no. 1 (1997): 7–8. See also Danielson, *Cuban Medicine*, 73.

8 See GMCR 1, no. 3 (1896): 82; and GMCR 5, no. 8 (1901): 201–3.

9   See Luis Felipe González Flores, *Historia de la influencia extranjera en el desen-volvimiento educacional y científico de Costa Rica* (San José: Editorial Costa Rica, 1976), 71; GMCR 1, no. 4 (1896): 122–34; GMCR 1, no. 5 (1896): 164–73; "Un nuevo parásito intestinal en Costa Rica," GMCR 4, no. 10 (1900): 251–52; and Láchner Sandoval, "Apuntes de higiene," 217.

10   See Centro de Investigaciones Históricas de América Central, "El Censo Municipal de San José, 1904."

11   Rockefeller Foundation Archives (hereafter RFA), "Henry Carter to Ernst Meyer," record group 5, series 1.2, box 6, folder 96, Rockefeller Archive Center, North Tarrytown, N.Y., 3.

12   See Aristides A. Moll, *Aesculapius in Latin America* (Philadelphia, Pa.: W. B. Saunders Company, 1944), 138.

13   See "Rasgos biográficos del Dr. don José María Jiménez Oreamuno," GMCR 2, no. 2 (1897): 104.

14   On Flores, see GMCR 7, no. 2 (1902): 59. On Céspedes's sanitary code, see GMCR 7, no. 1 (1902): 3.

15   See GMCR 4, no. 5 (1899): 167; Centro de Investigaciones Históricas, "Censo, 1904"; and Dobles Segreda, *Medicina e higiene*, 411–15.

16   GMCR 4, no. 11 (1900): 266. The calculation has been made by comparing Dobles Segreda's index of place of study of incorporated physicians with the names of those reporting as district physicians in the 1899 volumes of the official newsheet, *La Gaceta*. An index of these reports can be found in *Indice de las publicaciones contenidas en "La Gaceta" oficial de 1899,* first semester, second semester.

17   For an example of the board's stalling tactics, see GMCR 1, no. 2 (1896): 27–28; and Láchner Sandoval, "Apuntes de higiene," 217.

18   See GMCR 4, no. 12 (1900): 296–97. His 1898 Montpellier thesis on the treatment of tuberculosis is cited in Dobles Segreda, *Medicina e higiene*, 14.

19   Carlos Durán, "Algunas observaciones," 56–61. The locations of the physicians' offices have been assembled from the *Directorio comercial de San José, 1898* (San José: Imprenta Greñas, 1898), 9–77.

20   Antonio Giustiniani, "La fiebre amarilla," GMCR 4, no. 1 (1899): 14–15. See Stanley Joel Reiser, "The Science of Diagnosis: Diagnostic Technology," in *Companion Encyclopedia of the History of Medicine*, ed. W. F. Bynum and Roy Porter (London: Routledge, 1993), 2:834–39.

21   César Borja, "Memorias Clínicas," GMCR 1, no. 3 (1896): 96.

22   See GMCR 5, no. 10 (1901): 259–60.

23   Luis Ros Pochet, "Estudio crítico de los casos ginecológicos ocurridos en mi práctica en esta República," GMCR 1, no. 10 (1897): 299.

24   José María Soto Alfaro, "Hidroamnios hidrocéfalo," GMCR 1, no. 1 (1896): 5.

25   Carlos Pupo Pérez, "Notas sobre algunos casos de fiebre puerperal y su tratamiento," GMCR 8, no. 7 (1904): 103.

26   See GMCR 5, no. 10 (1901): 260.

27   Ros Pochet, "Estudio crítico," 305; "El Dr. Rafael Angel Calderón Guardia,"

Revista Médica (Costa Rica) 5, no. 110 (1943): 473; and Dobles Segreda, *Medicina e higiene,* 11–13.

28 See González Flores, *Historia de la influencia extranjera,* 95. A prickly obituary of Bansen can be found in *GMCR* 6, no. 6 (1902): 120–21.

29 RFA, "Carter to Meyer," 3.

30 Paulina Malavassi, "Entre la marginalidad social y los orígenes de la salud pública: Leprosos, curanderos y facultativos en el valle Central de Costa Rica, 1784–1845" (master's thesis, Universidad de Costa Rica, 1998), 131–65.

31 See Carlos Eduardo González Pacheco, *Hospital San Juan de Dios: 150 años de historia* (San José: Editorial Nacional del Seguro Social, 1995), 48.

32 Guenter B. Risse, *Mending Bodies, Saving Souls: A History of Hospitals* (New York: Oxford University Press, 1999), 5. To give an example of such "miniaturization," whereas Buenos Aires at this time saw the creation of its first hospitals for the different foreign communities and others for children, Costa Rica's San Juan de Dios acquired separate pavilions for foreigners and children within the same hospital complex.

33 See Carlos Andrés Escudé, "Health in Buenos Aires in the Second Half of the Nineteenth Century," in *Social Welfare, 1850–1950: Australia, Argentina, and Canada Compared,* ed. D. C. M. Platt (London: Macmillan Publishers Ltd., 1989), 60–70.

34 See González Pacheco, *Hospital San Juan de Dios,* 49, 69.

35 Ibid., 66–99.

36 Ibid., 117–19.

37 Ibid., 118.

38 See "Informe del Hospital San Juan de Dios a la Junta de Caridad, 1895," *GMCR* 1, no. 3 (1896): 78–85; and González Pacheco, *Hospital San Juan de Dios,* 140.

39 Láchner Sandoval, "Apuntes de higiene," 205.

40 Cited in "Informe del Hospital San Juan de Dios a la Junta de Caridad, 1902," *GMCR* 7, no. 10 (1903): 268–74.

41 See George Palmer Putnam, *The Southland of North America: Rambles and Observations in Central America during the Year 1912* (New York: G. P. Putnam and Sons, 1913), 27.

42 See Láchner Sandoval, "Apuntes de higiene," 205–6; and Trino Echavarría Campos, *Historia y geografía del Cantón de San Ramón* (San José: Imprenta Nacional, 1966), 26.

43 See Aviva Chomsky, *West Indian Workers and the United Fruit Company in Costa Rica, 1870–1940* (Baton Rouge: Louisiana State University Press, 1996), 89–109.

44 See *GMCR* 5, no. 6 (1901): 154.

45 For Limón in 1875, see Archivos Nacionales de Costa Rica (hereafter ANCR), Policía 5532, 5533; for Naranjo in 1895, see ANCR, Policía 514; and for Escazú in 1902, see ANCR, Policía 840.

46 See ANCR, Policía 1308, ff. 1–2. For a similar case in Grecia in 1896, see ANCR, Policía 3757.

47 ANCR, Policía 5091, f. 2v. For more on the same incident, see ANCR, Policía
    5279.

48 See Departamento Nacional de Estadísticos, *Resumenes estadísticos, 1883–1893*
    (San José: Tipografía Nacional, 1895), 97; and *GMCR* 5, no. 6 (1901): 154.

49 Láchner Sandoval, "Apuntes de higiene," 194–95. For birth statistics, see
    Robles Soto, "Patrones de población," 45.

50 See Teresa A. Meade, *"Civilizing" Rio: Reform and Resistance in a Brazilian
    City, 1889–1930* (University Park: Pennsylvania State University Press, 1997),
    104–5.

51 Sidney Chalhoub, *Cidade febril: Cortiços e epidemias na Corte imperial* (Rio de
    Janeiro: Companha das letras, 1996), 97–163; Jeffrey Needell, "The *Revolta
    Contra Vacina* of 1904: The Revolt against 'Modernization' in Belle-Epoque Rio
    de Janeiro," *Hispanic American Historical Review* 67, no. 2 (1987): 244; Nancy
    Leys Stepan, *Beginnings of Brazilian Science: Oswaldo Cruz, Medical Research, and
    Policy, 1890–1920* (New York: Science History Publications, 1981); 51; and
    Carl J. Murdock, "Physicians, the State, and Public Health in Chile, 1881–
    1891," *Journal of Latin American Studies* 27 (1995): 557.

52 See Ricardo Campos Marín, "Vacunadores en Guerra: La lucha por el monop-
    olio profesional de la vacunación antivariólica en España, 1870–1900" (paper
    presented at the Symposium on Practices of Healing in Latin America and
    Spain, New York University, April 2001). A critical view of vaccination can be
    found in David Arnold, "Smallpox and Colonial Medicine in Nineteenth-
    Century India," in *Imperial Medicine and Indigenous Societies,* ed. David Arnold
    (Manchester: Manchester University Press, 1988), 54–55. See also Juan José
    Marín Hernández, "De curanderos a médicos: Una aproximación a la historia
    de la medicina en Costa Rica, 1800–1949," *Revista de Historia* (Costa Rica) 32
    (1995): 70–72.

53 See Stepan, *Beginnings of Brazilian Science,* 90; and Murdock, "Physicians, the
    State, and Public Health in Chile," 553.

54 See Láchner Sandoval, "Apuntes de higiene," 195.

55 See ANCR, Policía 956.

56 See, for example, the report of Miguel Dobles, the district physician in Barba,
    in *GMCR* 11, no. 1 (1904): 6.

57 See *Indice de las publicaciones contenidas en la Gaceta, año de 1908,* first semester.
    On salaries, see Carlos Luis Fallas Monge, *El movimiento obrero en Costa Rica,
    1830–1902* (San José: Editorial Universidad Estatal a Distancia, 1983), 338–
    39.

58 Two were unknown. Again, the data are based on a comparison of Dobles
    Segreda's list of the country of study of physicians who incorporated in the
    faculty, with district physician reports from the official paper. See *Indice de las
    publicaciones contenidas en la Gaceta, año de 1908,* first semester.

59 A list of state salaries can be found in ibid.

60 See Steven Palmer, "Getting to Know the Unknown Soldier: Official National-
    ism in Liberal Costa Rica, 1880–1900," *Journal of Latin American Studies* 25

Notes to Chapter Four

(1993): 45–72; Alvaro Quesada Soto, *La formación de la narrativa nacional costarricense (1890–1910): Enfoque histórico-social* (San José: Editorial de la Universidad de Costa Rica, 1986), 91–132; and Flora Ovares et al., *La casa paterna: Escritura y nación en Costa Rica* (San José: Editorial de la Universidad de Costa Rica, 1993), 51–87.

61 See Robert Darnton, "Workers Revolt: The Great Cat Massacre of the Rue Saint-Séverin," in *The Great Cat Massacre and Other Episodes in French Cultural History*, ed. Robert Darnton (New York: Vintage Books, 1985), 88 n. 21.

62 *GMCR* 14, no. 2 (1909): 21–22.

63 Carlos Pupo Pérez, "Notas sobre algunos casos de fiebre puerperal," *GMCR* 8, no. 7 (1904): 99–104, and *GMCR* 8, no. 8 (1904): 125–30.

64 See *Indice de la Gaceta, año de 1908*.

65 See *GMCR* 14, no. 16 (1910): 182; and Chomsky, *West Indian Workers*, 89–109.

66 Putnam, *The Southland of North America*, 18.

67 Ibid., 27, 29.

68 RFA, "Carter to Meyer, record group 5, series 1.2, box 6, folder 96, 2–3.

69 Jaime Benchimol, *Dos micróbios aos mosquitos: Febre amarela e a revoluçao pasteuriana no Brasil* (Rio de Janeiro: Editorial Fiocruz, 1999), 299–344.

70 González Leandri, *Curar, persuadir, gobernar*, 51.

71 Marcos Cueto, "Indigenismo and Rural Medicine in Peru: The Indian Sanitary Brigade and Manuel Núñez Butrón," *Bulletin of the History of Medicine* 65 (1991): 41, 34.

Chapter 5. Other Healers: Survival, Revival, and Public Endorsement

1 Vicente Láchner Sandoval, "Apuntes de higiene pública: Organismos, institutos y profesiones en relación con este ramo," in *Revista de Costa Rica en el siglo XIX* (San José: Imprenta Nacional, 1902), 216.

2 See Gonzalo González González, "Algunos datos sobre historia de la farmacia y la medicina en Costa Rica," *Revista de la Universidad de Costa Rica* 1 (September 1945): 67; and República de Costa Rica, *Censo general de la República de Costa Rica* (1892) (San José: Tipografía Nacional, 1893), lxxxix. This preponderance of foreigners, and particularly Frenchmen, in the pharmaceutical profession was also typical of late-nineteenth-century Brazil; see Lycurgo de Castro Santos Filho, *História geral da medicina brasileira* (São Paulo: Editoria de Universidade de São Paulo, 1977–1991), 2:372.

3 See Grace Aguilar, "Colegio de farmacéuticos de Costa Rica, 1902–1996," in *Centenario de la Facultad de Farmacia*, ed. Patricia Fumero Vargas (San José: Editorial de la Universidad de Costa Rica, 1997), 57–59.

4 See González González, "Algunos datos," 67–68; and Aguilar, "Colegio de farmacéuticos," 57–64.

5 Juan Gómez A., "José C. Zeledón," in *Homenaje a don José C. Zeledón* (San José: Imprenta Trejos Hermanos, 1924), 69, 68–73; Fausto Coto Montero, *Home-*

naje a doña Amparo de Zeledón (San José: Imprenta Nacional, 1951); and *Recuerdo del cincuagésimo aniversario de la Botica Francesa (1868–1918)* (San José: Imprenta Alsina, 1918), 11–41.

6 For an analysis of a particularly extreme war between the two groups over who was responsible for the spreading addiction to heroin among young male artisans in San José in 1929, see Steven Palmer, "Pánico en San José: El consumo de heroína, la cultura plebeya y la política social en 1929," in *El paso del cometa: Estado, política social y culturas populares en Costa Rica (1800–1950)*, ed. Iván Molina Jiménez and Steven Palmer (San José: Plumsock Mesoamerican Studies, 1994), 193–201.

7 See República de Costa Rica, *Censo (1892)*, xciii; and Edgar Cabezas Solera, *La medicina en Costa Rica hasta 1900* (San José: Editorial Nacional de Salud y Seguro Social, 1990), 140.

8 Cited in *Directorio comercial de San José, 1898* (San José: Imprenta Greñas, 1898), 1.

9 *La Prensa Libre*, 26 June 1995, 3.

10 Martin Kaufman, "Homeopathy in America: The Rise and Fall and Persistence of a Medical Heresy," in *Other Healers: Unorthodox Medicine in America*, ed. Norman Gevitz (Baltimore, Md.: Johns Hopkins University Press, 1988), 99.

11 Ibid.

12 See Norman Gevitz, "Unorthodox Medical Theories," in *Companion Encyclopedia of the History of Medicine*, ed. W. F. Bynum and Roy Porter (London: Routledge, 1993), 604–7.

13 See David Sowell, "Miguel Perdomo Neira: Healing, Culture, and Power in the Nineteenth-Century Andes," *Anuario Colombiano de Historia Social y de la Cultura* 24 (1997): 175.

14 In Chile and Mexico, it was introduced by Spanish practitioners in the 1850s; Cuba had a journal of homeopathy between 1856 and 1858, and Argentina and Colombia saw virulent disputes between regulars and homeopaths in the 1860s. See Santos Filho, *História geral*, 2:388–95; and Aristides A. Moll, *Aesculapius in Latin America* (Philadelphia, Pa.: W. B. Saunders Company, 1944), 472.

15 See Carlos Hernández Rodríguez, "Herbolarios, empíricos y farmacéuticos: Contribución a la historia de la farmacia en Costa Rica," in *Centenario de la Facultad de Farmacia, Universidad de Costa Rica, 1897–1997*, ed. Patricia Fumero (San José: Editorial de la Universidad de Costa Rica, 1998), 131; and German Tjarks et al., "La epidemia de cólera de 1856 en el Valle Central: Análisis y consecuencias demográficas," *Revista de Historia* (Costa Rica) 3 (1978): 122.

16 See *GMCR* 4, no. 7 (1900): 204; Santos Filho, *História geral*, 2:395; and Francisco de Asis Flores y Troncoso, *Historia de la Medicina en México desde la época de los indios hasta el presente* (1886–1888; reprint, Mexico City: Instituto Mexicano de Seguro Social, 1982), 2:278–79. In Brazil, the government even approved the creation of a chair in homeopathy at the Rio Faculty of Medicine, only to back down when many on the faculty threatened to resign.

17 Gregorio Quesada, *La homeopatía en Costa Rica* (San José: Imprenta de Avelino Alsina, 1905), 3, 38–40; and Genaro Peralta F., *Guía-directorio la ciudad de San José, 1905* (San José: Imprenta de Antonio Lehmann, 1905), 81.

18 See Carmel Goldwater, "Traditional Medicine in Latin America," in *Traditional Medicine and Health Care Coverage: A Reader for Health Care Administrators and Practitioners,* ed. Robert H. Bannerman et al. (Geneva: World Health Organization, 1983), 46–47. See also David J. Hess, *Spirits and Scientists: Ideology, Spiritism, and Brazilian Culture* (University Park, Pa.: Penn State University Press, 1991), 201–10.

19 Similar currents in spiritism, traceable to Kardec's influence among Latin American elites in the mid–nineteenth century, have been documented in Puerto Rico and Mexico. See Joan D. Koss, "Religion and Science Divinely Related: A Case History of Spiritism in Puerto Rico," *Caribbean Studies* 16, no. 1 (April 1976): 23–43; and Kaja Finkler, *Spiritualist Healers in Mexico: Success and Failure of Alternative Therapeutics* (New York: Praeger, 1985), 19–20. In Mexico, the first famous cases of spiritism had strong Catholic expressions, particularly the touring trance healer Roque Rojas and Damiana Oviedo, who was declared the incarnation of Christ and founded a number of healing temples; see Isabel Lagarriga Attias, *Medicina tradicional y espiritismo: Los espiritualistas trinitarios marianos de Jalapa, Veracruz* (Mexico City: Sociedad de Estudios Paranormales, 1975), 23–26.

20 Roberto Brenes Mesén, *El misticismo como instrumento de la investigación de la verdad* (San José: Repertorio Americano, 1921). On Brenes Mesén's publications and his tenure at the Colegio de Señoritas, see Constantino Láscaris, *Desarrollo de las ideas en Costa Rica,* 2d ed. (San José: Editorial Costa Rica, 1975), 423–26. On his role in Costa Rica's "Scopes' Trial," a 1907 scandal over the teaching of evolutionism in the public schools that pitted modernists like Brenes Mesén against Catholic ideologues, see Iván Molina Jiménez, *La ciudad de los monos: Roberto Brenes Mesén, los católicos heredianos y el conflicto cultural de 1907 en Costa Rica* (San José: Editorial de la Universidad de Costa Rica, 2001).

21 Cited in Archivos Nacionales de Costa Rica (hereafter ANCR), Policía 5541, ff. 46–v.

22 ANCR, Policía 5541, ff. 2–v.

23 See Trino Echavarría Campos, *Historia y geografía del Cantón de San Ramón* (San José: Imprenta Nacional, 1966), 26.

24 See ANCR, Policía 3494, ff. 3, 5.

25 See ANCR, Policía 3387.

26 See ANCR, Policía 2262.

27 See Steven Palmer, "Prolegómenos a toda futura historia de San José, Costa Rica," *Mesoamérica* 31 (1996): 210–13.

28 See ANCR, Policía 3637. Thanks to Patricia Alvarenga for bringing this document to my attention.

29 For a common male healer who displayed similar tendencies, see the case of Nicomedes Sáenz, ANCR, Policía 3480.

30 See ANCR, Policía 1605, ff. 1–3v, 22.

31 See ANCR, Policía 3185, ff. 1–1v, 8, 14–14v.

32 See Joseph W. Bastien, *Healers of the Andes: Kallawaya Herbalists and Their Medicinal Plants* (Salt Lake City: University of Utah Press, 1987), 21–24.

33 On the Guatusos, see Marc Edelman, "A Central American Genocide: Rubber, Slavery, Nationalism, and the Destruction of the Guatusos-Malekus," *Comparative Studies in Society and History* 40, no. 2 (1998): 356–90.

34 William M. Gabb, "On the Indian Tribes and Languages of Costa Rica," *Proceedings of the American Philosophical Society* 14 (1875): 483–601; and Alanson Skinner, "Notes on the Bribri of Costa Rica," *Indian Notes and Monographs* 6, no. 3 (1920): 44.

35 Doris Stone, *Los tribus talamanqueños de Costa Rica* (San José: Editorial Antonio Lehmann, 1961), 93–107.

36 Jeffrey Casey Gaspar, "El ferrocarril al Atlántico en Costa Rica, 1871–74," *Anuario de Estudios Centroamericanos* (Costa Rica) 2 (1976): 318–27.

37 Miguel Angel Sabater Reyes, "Los primeros médicos chinos en Cuba," *Boletín del Archivo Nacional* (Cuba), no. 11 (1988): 23–29.

38 Cited in *Diario de Costa Rica*, 12 June 1925, 4.

39 See Arodys Robles Soto, "Patrones de población en Costa Rica, 1860–1930," *Avances de Investigación* (Centro de Investigaciones Históricas, Universidad de Costa Rica) 14 (1986): 13; and Aviva Chomsky, *West Indian Workers and the United Fruit Company in Costa Rica, 1870–1940* (Baton Rouge: Louisiana State University Press, 1996), 34.

40 See Richard B. Sheridan, *Doctors and Slaves: A Medical and Demographic History of Slavery in the British West Indies, 1680–1834* (Cambridge: Cambridge University Press, 1985), 79.

41 See Carmen Murillo Chaverri, *Identidades de hierro y humo: La construcción del ferrocarril al Atlántico, 1870–1890* (San José: Editorial Porvenir, 1995), 125.

42 Chomsky, *West Indian Workers*, 191–93.

43 Cited in ANCR, Gobernación 2660, ff. 5–5v.

44 Ibid., ff. 19, 17.

45 See ANCR, Policía 3637.

46 See ANCR, Policía 1605.

47 ANCR, Policía 4730.

48 See Moll, *Aesculapius in Latin America*, 87.

49 Sowell, "Miguel Perdomo Neira," 169–70. Notably, despite the deregulated medical environment of Colombia in the 1870s, the Perdomo Neira tumult erupted when the popular healer decided to challenge physicians and surgeons in their capital city stronghold. A similar dynamic is visible in the last-minute commutation by wiser Spanish authorities of a death sentence handed down by a military court against Má Dolores, a popular Cuban *santera* of the 1870s accused of being an independence conspirator; see Lydia Cabrera, *La medicina popular de Cuba: Médicos de antaño, curanderos, santeros y paleros de hogaño* (Miami, 1984), 140–41.

Notes to Chapter Five

50 Domingos José Goncalves de Magalhães, "Uprising in Maranhão," in *The Brazil Reader: History, Culture, Politics,* ed. Robert M. Levine and John J. Crocitti (Durham, N.C.: Duke University Press, 1999), 72. On Tomochí, see Friedrich Katz, *The Life and Times of Pancho Villa* (Stanford, Calif.: Stanford University Press, 1995), 21–27. On Canudos and Contestado, see Todd A. Diacon, *Millenarian Vision, Capitalist Reality: Brazil's Contestado Rebellion, 1912–1916* (Durham, N.C.: Duke University Press, 1991), 1–3.

51 See ANCR, Policía 4721, f. 1v; ANCR, Policía, 5419, ff. 1–2; ANCR, Policía 5534, and ANCR, Policía 5167, f. 1.

52 See Láchner Sandoval, "Apuntes de higiene," 217; and Cabezas Solera, *La medicina en Costa Rica,* 187.

53 See, for example, the case of Rafael Avila in ANCR, Policía 1801.

54 Láchner Sandoval, "Apuntes de higiene," 217.

55 Ross Danielson, *Cuban Medicine* (New Brunswick, N.J.: Transaction Books, 1979), 73.

56 Cited in República de Costa Rica, "Informe de la Subsecretaría de Policía, higiene y salud pública," in *Memoria de Gobernación y Policía correspondiente al año 1923* (San José: Imprenta Nacional, 1924), 265. Ricardo González Leandri has noted a similar dynamic impeding the realization of a functional professional medical monopoly in the Argentine provinces during the second half of the nineteenth century *Curar, persuadir, gobernar: La construcción histórica de la profesión médica en Buenos Aires, 1852–1886* (Madrid: Consejo Superior de Investigaciones Científicas-Centro de Estudios Históricos, 1999), 47–55.

57 Benjamín de Céspedes, *Higiene de la infancia* (San José: Tipografía Nacional, 1900), 8, 233–34.

Chapter 6. Midwives of the Republic

1 "Lord have mercy, Christ have mercy, God the Father of Heaven have mercy on us." The description is from Luisa González, *A ras del suelo,* 9th ed. (San José: Editorial Costa Rica, 1989), 42–43.

2 A recent anthropological study of the transformation of childbirth after a state training program for empirical midwives in Costa Rica in the 1960s supposes that this was the origin of the introduction of a biomedical model of pregnancy and birthing in rural areas. Gwynne L. Jenkins, "Changing Roles and Identities of Midwives in Rural Costa Rica," *Medical Anthropology* 20 (2001): 409–44.

3 Fine and provocative explorations of this theme can be found in Susan K. Besse, *Restructuring Patriarchy: The Modernization of Gender Inequality in Brazil, 1914–1940* (Chapel Hill: University of North Carolina Press, 1996); and Alexandra Minna Stern, "Reasonable Mothers and Normal Children: Eugenics, Nationalism, and Welfare in Post-revolutionary Mexico, 1920–1940," *Journal of Historical Sociology* 12, no. 4 (1999): 369–97.

4 Archivo General de la Nación (Mexico City), Protomedicato, 3:16; cited in John Tate Lanning, *The Royal Protomedicato: The Regulation of the Professions in the*

Spanish Empire, ed. John Jay TePaske (Durham, N.C.: Duke University Press, 1985), 303.

5   Luz María Hernández Sáenz, "Learning to Heal: The Medical Profession in Colonial Mexico, 1767–1831" (Ph.D. diss., University of Arizona, 1993), 372–57. Sandra Orellana claims that in the indigenous highlands of colonial Guatemala, midwifery was probably a calling—that women had epiphanies that led them to devote themselves to the art *Indian Medicine in Highland Guatemala: The Pre-Hispanic and Colonial Periods* (Albuquerque: University of New Mexico Press, 1987), 70–71.

6   Informe del Dr. José Antonio Ríos, Santiago, 8 July 1790; cited in Lanning, *Royal Protomedicato,* 305–6. On the other hand, of the twenty-four women who practiced midwifery in early-nineteenth-century Mexico City, eight were *españolas,* five were *castas,* and eleven were *indias;* see Hernández Sáenz, "Learning to Heal," 370.

7   See Archivos Nacionales de Costa Rica (hereafter ANCR), Juzgado Civil y del Crimen, Guanacaste, expediente 597, f. 1; cited in Eugenia Rodríguez Sáenz, " 'Tiyita, bea lo que me han echo': Estupro e incesto en Costa Rica (1800–1850)," in *El paso del cometa: Estado, política social y culturas populares en Costa Rica (1800–1950),* ed. Iván Molina Jiménez and Steven Palmer (San José: Plumsock Mesoamerican Studies, 1994), 29. See also Carlos Martínez Durán, *Las ciencias médicas en Guatemala: Orígen y evolución,* 3d ed. (Guatemala City: Editorial Universitaria, 1964), 464.

8   See Lycurgo de Castro Santos Filho, *História geral de medicina brasileira* (São Paulo: Editora de Universidade de São Paulo, 1977–1991), 2:329; Juan B. Lastres, *Historia de la medicina peruana* (Lima: Imprenta Santa María, 1951), 3:170, 187; and Lanning, *Royal Protomedicato,* 306.

9   See Irvine S. L. Loudon, "Childbirth," in *Companion Encyclopedia of the History of Medicine,* ed. W. F. Bynum and Roy Porter (London: Routledge, 1993), 1051; Richard B. Sheridan, *Doctors and Slaves: A Medical and Demographic History of Slavery in the British West Indies, 1680–1834* (Cambridge: Cambridge University Press, 1985), 299; and Ricardo Archila, *Historia de la medicina en Venezuela* (Mérida, Mexico: Universidad de los Andes, 1966), 76.

10 See Edgar Cabezas Solera, *La medicina en Costa Rica hasta 1900* (San José: Editorial Nacional de Salud y Seguro Social, 1990), 140; Aristides A. Moll, *Aesculapius in Latin America* (Philadelphia, Pa.: W. B. Saunders Company, 1944), 340; and Vicente Láchner Sandoval, "Apuntes de higiene pública: Organismos, institutos y profesiones en relación con este ramo," in *Revista de Costa Rica en el siglo XIX* (San José: Imprenta Nacional, 1902), 222.

11 See Santos Filho, *Historia geral,* 1:231; and Lastres, *Historia de la medicina peruana,* 3:186.

12 Silvia Marina Arrom, *The Women of Mexico City, 1790–1857* (Stanford, Calif.: Stanford University Press, 1985), 198. For examples of increased schooling under the supervision of titled foreign midwives in other parts of Latin America, see Santos Filho, *Historia geral,* 2:327–28; Lanning, *Royal Protomedicato,*

309–20; Hernández Sáenz, "Learning to Heal," 360–61; Moll, *Aesculapius in Latin America*, 106; and Pedro Lantaro Ferrer, *Historia general de la medicina en Chile* (Talca, Chile: Imprenta Talca, 1904), 356–57.

13 Judith Walzer Leavitt, *Brought to Bed: Childbearing in America, 1750–1950* (New York: Oxford University Press, 1986), 36–63.

14 See Martínez Durán, *Las ciencias médicas en Guatemala*, 444; Lanning, *Royal Protomedicato*, 318–20; Francisco de Asis Flores y Troncoso, *Historia de la Medicina en México desde la época de los indios hasta el presente* (1886–1888; reprint, Mexico City: Instituto Mexicano de Seguro Social, 1982), 2:401; and Santos Filho, *Historia geral*, 1:231.

15 See Leavitt, *Brought to Bed*, 117–27; and Santos Filho, *Historia geral*, 2:330.

16 República de Costa Rica, *Censo general de la República de Costa Rica (27 de noviembre de 1864)* (San José: Imprenta Nacional, 1868), 89.

17 González, *A rás del suelo*, 44–45. In the 1920s in Brazil, Dain Borges reports that postparturients might take a special infusion of herbs in wine and broth (*The Family in Bahia, Brazil, 1870–1945* [Stanford, Calif.: Stanford University Press, 1992], 75).

18 See *Gaceta Médica de Costa Rica* (hereafter GMCR) 5, no. 10 (1901): 259; and Carlos Pupo Pérez, "Notas sobre algunos casos de fiebre puerperal," GMCR 8, no. 7 (1904): 103.

19 González, *A ras del suelo*, 34.

20 Ibid., 34–35.

21 The town of Escazú, a former Indian village on the outskirts of San José, was famous for its concentration of women sorcerers, and well into the 1920s was known as the residence of clandestine witches who were called on to heal or make ill. See Abelardo Bonilla, "Rumbo a Escazú," *Diario de Costa Rica*, 1 May 1929, illustrated supplement, 5–7. For an extended catalog of such sorcery in the Peruvian context, see Hermilio Valdizán and Angel Maldonado, *La medicina popular peruana: Contribución al "folk-lore" médico del Perú* (Lima: Imprenta Torres Aguirre, 1922), 1:129–242.

22 Julyan G. Peard has documented a similar perception of ideological challenge among doctors in Bahia at about this time in *Race, Place, and Medicine: The Idea of the Tropics in Nineteenth-Century Brazilian Medicine* (Durham, N.C.: Duke University Press, 1999), 117–23.

23 See Láchner Sandoval, "Apuntes de higiene," 218.

24 Cited in GMCR 5, no. 10 (1901): 260.

25 Loudon, "Childbirth," 1054.

26 See Robert A. Nye, *Crime, Madness, and Politics in Modern France: The Medical Concept of National Decline* (Princeton, N.J.: Princeton University Press, 1984), 132–69; and Allan M. Brandt, *No Magic Bullet: A Social History of Venereal Disease in the United States since 1880* (New York: Oxford University Press, 1987), 7–8.

27 See República de Costa Rica, *Memoria de Gobernación y Policía correspondiente a los años de 1907 y 1908* (San José: Imprenta Nacional, 1909), lxvii. For other

prominent examples of this anxiety, see República de Costa Rica, *Memoria de Gobernación, Policía y Fomento, 1902–1903* (San José: Tipografía Nacional, 1903), xli–xlii; and Carlos Pupo Pérez, *Nuestras enfermedades evitables: Principios de higiene que nadie debe ignorar* (San José: Imprenta Alsina, 1913), 21.

28 See Héctor Pérez Brignoli, "El crecimiento demográfico de América Latina en los siglos XIX y XX: Problemas, métodos y perspectiva," *Avances de Investigación* (Centro de Investigaciones Históricas, Universidad de Costa Rica) 48 (1989): 12–14.

29 See Arodys Robles Soto, "Patrones de población en Costa Rica, 1860–1930," *Avances de Investigación* (Centro de Investigaciones Históricas, Universidad de Costa Rica) 14 (1986), 13.

30 See Bienvenido Ortíz Cartín, *Copilación de leyes, decretos y circulares referentes a medicina e higiene del año 1821 hasta 1920* (San José: Tipografía Nacional, 1924), 99.

31 Donna J. Guy, *Sex and Danger in Buenos Aires: Prostitution, Family, and Nation in Argentina* (Lincoln: University of Nebraska Press, 1990), 85; and Brandt, *No Magic Bullet*, 31–32.

32 Cited in "Mensaje del Señor Presidente de la República presentado al Congreso Constitucional, 1908," in *Mensajes presidenciales, 1896–1916,* ed. Carlos Meléndez Chaverri (San José: Academia de Geografía e Historia, 1983), 41. See also "Mensaje del Presidente de la República al Congreso Constitucional (1929)," in *Mensajes presidenciales, 1928–1940* (San José: Academia de Geografía e Historia, 1987), 31.

33 The eugenic sublation of Alberdi was not unique to Costa Rica. It was explicitly articulated in 1931 by Gonzalo Bosch, a prominent Argentine psychiatrist and one of the founders of the Argentine League of Mental Health: "Alberdi would say: To Govern is to Populate, a concept typical of his era; we, today, would say: To Govern is to Select" (cited in Mariano Ben Plotkin, "Freud, Politics, and the Portenos: The Reception of Psychoanalysis in Buenos Aires, 1910–1943," *Hispanic American Historical Review* 77, no. 1 (1997): 51.

34 See Angela Acuña de Chacón, *La mujer costarricense a través de cuatro siglos* (San José: Imprenta Nacional, 1969–1970), 1:275–77; and Francisco J. Rucavado, "Reseña sobre los trabajos realizados por la Facultad de Medicina de Costa Rica," GMCR 4, no. 6 (1900): 180.

35 Benjamín de Céspedes, *Higiene de la infancia* (San José: Tipografía Nacional, 1900), 7.

36 See "Discurso del Dr. F. J. Rucavado," GMCR 5, no. 4 (1900): 71; and GMCR 5, no. 7 (1902), 139.

37 Cited in ANCR, Municipal 9407.

38 Cited in ANCR, Municipal 4361. For other candidates, see ANCR, Municipal 4360.

39 See GMCR 6, no. 7 (1902): 139.

40 See GMCR 8, no. 1 (1902): 4. On the normal school students and fellowships, see Steven Palmer and Gladys Rojas Chaves, "Educating Señorita: Teacher

Training, Social Mobility, and the Birth of Costa Rican Feminism," *Hispanic American Historical Review* 78, no. 1 (1998): 62–70.

41 See *GMCR* 12, no. 6 (1908): 153.

42 Cited in ANCR, Policía, 514, f. 1v.

43 Francisco J. Rucavado, *Lecciones del Primero y del Segundo Curso: Escuela de Obstetricia de Costa Rica* (San José: Tipografía Nacional, 1903). On the faculty discussions, see *GMCR* 6, no. 5 (1901): 106. On the prophysician orientation of the school, see also *Reglamento de la Escuela de Obstetricia de la Facultad de Medicina de la República de Costa Rica* (San José: Imprenta María v. de Lines, 1907), 14.

44 See *GMCR* 7, no. 4 (1903): 102–4.

45 Cited in *GMCR* 6, no. 7 (1902): 139. On the number of students, see *GMCR* 7, no. 4 (1903): 83.

46 *GMCR* 7, no. 2 (1902): 27–30.

47 "Nuestros métodos para amamantar al niño," *GMCR* 8, no. 1 (1902): 4–8.

48 Ibid., 4.

49 Cited in *GMCR* 7, no. 6 (1903): 179; and *GMCR* 7, no. 7 (1903): 190.

50 For Villalobos's figures, see "Informe del trabajo," ANCR, Municipal 3260. In 1909, 131 women were attended in the Maternidad, almost all of them from the capital; see *GMCR* 9, no. 4 (1910): 57. On the number of births in San José in that year, see Robles Soto, "Patrones de población," 45.

51 See Tulio von Bulow, "Apuntes para la historia de la medicina en Costa Rica durante la colonia (4a parte)," *Revista de los Archivos Nacionales* (Costa Rica) 9, nos. 11–12 (1945): 577. The cost of the textbook is from *GMCR* 6, no. 5 (1901): 106.

52 On these projects, see Steven Palmer, "Adiós *laissez-faire:* La política social en Costa Rica, 1880–1940," *Revista de Historia de América* 124 (1999): 99–117; *La Gota de Leche: Memoria relativa a la actuación del año 1913–1914* (San José: Tipografía Nacional, n.d.).

53 Anne-Emanuelle Birn has proposed that the traditional parteras retrained by the Rockefeller Foundation in Mexico in the late 1920s and 1930s subsequently lost much of their authority within the community. Another study of the African American "granny midwives" of the U.S. South, retrained and licensed by county health departments in the 1920s, claims the opposite: that their new secular license was easily combined with the mandate from the supreme authority that they had acquired on the day they got the "call" and that the combination augmented their prestige. Something similar is asserted in a study of Hispanic midwives trained in New Mexico in the 1940s. Although the midwives considered here do not belong in the same category (other than the first graduating class of three elderly widows), it is worth noting that biomedical training did not necessarily lead to a loss of a midwife's stature in the eyes of birthing women. Anne-Emanuelle Birn, "A Revolution in Rural Health? The Struggle over Local Health Units in Mexico, 1928–1940," *Journal of the History of Medicine* 53, no. 1 (January 1998): 58–59; Beatrice Bell

Mongeau, "The 'Granny' Midwives: A Study of a Folk Institution in the Process of Social Disintegration" (Ph.D. diss., University of North Carolina, 1973), 44–48; and Fran Leeper Buss, *La Partera: Story of a Midwife* (Ann Arbor: University of Michigan Press, 1980), 118.

54 Kristin Ruggiero, "Honor, Maternity, and the Disciplining of Women: Infanticide in Late-Nineteenth-Century Buenos Aires," *Hispanic American Historical Review* 72, no. 3 (1992): 353–73. Ruggiero's contention seems to rest on the fact that pregnant women who committed infanticide had evaded midwives at the moment of giving birth and hid their subsequent act from them—the questionable implication being that infanticide would have been considered a legitimate act within authentically autonomous women's networks.

55 Celia Davies, "The Health Visitor as Mother's Friend: A Woman's Place in Public Health, 1900–1914," *Social History of Medicine* 1, no. 1 (April 1988): 39–59; and Leavitt, *Brought to Bed*, 3–12.

56 Seth Koven and Sonya Michel, "Womenly Duties: Maternalist Politics and the Origins of the Welfare State in France, Germany, Great Britain, and the United States, 1880–1920," *American Historical Review* 95, no. 4 (1990): 1107.

57 See Palmer and Rojas, "Educating Señorita," 76–81.

58 Mario Samper, ed. *El censo de población de 1927: Creación de una base nominal computarizada* (San José: Oficina de Publicáciones de la Universidad de Costa Rica, 1991), 82.

59 See *GMCR* 13, no. 8 (1909): 468; *GMCR* 15, no. 7 (1911): 49; Carlos Eduardo González Pacheco, *Hospital San Juan de Dios: 150 años de historia* (San José: Editorial Nacional del Seguro Social, 1995), 135–38; and Escuela de Enfermería y Obstetricia del Colegio de Médicos y Cirujanos Anexa al Hospital San Juan de Dios, *Graduación 1947–1948* (San José: Imprenta Nacional, 1949). Some forty years later than Florence Nightingale's pioneering efforts at St. Bartholomew's in London, Costa Rica's School of Nursing was near the front of the Latin American pack: the first school was established in 1897 under the direction of Argentina's first woman physician, Cecilia Grierson, with other schools following in Havana (under the United States Army in 1899), Montevideo (1904–1911), Peru (1910–1913), Bolivia and Brazil (1917), Ecuador (1927), and Paraguay (1929); see Brian A. Smith, *A History of the Nursing Profession* (London: Heinemann, 1960), 23–27; and Moll, *Aesculapius in Latin America*, 346–48.

60 Created in 1930, its first boards of directors included the philanthropist, leading pharmaceutical merchant, and curandera Amparo de Zeledón, as well as the educator of radical political persuasion María Isabel Carvajal (more famous as a writer under the pseudonym Carmen Lyra); Carvajal soon resigned, and by 1933 the entire eight-person directorate was male, most prominent among them the politically influential Luis Felipe González Flores and the physician Mario Luján; see República de Costa Rica, "Informe del Presidente del Patronato Nacional de la Infancia," *Memoria de Gobernación, Policía, Trabajo y Previsión Social correspondiente al año 1932* (San José: Imprenta Nacional,

1934), 183; and *Patronato Nacional de la Infancia: 10 años de labor, 1930–1940* (San José: n.p., n.d.).

Chapter 7. Hookworm Disease and the Popularization of Biomedical Practice

1   Juan José Ulloa Giralt, *Algunas observaciones sobre la tosferina* (San José: Imprenta Nacional, 1898): cited in Luis Dobles Segreda, *Medicina e higiene*, vol. 9 of *Índice bibliográfico de Costa Rica* (San José: Imprenta Lehmann, 1927–1936), 15–16.

2   "A District Laboratory in Costa Rica," Rockefeller Foundation Archives (hereafter RFA), record group 5, series 2, box 29, folder 176, Rockefeller Archive Center, North Tarrytown, New York.

3   By quickly accepting the Rockefeller Foundation's offer to establish a hookworm mission under the purview of their government, Costa Rica became, in April 1914, the first Latin American country to agree to collaborate with the newly created Rockefeller Foundation, the international arm of Rockefeller philanthropy.

4   Among the earlier generation of studies working from a cultural imperialist or dependency theory perspective, see Edward H. Berman, *The Influence of the Carnegie, Ford, and Rockefeller Foundations on American Foreign Policy: The Ideology of Philanthropy* (Albany: State University of New York Press, 1983), E. Richard Brown, *Rockefeller Medicine Men: Medicine and Capitalism in America* (Berkeley: University of California Press, 1979); and Soma Hewa, "The Hookworm Epidemic on the Plantations in Colonial Sri Lanka," *Medical History* 38, no. 1 (1994): 167–83. Studies that broke the mold through more dynamic readings of the foundation's relations with host countries are Mary Brown Bullock, *An American Transplant: The Rockefeller Foundation and Peking Union Medical College* (Berkeley: University of California Press, 1980); John Ettling, *Germ of Laziness: Rockefeller Philanthropy and Public Health in the New South* (Cambridge: Harvard University Press, 1981); Marcos Cueto, ed., *Missionaries of Science: The Rockefeller Foundation in Latin America* (Bloomington: Indiana University Press, 1994); and Anne-Emanuelle Birn, "A Revolution in Rural Health? The Struggle over Local Health Units in Mexico, 1928–1940," *Journal of the History of Medicine* 53, no. 1 (January 1998): 43–76. See also Christian Brannstrom, "Polluted Soil, Polluted Souls: The Rockefeller Hookworm Eradication Campaign in São Paulo, Brazil, 1917–1926," *Historical Geography* 25 (1997): 25–45.

5   See chapter 3; and Christopher Abel, "External Philanthropy and Domestic Change in Colombian Health Care: The Role of the Rockefeller Foundation, ca. 1920–1950," *Hispanic American Historical Review* 75, no. 3, 351.

6   See Ettling, *Germ of Laziness*, 189.

7   Belisário Penna began a Brazilian initiative to treat hookworm in late 1917, while other Rockefeller projects were already underway in Brazil; on the ambitious scope of Penna's campaign against hookworm disease, see the superb study of Gilberto Hochman, *A era do saneamento: As bases da política de saúde pública no Brasil* (São Paulo: Editora Hucitec, 1998), 71–79. See also Nísia

Trinidade Lima and Narra Britto, "Salud y nación: Propuesta para el saneamiento rural. Un estudio de la revista *Saúde* (1918–1919)," in *Salud, cultura y sociedad en América Latina,* ed. Marcos Cueto (Lima: Instituto de Estudios Peruanos, 1966), 141; and Abel, "External Philanthropy," 351.

8 See Ettling, *Germ of Laziness,* 203; and John Farley, "Parasites and the Germ Theory of Disease," in *Framing Disease: Studies in Cultural History,* ed. Charles Rosenberg and Janet Golden (New Brunswick, N.J.: Rutgers University Press, 1992), 33–49.

9 See Andrew Cunningham, "Transforming Plague: The Laboratory and the Identity of Infectious Diseases," in *The Laboratory Revolution in Medicine,* ed. Andrew Cunningham and Perry Williams (Cambridge: Cambridge University Press, 1992).

10 See Ettling, *Germ of Laziness,* 22–25.

11 Juan César García, *Pensamiento social en salud en América Latina* (Mexico City: Interamericana McGraw Hill/Organización Panamericana de Salud, 1994), 112–13.

12 Marcos Cueto, "Nacionalismo y ciencias médicas: Los inicios de la investigación biomédica en el Perú, 1900–1950," *Quipu* 4, no. 3 (1987): 330.

13 See Marshall C. Eakin, "The Origins of Modern Science in Costa Rica: The Instituto Físico-Geográfico Nacional, 1887–1904," *Latin American Research Review* 34, no. 1 (1999): 134.

14 Abel, "External Philanthropy," 351.

15 Gerardo Jiménez, "El cansancio," 205; and Mauro Fernández, *La anquilostomiasis y la agricultura* (San José: Imprenta de Avelino Alsina, 1907), 5–9.

16 Facultad de Medicina to Ministro de Gobernación y Policía, 17 August 1907, Archivos Nacionales de Costa Rica (hereafter ANCR), Policía 1907.

17 See *Gaceta Médica de Costa Rica* (hereafter GMCR), xii, no. 2 (1908), 128–29.

18 See Steven Palmer, "Confinement, Policing, and the Emergence of Social Policy in Costa Rica, 1885–1935," in *The Birth of the Penitentiary in Latin America: Essays on Criminology, Prison Reform, and Social Control, 1830–1940,* ed. Carlos Aguirre and Ricardo Salvatore (Austin: University of Texas Press, 1996), 224–53; and Dobles Segreda, *Medicina e higiene,* 78.

19 In 1902, he was named to an emergency health commission established to combat a smallpox outbreak in the Ipis region of San José province; in 1904, he drew up a proposal to create a tuberculosis sanatorium; and in 1907, he was sent to serve as official monitor of an outbreak of typhoid in Grecia. See Dobles Segreda, *Medicina e higiene,* 393; GMCR 6, no. 9 (1902): 173; and GMCR 11, no. 11 (1907): 210–12.

20 See "Informe," *Gaceta Oficial,* 27 October 1908, 477–79.

21 Jiménez, "El cansancio," 205.

22 There was no agreed-on distinction between the two states—something that was often fudged in order to justify hookworm crusading in areas that might not have needed to be "cured" on purely medical grounds; see Ettling, *Germ of Laziness,* 3–4, 210.

Notes to Chapter Seven

281

23   See *GMCR* 12, no. 11 (1908): 345–46.

24   See *GMCR* 14, no. 2 (1909): 21–22.

25   See "Informe presentado por la delegación de la República de Costa Rica," *Actas de la Cuarta Conferencia Sanitaria Internacional de las Repúblicas Americanas* (Washington, D.C.: Unión Panamericana, 1910), 133.

26   See "Láchner a Policía," 13 September 1911, ANCR, Policía 5969; "Durán to Gobernación," 25 September 1911, ANCR, Policía 5969.

27   See ANCR, Policía 5969.

28   See "Jiménez to White," 1914, RFA, record group 5, series 1.2, box 6, folder 87.

29   "Médico de Pueblo de San Mateo a Gobernación," 5 March 1911, ANCR, Policía 5969; and "Jiménez to Gobernación," 9 March 1911, ANCR, Policía 5969.

30   "Láchner to Gobernación," 13 September 1911, ANCR, Policía 5969; and "Durán to Gobernación," 25 September 1911, ANCR, Policía 5969. See also ANCR, Policía 4627, ff. 6–6v.

31   ANCR, Policía 4627, ff. 1–3.

32   See "Hookworm Campaign in Costa Rica," RFA, record group 5, series 2, box 28, folder 168, 1; and "Jiménez to White," 28 May 1914, RFA, record group 5, series 1.2, box 6, folder 87, 3–4.

33   "Chacón to Policía," 26 July 1911, ANCR, Policía 5969.

34   "Jiménez to White," 28 May 1914, RFA, record group 5, series 1.2, box 6, folder 87, 4.

35   "Jiménez to White," 28 May 1914, RFA, record group 5, series 1.2, box 6, folder 87, 1.

36   "Carter to White," 27 July 1914, RFA, record group 5, series 1.2, box 6, folder 96; and "White to Rose," 25 May 1914, RFA, record group 5, series 1.2, box 6, folder 87, 2.

37   Ettling, *Germ of Laziness,* 168; on Stiles's fate, 200–2.

38   "Rose to White," 5 October 1914, 10 October 1914, RFA, record group 5, series 1.2, box 6, folder 88; and Luis Felipe González Flores, *Historia de la influencia extranjera en el desenvolvimiento educacional y científico de Costa Rica* (San José: Editorial Costa Rica, 1976), 160.

39   Judith Walzer Leavitt, *The Healthiest City: Milwaukee and the Politics of Health Reform* (Princeton, N.J.: Princeton University Press, 1982).

40   Gerardo Morales, *Cultura oligárquica y nueva intelectualidad en Costa Rica, 1880–1914* (San José: Editorial de la Universidad Autónoma, 1993), 146–74.

41   For a basic biography and a selection of his writings, see Juan Bautista Frutos Verdesia, *Dr. Solón Núñez Frutos* (San José: Ministerio de Cultura, Juventud y Deportes, 1979). On the importance of his youthful anarchism, see Alvaro Quesada Soto, *La voz desgarrada: La crisis del discurso oligárquico y la narrativa costarricense (1917–1919)* (San José: Editorial de la Universidad de Costa Rica, 1988), 167–68.

42   For defenses of Schapiro by Núñez, see República de Costa Rica, *Memoria de Salubridad Pública y Protección Social correspondiente al año 1927* (San José: Im-

prenta Nacional, 1928), xi; and República de Costa Rica, *Memoria de la Secretaría de Salubridad Pública y Protección Social correspondiente a los años de 1930–1931* (San José: Imprenta Nacional, 1932), 8.

43 Lynn Marie Morgan, *Community Participation in Health: The Politics of Primary Care in Costa Rica* (New York: Cambridge University Press, 1993), 18–19, 83; and E. Richard Brown, "Public Health and Imperialism: Early Rockefeller Programs at Home and Abroad," *American Journal of Public Health* 66, no. 9 (September 1976): 900.

44 "Schapiro to Ferrell," 8 July 1915, RFA, record group 5, series 1.2, box 7, folder 107. For a good overview of the manner in which the campaign was undertaken, see República de Costa Rica, "Informe de la Subsecretaría de Higiene y Salubridad Pública," in *Memoria de Gobernación y Policía correspondiente al año 1923* (San José: Imprenta Nacional, 1924), 257–81.

45 "Carter to Ferrell," 3 December 1914, RFA, record group 5, series 1.2, box 7, folder 104. See also Ettling, *Germ of Laziness*, 158–67.

46 See "Hookworm Campaign in Costa Rica," RFA, record group 5, series 2, box 28, folder 168, 5.

47 See República de Costa Rica, "Informe annual del Departamento de Anky-lostomiasis, 1919," in *Memorias de Gobernación y Policía, 1919* (San José: Imprenta Nacional, 1920), 220.

48 For examples of each from the campaign in the Canton of Jiménez in 1917, see ANCR, 6475, ff. 119–24.

49 "Conferencia con las autoridades y personas influyentes de la localidad," RFA, record group 5, series 2, box 29, folder 175.

50 "Schapiro to Rose," 30 September 1915, RFA, record group 5, series 1, box 7, folder 107.

51 "Schapiro to Rose," 22 May 1916, RFA, record group 5, series 1.2, box 29, folder 451.

52 See Ettling, *Germ of Laziness*, 157.

53 On the tradition, see Francisco Enríquez, "Diversión pública y sociabilidad en las comunidades cafetaleras de San José: El caso de Moravia (1890–1930)" (master's thesis, University of Costa Rica, 1998).

54 "Schapiro to Ferrell," 4 August 1917, RFA, record group 5, series 1.2, box 29, folder 702. On the inauguration of lab in San Rafael de Heredia that drew an enthusiastic gathering of one thousand, see "Schapiro to Ferrell," 30 July 1918, RFA, record group 5, series 1.2, box 63, folder 912.

55 República de Costa Rica, "Informe, 1919," 223. On the magic lanterns used in the canton of Jiménez in Cartago in 1917, see ANCR, 6475, folio 113. For a picture of a lecture audience outside of an unidentified parish church, with some 150 people all decked out in their best clothes, see "Report on Work for the Relief and Control of Hookworm Disease in Costa Rica, from December 23, 1914, to December 31, 1919," RFA, record group 5, series 2, box 28, folder 169, 15.

56 República de Costa Rica, "Departamento de Ankylostomiasis: Informe narrativo anual," in *Memorias de Gobernación y Policía, 1921* (San José: Imprenta Nacional, 1922), 274.

57 Ibid., 274.

58 República de Costa Rica, "Departamento de Ankylostomiasis," in *Memorias de Gobernación y Policía, 1922* (San José: Imprenta Nacional, 1923), 232–33.

59 "Relief and Control of Hookworm Disease in Costa Rica, 1914–1919," 17; and República de Costa Rica, "Informe anual del Departamento de Ankylostomiasis," *Memorias de Gobernación y Policía, año 1920* (San José: Imprenta Nacional, 1921); "Informe 1920," 268.

60 See ANCR, 6475, f. 28, Base de datos, censo de 1927. Thanks to Iván Molina Jiménez for this information.

61 *Instrucciones para la construcción de excusados* (San José: Tipografía Nacional, 1916); in RFA, record group 5, series 1, box 29, folder 450.

62 On the extent of literacy in Costa Rica, see Iván Molina Jiménez, "Clase, género y etnia van a la escuela: El aflabetismo en Costa Rica y Nicaragua (1880–1950)," in *Educando a Costa Rica: Alfabetización popular, formación docente y género (1880–1950),* ed. Iván Molina Jiménez and Steven Palmer (San José: Editorial Porvenir and Plumsock Mesoamerican Studies, 2000), 27–43.

63 See "Informe Anual, 1917," ANCR, Policía 6475, f. 30.

64 See República de Costa Rica, "Informe, 1919," 221.

65 See "Report on Work for the Relief and Control of Hookworm Disease," 8. This technique changed in 1921 to one single dose since it made it more likely that people would turn up at the lab; see República de Costa Rica, "Departamento de Ankylostomiasis [1921]," 229.

66 Cited in República de Costa Rica, "Informe, 1920," 268.

67 Cited in "A District Laboratory in Costa Rica," RFA, record group 5, series 2, box 29, folder 176.

68 Cited in "Schapiro to Rose," 21 September 1916, RFA, record group 5, series 1.2, box 29, folder 452.

69 Cited in República de Costa Rica, "Departamento de Ankylostomiasis [1921]," 229.

70 On syrup and castor oil supplements, see República de Costa Rica, "Informe, 1919," 221.

71 See Charles E. Rosenberg, *The Cholera Years: The United States in 1832, 1849, and 1866* (Chicago: University of Chicago Press, 1962), 66–67.

72 Cited in República de Costa Rica, "Informe, 1919," 220–21.

73 Cited in "Report on Work for the Relief and Control of Hookworm Disease," 13.

74 Ibid., 6.

75 Ibid., 24.

76 Cited in República de Costa Rica, "Informe, 1919," 220.

77 Ibid.

78 See "Schapiro to Ferrell," 26 February 1915, RFA, record group 5, series 1.2, box 27, folder 105.

79 Cited in "Report on Work for the Relief and Control of Hookworm Disease," 15.

80 See República de Costa Rica, "Departamento de Ankylostomiasis [1921]," 269, 272–73.

81 See República de Costa Rica, "Departamento de Ankylostomiasis [1922]," 233.

82 Cited in República de Costa Rica, "Subsecretaría de Policía, Higiene y Salud Pública," in *Memoria de Gobernación y Policía correspondiente al año 1923* (San José: Imprenta Nacional, 1924), 261; and República de Costa Rica, "Departamento de Ankylostomiasis [1921]," 231.

83 In 1919, Schapiro explained that "if at the termination of a reasonable period the householder has failed to provide himself with suitable latrine accommodation, a written police order is issued compelling him to make such provision. Recourse to coercion is had, however, only after every means of persuasion has failed" "Report on Work for the Relief and Control of Hookworm Disease," 17.

84 Cited in "Informe Anual, 1917."

85 Cited in República de Costa Rica, "Departamento de Ankylostomiasis [1922]," 231. See also "Informe, 1920," 274.

86 See Steven Palmer and Gladys Rojas Chares, "Educating Señorita: Teacher Training, Social Mobility, and the Birth of Costa Rican Feminism," *Hispanic American Historical Review* 78, no. 1 (1998): 70–76.

87 Cited in República de Costa Rica, 274.

88 See "Departamento de Ankylostomiasis [1921]," 232.

89 Ibid., 233.

90 "Letter to Physicians," 6 May 1915, RFA, record group 5, series 1, box 7, folder 106.

91 Cited in ANCR, Policía 6475, f. 27.

92 Cited in República de Costa Rica, "Departamento de Ankylostomiasis [1922]," 227.

93 Abel, "External Philanthropy," 352.

94 See "Report of an Inspection made by Dr. F. F. Russell (Costa Rica)," RFA, record group 5, series 2, box 41, folder 244, 10.

95 See Steven Palmer, "Central American Encounters with Rockefeller Public Health, 1914–1921," in *Close Encounters of Empire: Writing the Cultural History of U.S.–Latin American Relations*, ed. Gilbert M. Joseph, Catherine C. LeGrand, and Ricardo D. Salvatore (Durham, N.C.: Duke University Press, 1998), 317–21.

96 "Circular from Depto San Esc to heads of Juntas de Educación," 21 July 1915, RFA, record group 5, series 1.2, box 7, folder 107.

97 "Schapiro to Rose," 22 May 1916, RFA, record group 5, series 1.2, box 29, folder 451.

98 Cited in "Informe Anual, 1917," f. 22.

99 Cited in "Report on Work for the Relief and Control of Hookworm Disease,"
15.

100 Louis Schapiro, *Misión del maestro de escuela en el servicio de inspección sanitaria
escolar* (San José: Tipografía Nacional, 1915), 3.

101 See República de Costa Rica, *Memoria de la Secretaría de Salubridad Pública,
1930–1931,* 13–14.

102 Solón Núñez, *Mi catecismo higiénico* (San José: Imprenta Nacional, 1926), 5.

103 See "Report on Work for the Relief and Control of Hookworm Disease," 22;
"Hookworm Campaign in Costa Rica," RFA, record group 5, series 2, box 28,
folder 168, 2; and "Schapiro to Rose," 23 December 1915, RFA, record group
5, series 1.2, box 7, folder 107.

104 Cited in "Hookworm Campaign in Costa Rica," RFA, record group 5, series 2,
box 28, folder 168, 2.

105 See "Report of an Inspection made by Dr. F. F. Russell," 2.

106 See "Report on Work for the Relief and Control of Hookworm Disease," 12,
23.

107 See República de Costa Rica, *Memoria de Gobernación y Policía, año 1920,* xxii.

108 See "Hookworm Campaign in Costa Rica," RFA, record group 5, series 2, box
28, folder 168, 4.

109 See República de Costa Rica, *Memoria, 1920,* vi.

110 See República de Costa Rica, "Departamento de Ankylostomiasis [1921],"
266.

111 See República de Costa Rica, "Departamento de Ankylostomiasis [1922],"
227, 231.

112 Cited in "Conference with Cabinet," RFA, record group 5, series 2, box 29,
folder 177, 1–2.

113 See ANCR, Congreso, 13.114, f. 1; and República de Costa Rica "Subsecretaría
de Policía Higiene y Salud Pública, 1922," *Memora de Gobernación y Policía
correspondiento al año 1922* (San José: Imprenta Nacional, 1923), 213.

114 See Carmelo Mesa-Lago, *Social Security in Latin America: Pressure Groups, Stratification, and Inequality* (Pittsburgh, Pa.: University of Pittsburgh Press, 1978),
116, 165; and Aristides A. Moll, *Aesculapius in Latin America* (Philadelphia, Pa.:
W. B. Saunders Company, 1944), 425. It should be noted that Argentina in
particular had a highly efficient and autonomous National Department of
Health, which had grown out of the explosive urbanization in Buenos Aires,
and that many other Latin American countries that had already developed
national health bodies followed hard on the heels of Costa Rica in raising
them to ministerial status, most doing so before 1935. Still, especially in Central American terms, the country was quite precocious.

115 "Report of Quarter Ending March 31, 1915," RFA, record group 5, series 1.2, box
7, folder 106; and Benedict Anderson, *Imagined Communities: Reflections on the
Origin and Spread of Nationalism,* 2d ed. (London: Verso Editions, 1991), 35–36.

Chapter 8. The Magician versus the Monopolists:
The Popular Medical Eclecticism of Professor Carbell

1   The information on his arrival with the carnival comes from a later newspaper article, "Decíase esta mañana que el Profesor Carbell había salido del pais," *La Nueva Prensa,* 11 June 1932, 6. Images of Costa Ricans "riding the worm" at this amusement park on New Year's Day 1932 can be seen in José María Arce, "Películas de San José, 1931–1934," Videoteca de la Escuela de Historia de la Universidad Nacional Autónoma, Heredia, Costa Rica.

2   The incident is re-created from a retrospective newspaper article, " 'Es falso que me haya declarado en rebeldía al no comparecer a declarar en el asunto de Carbell' nos dice el Dr. Antillón," *La Prensa Libre,* 8 April 1932, 5; and from the "Actas Municipales," session 8, 8 March 1932, and session 19, 3 May 1932, Archivos Nacionales de Costa Rica (hereafter ANCR), Municipal 11380. The faculty petition is found in ANCR, Salubridad Pública, 144, ff. 1.

3   Cited in ANCR, Salubridad Pública 144, ff. 1–2.

4   Roy Porter, *Health for Sale: Quackery in England, 1650–1850* (Manchester: Manchester University Press, 1989), 17.

5   The diploma is described by an adherent of Carbell's in "El Profesor Kendall y el Profesor Carbell," *La Nueva Prensa,* 16 March 1932, 3.

6   This is a composite portrait of Carbell's office from the testimony of patients and staff; see ANCR, Salubridad Pública 144. In 1938, Dr. Moreno Cañas charged four colones for a consultation to his enormous clientele; see Eduardo Oconitrillo, *Vida, muerte y mito del Dr. Moreno Cañas* (San José: Editorial Costa Rica, 1985), 18.

7   Cited in "Con el Profesor Carbell," *El Heraldo* (Puntarenas), 28 June 1932, 4. For a staged representation of Carbell as Christ, see his publicity photo, which appeared in newspaper advertisements and the frontispiece of his book on occult medicine, reproduced on p. 204 (Carlos Carballo Romero, *Hacia allá: Breve estudio sobre la medicina de hoy y de mañana, en relación con las fuerzas ocultas de la Naturaleza* [San José: Editorial Aurora, 1932]).

8   See ANCR, Salubridad Pública 144, f. 5.

9   Cited in ibid., ff. 2v–3.

10   Cited in ibid., ff. 22v, 18.

11   See ibid., ff. 13, 23.

12   This was confirmed in a personal communication with pharmacist Fernando Cerdas, who observed the lines as a boy.

13   Cited in ANCR, Salubridad Pública 144, f. 14v.

14   See ibid., f. 29v; and Erwin H. Ackerknecht, *A Short History of Medicine,* 2d ed. (Baltimore, Md.: Johns Hopkins University Press, 1982), 61.

15   Carballo Romero, *Hacia allá,* 47–56, 66–79; and ANCR, Salubridad Pública 144, 13v, 9–10v.

16   See ANCR, Salubridad Pública 144, ff. 18, 30–30v, 32v.

17 See James Dow, *The Shaman's Touch: Otomi Indian Symbolic Healing* (Salt Lake City: University of Utah Press, 1986), 6–9.

18 James Dow, "Curandero/Curandeiro," in vol. 2 of *Encyclopedia of Latin American History and Culture,* ed. Barbara Tenenbaum (New York: Charles Scribner's and Sons, 1995), 344.

19 James Dow hangs on to this anthropological mark of authenticity in his description of the urban curandero, claiming they "usually charge modest fees or accept only donations" ("Curandero/Curandeiro," 346).

20 See Eduardo Oconitrillo, *Julio Acosta: El hombre de la providencia* (San José: Editorial Costa Rica, 1994), 154, and Eduardo Oconitrillo, *Los Tinoco (1917–1919)* (San José: Editorial Costa Rica, 1982), 15. The one former president who did not support the regime was Ricardo Jiménez.

21 See Bienvenido Ortíz Cartín, *Copilación de leyes, decretos y circulares referentes a medicina e higiene del año 1821 hasta 1920* (San José: Tipografía Nacional, 1924), 45–46.

22 See Oconitrillo, *Julio Acosta,* 154.

23 The rough calculations are based on Vicente Láchner Sandoval, "Apuntes de higiene pública: Organismos, institutos y profesiones en relación con este ramo," in *Revista de Costa Rica en el siglo XIX* (San José: Imprenta Nacional, 1902), 189–222; "Report of an Inspection made by Dr. F. F. Russell (Costa Rica), Rockefeller Foundation Archives (hereafter RFA), record group 5, series 2, box 41, folder 244, Rockefeller Archive Center, North Tarrytown, N.Y.; and Luis Dobles Segreda, *Medicina e higiene,* vol. 9 of *Indice bibliográfico de Costa Rica* (San José: Imprenta Lehmann, 1927–1936), 384–402.

24 See "Nómina de médicos de Costa Rica que actualmente ejercen," *Revista Médica* (Costa Rica) 11, no. 16 (1935): 426–31; and Pablo Luros, "Nuestro problema médico-hospitalario," *Revista Médica* (Costa Rica) 9, no. 189 (1950): 22. Although the data are sketchy, similar tendencies can be detected in other Latin American countries. In Peru, the average number of medical school graduates rose from about thirty per year between 1900 and 1912, to forty or more per year between 1923 and 1940. The latter year marked a real takeoff, with enrollment in San Marcos jumping from five hundred to almost three thousand by 1952. After Argentina and Uruguay, Cuba had the greatest ratio of medical doctors to populace in Latin America during this era. In 1934, of Cuba's 2,542 physicians, 1,200 lived in the city of Havana—almost exactly the same proportion (47 percent) as in Costa Rica's capital, although Cuba's physician to populace ratio was significantly smaller at 1 to 450, as was the national ratio at 1 to 1,559. The number of new physicians incorporating in Cuba continued to rise rapidly over the next fifteen years, but only at the same rate as the population, and the physician-populace ratio remained roughly the same. Even so, the proportion was considered extremely disadvantageous for the profession, which suffered from chronic underemployment and low wages—a situation that led to radical medical unrest there in the 1930s. See Cyrille Dechamp and Moíses Poblete Troncoso, *El problema médico y la asistencia*

mutualista en Cuba (Havana, 1934), 28–29; cited in Ross Danielson, *Cuban Medicine* (New Brunswick, N.J.: Transaction Books, 1979), 111.

25 For a composite portrait of this generation, see Carlos Eduardo González Pacheco, *Hospital San Juan de Dios: 150 años de historia* (San José: Editorial Nacional del Seguro Social, 1995), 189–227. See also Oconitrillo, *Vida, muerte y mito;* and Manuel Picado Chacón, *Dr. Clodomiro Picado: Vida y obra* (San José: Editorial de la Universidad de Costa Rica, 1980).

26 Cited in Dobles Segreda, *Medicina e higiene,* 362–63.

27 Many of the publications from the conference are listed in ibid., 309–23.

28 See Rockefeller Foundation, *Directory of Fellowship Awards, 1917–1950* (n.p., n.d.).

29 Luros, "Nuestro problema médico-hospitalario," 20–21.

30 See *Gaceta Médica de Costa Rica* (hereafter GMCR) 16 (1915): 182; José Enrique Sotela, *Reseña histórica de la anestesia en Costa Rica* (San José: Editorial Nacional de Salud y Seguro Social, 1997), 35; and González Pacheco *Hospital San Juan de Dios,* 190.

31 See González, *Hospital San Juan de Dios,* 156.

32 Emilio Roig de Leuchsenring, *Médicos y medicina en Cuba: Historia, biografía y costumbrismo* (Havana: Museo Histórico de las Ciencias Médicas "Carlos J. Finlay," 1965), 197–212.

33 "Clínica Victory-Pacheco," single ad sheet, Biblioteca Nacional de Costa Rica; and Charles D. Ameringer, *A Political Biography of José Figueres of Costa Rica* (Albuquerque: University of New Mexico Press, 1978), 5.

34 Cited in República de Costa Rica, "Informe del Director del Servicio de Asistencia Pública," in *Memoria de Gobernación y Policía correspondiente al año 1923* (San José: Imprenta Nacional, 1924), 277. See also Allan M. Brandt, *No Magic Bullet: A Social History of Venereal Disease in the United States since 1880* (New York: Oxford University Press, 1987), 40.

35 Cited in República de Costa Rica, "Informe del Director," 277; and ANCR, Salubridad Pública 46. Popular logic apparently associated the cutaneous and mucoid manifestations of venereal disease with bad or rotten blood, and so categorized syphilis along with all skin diseases whose origin was difficult to explain; see Hermilio Valdizán and Angel Maldonado, *La medicina popular peruana: Contribución al "folk-lore médico del Perú* (Lima: Imprenta Torres Aguirre, 1922), 2:434. This was a curious inversion of the syphilophobia that wracked Georgian England, when people feared that any symptom, from a twitch to a running sore, was a sign of venereal disease; see Porter, *Health for Sale,* 151.

36 Carlos Pupo Pérez, *Medios para desarrollar la medicina científica en Costa Rica* (San José: Imprenta Gutenberg, 1932), 15–16.

37 Cited in República de Costa Rica, *Memoria de Salubridad Pública y Protección Social correspondiente al año 1927* (San José: Imprenta Nacional, 1928), xxxi; and Solón Núñez, *La tosferina* (San José: Imprenta Nacional, 1923), 8.

38 "Informe anual del Pres. Del Colegio de Farmacéuticos, Horacio Acosta García, dic., 1925"; cited in María Cecilia Brenes Jiménez, "Estudios sobre historia

de la farmacia en Costa Rica, período 1917–1926" (Licenciatura Thesis, University of Costa Rica, 1969), 192.

39   Daniel Acuña, *Cartilla médica del hogar indispensable a las familias del campo* (San José: Imprenta Alsina, 1926); cited in Dobles Segreda, *Medicina e higiene*, 185–86. See also ANCR, Salubridad Pública 136.

40   Carlos Luis Fallas, *Marcos Ramírez (aventuras de un muchacho)* (San José: Imprenta Falcóm, 1952), 144, 173.

41   Mario Samper, ed. *El censo de la población de 1927: Creación de una base nominal computarizada* (San José: Oficina de Publicaciones de la Universidad de Costa Rica, 1991).

42   See Steven Palmer, "Pánico en San José: El consumo de heroína, la cultura plebeya y la política social en 1929," in *El paso del cometa: Estado, política social y culturas populares en Costa Rica (1800–1950),* ed. Iván Molina Jiménez and Steven Palmer (San José: Plumsock Mesoamerican Studies and Editorial Porvenir, 1994), 193–99.

43   See *GMCR* 11, no. 6 (1907): 110; and RFA, record group 5, series 1.2, box 7, folder 103.

44   Facultad de Cirugía Dental, *Documentación de la labor realizada por la Facultad de Cirugía Dental de Costa Rica contra las leyes que autorizen a los empíricos para ejercer la profesión en el país* (San José, 1933); cited in Dobles Segreda, *Medicina e higiene*, 301.

45   Cited in *La Tribuna,* 12 June 1924, 4.

46   See República de Costa Rica, "Informe de la Subsecretaria de Higiene y Salud Pública," in *Memoria de Gobernación y Policía, 1926* (San José: Imprenta Nacional, 1928), 549.

47   Evidence of the arrival of osteopathy in the country is Alejandro Vargas Araya, *Sinopsis de Osteopatía* (San José, 1921); cited in Dobles Segreda, *Medicina e higiene,* 151–52.

48   See ANCR, Salubridad Pública 142.

49   See Francisco Enríquez, "El Curandero de Moravia," *Actualidades del CIHAC* (Centro de Investigaciones Históricas de América Central, Universidad de Costa Rica) 1, no. 5 (1994): 1–2.

50   República de Costa Rica, *Leyes, decretos y reglamentos de carácter sanitario, 1923–1935* (San José: Imprenta Nacional, 1935), 20–21.

51   *Código de Moral Médica de la Facultad de Medicina de la República de Costa Rica* (San José: Imprenta Ernesto Ortiz, 1932); cited in Dobles Segreda, *Medicina e higiene,* 276.

52   See Dobles Segreda, *Medicina e higiene,* 385.

53   Cited in "Yo creo que Costa Rica es un País donde sólo se puede realizar algo por la fuerza," *La Nueva Prensa,* 1 November 1931, 4.

54   Cited in ANCR, Salubridad Pública 144, ff. 13–14.

55   Ibid., ff. 15, 30.

56   Ibid., f. 13v.

57   Indeed, Carbell may have been responding to the sexology that was just beginning to gain popularity in Latin America in the 1920s; see Mariano Ben

Plotkin, "Freud, Politics, and the Porteños: The Reception of Psychoanalysis in Buenos Aires, 1910–1943," *Hispanic American Historical Review* 77, no. 1 (1997): 58.

58 See Judith R. Walkowitz, *City of Dreadful Delight: Narratives of Sexual Danger in Late-Victorian London* (Chicago: University of Chicago Press, 1992), 171–77; and S. E. D. Shortt, "Physicians and Psychics: The Anglo-American Medical Response to Spiritualism, 1870–1890," *Journal of the History of Medicine and Allied Sciences* 39, no. 3 (July 1984): 339–55.

59 Carballo Romero, *Hacia allá,* 9, 11.

60 Ibid., 77–78.

61 Cited in " 'Es falso que me haya declarado en rebeldía," *Prensa Libre,* 8 April 1932, 5.

62 Cited in ANCR, Salubridad Pública 144, 13v; and Sotero Antillón, " 'Es falso que me haya declarado en rebeldía," 5. A classic treatment of "rough music" and popular culture is Natalie Zemon Davis, "The Reasons of Misrule: Youth Groups and Charivaris in Sixteenth-Century France," *Past and Present* 52 (1971): 41–75.

Chapter 9. Medical Populism: Dr. Calderón Guardia
and the Foundations of Social Security

1 On Calderón Guardia's "response to the pressures of the popular sectors," see Manuel Rojas Bolaños, *Lucha social y guerra civil en Costa Rica* (San José: Editorial Porvenir, 1989), 44–45. See also the lucid contextual discussions of José Manuel Cerdas Albertazzi, "La cuestión social y las condiciones de vida de los obreros de Costa Rica (1930–1960)," *ABRA* (Costa Rica) 21–22 (1995): 59–95; and José Manuel Cerdas Albertazzi, "Salud y caja costarricense de Seguro Social," in *El significado de la legislación social de los cuarenta en Costa Rica,* ed. Jorge Mario Salazar Mora (San José: Ministerio de Educación Pública, 1993), 267–87.

2 Mark Rosenberg, *Las luchas por el seguro social en Costa Rica* (San José: Editorial Costa Rica, 1983), esp. 15–54. See also Carlos Monge Alfaro, *Nuestra historia y los seguros* (San José: Editorial Costa Rica, 1974); and Jorge Mario Salazar Mora, *Política y reforma en Costa Rica, 1914–1958* (San José: Editorial Porvenir, 1981). For a cogent revisionist view of state mediation and the development of social policy, see Carlos Hernández Rodríguez, "Trabajadores, empresarios y Estado: La dinámica de clase y los límites institucionales del conflicto, 1900–1943," *Revista de Historia* (Costa Rica) 27 (1993): 51–86. See also Carlos Monge Alfaro, *Nuestra historia y los seguros* (San José: Editorial Costa Rica, 1974).

3 Patricio V. Marquez and Daniel J. Joly, "A Historical Overview of the Ministries of Public Health and the Medical Programs of the Social Security Systems in Latin America," *Journal of Public Health Policy* 7, no. 3 (1986): 390; Carmelo Mesa-Lago, *Social Security in Latin America: Pressure Groups, Stratifications, and*

Inequality (Pittsburgh, Pa.: University of Pittsburgh Press, 1978); and James M. Malloy, *The Politics of Social Security in Brazil* (Pittsburgh, Pa.: University of Pittsburgh Press, 1979). It would seem that the historical dimensions of Latin American social policy are no longer on the agenda of contemporary scholars, if a recent review of new books on the topic is any indication; see Margaret S. Sherraden, "Social Policy in Latin America: Questions of Growth, Equality, and Political Freedom," *Latin American Research Review* 30, no. 1 (1995): 176–90.

4   See Alan Knight, "Populism and Neo-populism in Latin America, especially Mexico," *Journal of Latin American Studies* 30 (1998): 223–28.

5   See Eduardo Oconitrillo, *El Bellavistazo* (San José: Editorial Costa Rica, 1983).

6   See advertisement, *La Prensa Libre*, 2 May 1932, 2; and Jorge Volio, "Prólogo," Carlos Carballo Romero, *Hacia allá: Breve estudio sobre la medicina de hoy y de mañana, en relación con las fuerzas ocultas de la Naturaleza* (San José: Editorial Aurora, 1932, n.p.

7   In 1926, Volio had declared himself in rebellion against the Jiménez government and headed for the frontier with Nicaragua, presumably to prepare an invasion; Jiménez had had Volio delicately arrested, tried, and then packed off to European exile and treatment in a mental institution. See Vladimir de la Cruz, *Las luchas sociales en Costa Rica, 1870–1930* (San José: Editorial Costa Rica, 1980), 60–61; Victoria Ramírez, *Jorge Volio y la revolución viviente* (San José: Editorial Guayacan, 1989); Oconitrillo, *El Bellavistazo;* and Jorge Mario Salazar Mora, *Crisis liberal y Estado reformista, 1914–1949* (San José: Editorial Universidad de Costa Rica, 1995), 158.

8   Cited in "Un interesante libro del Profesor Carbell," *La Prensa Libre*, 26 April 1932, 5.

9   Carlos Carballo Romero, *Hacia allá: Breve estudio sobre la medicina de hoy y de mañana, en relación con las fuerzas ocultas de la Naturaleza* (San José: Editorial Aurora, 1932), 5–7, 10–11, 43–49, 78–89.

10   Carballo Romero, *Hacía allá*, 6–7, 26, 43, 89–100.

11   See Eduardo Oconitrillo, *Vida, muerte y mito del Dr. Moreno Cañas* (San José: Editorial Costa Rica, 1985), 127–32. The film was recently restored and screened by the Instituto Costarricense del Cine. "Centro de Estudios Moreno Cañas presenta 'Anales Médicos de Costa Rica: Un caso de *geno recurvatum con anquilosis* por Dr. Ricardo Moreno Cañas,' " (original date of production unknown; restored print, 1995).

12   See *La Nueva Prensa*, 12 May 1932, 4.

13   Presumably, Cuba was spared so that Carbell might be considered a national when called on to play a directive role in the new polity (or in that which would be formed in order to better prepare for the apocalypse). Yucatán had a great deal of importance as a center of theosophist and spiritist thought that, moreover, had supernatural geographic worth.

14   Cited in "Costa Rica y su profesía: Una interesante conferencia por radio del Eminente Profesor Carbell," *La Nueva Prensa*, 16 June 1932, 4.

15   See Steven Palmer, "Getting to Know the Unknown Soldier: Official National-
      ism in Liberal Costa Rica, 1880–1900," *Journal of Latin American Studies* 25
      (1993): 45–72. A classic, contemporary vision inspired by Oswald Spengler is
      Jorge Basadre, *La multitud, la ciudad y el campo en la historia del Perú [1929]*, 3d
      ed. (Lima: Mosca Azul, 1980).

16   It is of at least passing interest that in traditional occultist physiognomy, the
      will corresponds to the left side of the face. See José Sanfilippo B., "Ocultismo
      y medicina," *Boletín mexicano de historia y filosofía de la medicina* 12, nos. 71–74
      (1990): 50.

17   See Simón Bolívar, "Contestación de un americano meridional a un caballero
      de esta Isla [Carta de Jamaica de 6 de setiembre de 1815]," in vol. 1 of *Obras
      completas,* ed. Vicente Lecuna, 2d ed. (Havana: Editorial Lex, 1950), 171; and
      José Cecilio del Valle, "Sabios, capitalistas y obreros (discurso pronunciado en
      el acto de la instalación de la Sociedad Económica, por su Director, el 29 de
      noviembre de 1928)," in *Pensamiento vivo de José Cecilio del Valle,* ed. Rafael
      Heliodoro Valle, 2d ed. (San José: Editorial Universitaria Centroamericana,
      1971), 150, 160. A synthesis of this aspect of the philosophy of the important
      Mexican intellectual can be found in José Vasconcelos, *Indología: Una in-
      terpretación de la cultura ibero-americana* (Paris: Agencia Mundial de Librería,
      [1930]), 201–29. His controversial stay in Costa Rica is described in José
      Vasconcelos, *La Tormenta,* vol. 2 of *Memorias,* 2d ed. (Mexico City: Fondo de
      Cultura Económica, 1983), 929–39.

18   Augusto Sandino, "Manifiesto 'Luz y Verdad,' " in *El pensamiento vivo de San-
      dino,* ed. Sergio Ramírez (San José: Editorial Universitaria Centroamericana,
      1974), 213–14. On the spiritual and spiritist dimensions of Sandino's strug-
      gle, see Volker Wunderich, *Sandino: Una biografía política* (Managua: Editorial
      Nueva Nicaragua, 1995), 130–54.

19   Robert Darnton, *Mesmerism and the End of the Enlightenment in France* (Cam-
      bridge: Harvard University Press, 1968). One newspaper of the time noted
      how widespread the phenomenon of magicians and spiritists had become; see
      "La invasión de los pseudo-médicos," *La Prensa Libre,* 7 April 1932, 5. The end
      of the 1920s also witnessed a proliferation of other spiritualist sects in the
      country—for example, the attempt to form a local chapter of the liberal
      Catholic Church, and another effort to establish political spirituality accord-
      ing to formal rational categories; see José B. Acuña, *La Iglesia Católica Liberal
      (su historia, sus principios y sus fines)* (San José: Imprenta Alsina, 1927).

20   See Darnton, *Mesmerism,* 106–25; and Logie Barrow, "Socialism in Eternity:
      The Ideology of Plebeian Spiritualists, 1853–1913," *History Workshop* (Spring
      1980): 37–69.

21   See Francisco Enríquez, "El Curandero de Moravia," *Actualidades del CIHAC*
      (Centro de Investigaciones Históricas de América Central, Universidad de
      Costa Rica) 1, no. 5 (1994): 1–2.

22   On the secret police investigation, see "De nuevo en el tapete de la discusión el
      Profesor Carbell," *La Nueva Prensa,* 7 April 1932, 1.

23 "Cómo vio nuestro corresponsal en el Puerto la última aventura del profesor Carbell," *La Prensa Libre,* 30 June 1932, 7.

24 "Con el Profesor Carbell," *El Heraldo,* 28 June 1932, 4.

25 "Cómo vio nuestro corresponsal," *Prensa Libre,* 7.

26 Carballo Romero, *Hacía allá,* 89.

27 See Iván Molina Jiménez and Fabrice Lehoucq, *Urnas de lo inesperado: Fraude electoral y lucha política en Costa Rica (1901–1948)* (San José: Editorial de la Universidad de Costa Rica, 1999), 88. In Peru, by comparison, the proportion had stabilized at 13 percent between 1919 and 1930; see Marcos Cueto, *Excelencia científica en la periferia: Actividades científicas e investigación biomédica en el Perú, 1890–1950* (Lima: Tarea, 1989), 62.

28 See Francisco Guerra, *El médico político: Su influencia en la historia de Hispano-América y Filipinas* (Madrid: Afrodisio Aguado, 1975), 159–66. On Montero, see Cruz, *Las luchas sociales,* 99–101.

29 See Juan Dávila Cubero, *Viva Vargas! Historia del Partido Confraternidad Guanacasteca* (San José: Ediciones Guayacán, 1987), 44–105.

30 See Oconitrillo, *Vida, muerte y mito,* 127–32.

31 See Setha M. Low, "Dr. Moreno Cañas: A Symbolic Bridge to the De-medicalization of Healing," *Social Science and Medicine* 16, no. 5 (1982): 527.

32 Setha Low later reconsidered the earlier findings, but now determined that this "medicalization" of healing cults reflected the increasing power of the medical sector to control lives, even though the de-medicalizing impulse was still apparent. Low now posited a "medicalization/de-medicalization" and "secular/sacred" dialectic of Latin American healing cults. See Setha M. Low, "The Medicalization of Healing Cults in Latin America," *American Ethnologist* 15, no. 1 (1988): 136–55.

33 Rafael Angel Calderón Guardia, "Páginas autobiográficas del Dr. Calderón Guardia, presidente de la república." *Revista de los Archivos Nacionales* 6, nos. 11–12 (1942): 565.

34 See Jorge Mario Salazar Mora, *Calderón Guardia* (San José: Ministerio de Cultura, Juventud y Deportes, 1980), 20–27. On Mercier, see David A. Boileau, *Cardinal Mercier: A Memoir* (n.p.: Peeters, 1996).

35 D. J. Mercier, *Psicología: Vida orgánica y senstiva; Vida intelectiva o racional* (Buenos Aires: Ediciones Anaconda, 1942), 8.

36 Calderón Guardia, "Páginas autobiográficas," 566–67.

37 Rafael Angel Calderón Guardia, "Mensaje inaugural del Presidente Calderón Guardia, 8 mayo 1940," 247, and "El gobernante y el hombre frente al problema social costarricense [September 1942]," in *El pensamiento contemporaneo costarricense,* ed. Luis Demetrio Tinoco and Eugenio Rodríguez Vega (San José: Editorial Costa Rica, 1980).

38 See Paul W. Drake, *Socialism and Populism in Chile, 1932–1952* (Urbana: University of Illinois Press, 1978), 162.

39 See Guerra, *El médico político,* 169–70.

40 Ibid., 211.

41 Ibid., 232.

42 Ibid., 233; and Robert J. Alexander, *Juscelino Kubitschek and the Development of Brazil*, Ohio University, Monographs in International Studies, Latin America Series, no. 16, 31–71. Interestingly, in 1958 Kubitschek gave a presidential pardon to a famous spiritist surgeon from Minas Gerais who had been convicted of illegally practicing medicine. See David J. Hess, *Spirits and Scientists: Ideology, Spiritism, and Brazilian Culture* (University Park: Penn State University Press, 1991), 129.

43 See Michael L. Conniff, *Urban Politics in Brazil: The Rise of Populism, 1925–1945* (Pittsburgh, Pa.: University of Pittsburgh Press, 1981), 34–57. I might also mention in this regard François "Papa Doc" Duvalier, who had a distinguished career as a medical reformer and minister of health in Haiti before becoming the populist leader of the black masses in 1957.

44 See John Lee Anderson, *Che Guevara: A Revolutionary Life* (New York: Grove Press, 1997), 95–98, 120.

45 See Ana Cecilia Román Trigo, *Las finanzas públicas de Costa Rica: Metodología y fuentes (1870–1948)* (San José: Centro de Investigaciones Históricas de América Central, 1995), 77–79.

46 Cited in República de Costa Rica, *Memoria de Salubridad Pública y Protección Social correspondiente al año 1927* (San José: Imprenta Nacional, 1928), vi, lviii.

47 See Luis Dobles Segreda, "Reglamento del servicio técnico del Hospital San Juan de Diós," *Revista Médica* (Costa Rica) 2, no. 17 (1935): 453; and "Discurso del Dr. Peña Chavarría," *Revista Médica* (Costa Rica) 3, no. 21 (1936): 121–22.

48 See República de Costa Rica, *Memoria de la Secretaria de Salubridad Pública y Protección Social, año 1936* (San José: Imprenta Nacional, 1937), 54.

49 See Román Trigo, *Finanzas públicas de Costa Rica*, 79–80.

50 See República de Costa Rica, *Memoria, 1936*, 53.

51 Ibid., 28–29.

52 Ibid., 61.

53 See Héctor Pérez Brignoli, "El crecimiento demográfico de América Latina en los siglos XIX y XX: Problemas, métodos y perspectivas," *Avances de Investigación* (Centro de Investigaciones Históricas, Universidad de Costa Rica) 48 (1989): 12, graph 1; and Arodys Robles Soto, "Patrones de población en Costa Rica, 1860–1930," *Avances de Investigación* (Centro de Investigaciones Históricas, Universidad de Costa Rica) 14 (1986): 14, 49.

54 See *Memoria, 1936*, 29–30; and República de Costa Rica, *Memoria de la Secretaria de Salubridad Pública y Protección Social del año administrativo 1937* (San José: Imprenta Nacional, 1938), 222–32.

55 See *Memoria, 1936*, 29–30.

56 See *Memoria, 1937*, 222–32.

57 See *Memoria, 1936*, 28.

58 See *Memoria, 1937*, 194; and Joaquín Fermoselle Bacardí, "Resultado del esfuerzo sanitario y asistencial coordinados en la mortalidad infantil," *Revista Médica* (Costa Rica) 10, no. 104 (1942): 343.

59 Similar projects were piloted in other Latin American countries where the Rockefeller Foundation had established an influence. On Mexico, see Anne-Emanuelle Birn, "A Revolution in Rural Health? The Struggle over Local Health Units in Mexico, 1928–1940," *Journal of the History of Medicine* 53, no. 1 (January 1998): 43–76.

60 See *Memoria, 1937*, 8.

61 Cited in ibid., 7–8.

62 In Colombia, the French clinical model of medical education was similarly tenacious in the university, as it was in Argentina, much to the dismay of U.S. medical and public health reformers. See Marcos Cueto, "Visions of Science and Development: The Rockefeller Foundation's Latin American Surveys of the 1920s," in *Missionaries of Science: The Rockefeller Foundation in Latin America*, ed. Marcos Cueto (Bloomington: Indiana University Press, 1994), 7–13; and Emilio Quevedo, *Historia social de la ciencia en Colombia* 8:243–44.

63 See Pablo Luros, "Nuestro problema médico-hospitalario," *Revista Médica* (Costa Rica) 9, no. 189 (1950): 20–21.

64 Manuel Aguilar Bonilla, personal communication; and José Enrique Sotela, *Reseña histórica de la anestesia en Costa Rica* (San José: Editorial Nacional de Salud y Seguro Social, 1997), 9.

65 On this triste transition, see Ana Luisa Cerdas Albertazzi, "El surgimiento del enclave bananero en el Pacífico Sur," *Revista de Historia* (Costa Rica) 28 (1993): 117–59; and Ronny José Viales Hurtado, *Después del enclave: Un estudio de la región Atlántica costarricense, 1927–1950* (San José: Editorial de la Universidad de Costa Rica, 1998), 125–39.

66 See "Nómina de médicos de Costa Rica que actualmente ejercen," *Revista Médica* (Costa Rica) 11, no. 16 (1935): 426–31; and Luros, Nuestro problema médico-hospitalario," 22. Ironically, the same data show that in the areas of San José province outside the city and its plethora of practitioners, residents had the least access of almost anyone in the country to the services of a physician; in 1950, there were only four doctors serving a population of more than sixty thousand. That is, due to the pull of the capital, those who lived in its hinterland had poorer access to medical services than did other Costa Ricans residing in the hinterlands of urban and semiurban centers.

67 On the strategic importance of these sectors, see Victor Hugo Acuña Ortega, *Los orígenes de la clase obrera en Costa Rica: Las huelgas de 1920 por la jornada de ocho horas* (San José: Centro Nacional de Acción Pastoral, 1986), 9–13; and Cerdas Albertazzi, "La cuestión social," 63–68.

68 Mark Rosenberg, "Social Reform in Costa Rica: Social Security and the Presidency of Rafael Angel Calderón Guardia," *Hispanic American Historical Review* 61, no. 2 (1981): 279–84.

69 See *Revista Médica* (Costa Rica) 5, no. 110 (1943): 473.

70 See Steven Palmer, "Confinement, Policing, and the Emergence of Social Policy in Costa Rica, 1885–1935," in *The Birth of the Penitentiary in Latin America: Essays on Criminology, Prison Reform, and Social Control, 1830–1940*, ed. Car-

los Aguirre and Ricardo Salvatore (Austin: University of Texas Press, 1996), 242–46. Luis Felipe González Flores, *Paidofilaxis: Fundamentos sociales y científicos de la protección de la infancia* (San José: Imprenta Nacional, 1939.

71 What follows is taken principally from Rosenberg, *Las luchas por el seguro social,* 53–98.

72 Antonio Casas and Herman Vargas, "The Health System in Costa Rica: Toward a National Health Service," *Journal of Public Health Policy* 1, no. 3 (1980): 266.

73 See Yalena de la Cruz, *Guillermo Padilla Castro: Forjador de instituciones* (San José: ABC Ediciones, n.d.); and Yalena de la Cruz, *Los forjadores de la Seguridad Social en Costa Rica* (San José: Caja Costarricense de Seguro Social, 1994).

74 See Charles D. Ameringer, *A Political Biography of José Figueres of Costa Rica* (Albuquerque: University of New Mexico Press, 1978), 5.

BIBLIOGRAPHY

Newspapers
  Correo Nacional, 1929.
  Crónica de Costa Rica, 1858–1859.
  Diario de Costa Rica, 1923–1932.
  Gaceta Médica de Costa Rica, 1896–1918
  La Gaceta Médica, 1881, 1882.
  La Nueva Prensa, 1929–1932.
  La Prensa Libre, 1929–1932.
  Revista Médica (Costa Rica), 1933–1950.
  La Tribuna, 1929–1932.

Archives
Archivos Nacionales de Costa Rica. San José Guerra, Congreso, Gobernación, Policía, Municipal, and Salubridad Pública
Archivo General de la Nación, Mexico City Inquisición.
Centro de Investigaciones Históricas de América Central, "El Censo Municipal de San José de 1904," San José.
———. "El Censo de 1927," San José.
Rockefeller Foundation Archives, record groups 3–5, Rockefeller Archive Center, North Tarrytown, New York.

Films
Arce, José María. "Películas de San José, 1931–1934." Videoteca de la Escuela de Historia de la Universidad Nacional Autónoma. Heredia, Costa Rica.
Instituto Costarricense del Ciné, "Centro de Estudios Moreno Cañas presenta 'Anales Médicos de Costa Rica: Un caso de *geno recurvatum con anquilosis* por Dr. Ricardo Moreno Cañas." Original date of production unknown; restored print, 1995.

Published Primary Sources

Acuña, José B. *La Iglesia Católica Liberal (su historia, sus principios y sus fines)*. San José: Imprenta Alsina, 1927.

Actas de la Cuarta Conferencia Sanitaria Internacional de las Repúblicas Americanas. Washington, D.C.: Unión Panamericana, 1910.

Alfaro, Anastasio. *Arqueología criminal americana*. San José: Imprenta de Avelino Alsina, 1906.

Bolívar, Simón. *Obras completas*. Edited by Vicente Lecuna. 3 vols. 2d ed. Havana: Editorial Lex, 1950.

Brenes Mesén, Roberto. *El misticismo como instrumento de la investigación de la verdad*. San José: Repertorio Americano, 1921.

Calderón Guardia, Rafael Angel. "Páginas autobiográficas del Dr. Calderón Guardia, presidente de la república." *Revista de los Archivos Nacionales* 6, nos. 11–12 (1942): 561–76.

———. "Mensaje inaugural del Presidente Calderón Guardia, 8 mayo 1940." In Luis Demetrio Tinoco, ed. *El pensamiento contemporaneo costarricense*. San José: Editorial Costa Rica, 1980.

———. "El gobernante y el hombre frente al problema social costarricense [September 1942]." In Luis Demetrio Tinoco, ed. *El pensamiento contemporaneo costarricense*. San José: Editorial Costa Rica, 1980.

Carballo Romero, Carlos. *Hacia allá: Breve estudio sobre la medicina de hoy y de mañana, en relación con las fuerzas ocultas de la Naturaleza*. San José: Editorial Aurora, 1932.

Céspedes, Benjamín de. *Higiene de la infancia*. San José: Tipografía Nacional, 1900.

Departamento Nacional de Estadísticos. *Resúmenes estadísticos, 1883–1893*. San José: Tipografía Nacional, 1895.

Directorio comercial de San José, 1898. San José: Imprenta Greñas, 1898.

Durán, Francisco, ed. *Bitácora médica del Doctor Falcón: La medicina y la farmacia en el siglo XIX*. Mexico City: Universidad La Salle, 2000.

Fallas, Carlos Luis. *Marcos Ramírez (aventuras de un muchacho)*. San José: Imprenta Falcóm, 1952.

Fernández, León, ed. *Colección de documentos para la historia de Costa Rica*. 10 vols. San José: Imprenta Nacional, 1881–1907.

Fernández, Mauro. *La anquilostomiasis y la agricultura*. San José: Imprenta de Avelino Alsina, 1907.

Flores y Troncoso, Francisco de Asis. *Historia de la Medicina en México desde la época de los indios hasta el presente*. 4 vols. 1886–1888. Reprint, Mexico City: Instituto Mexicano de Seguro Social, 1982.

Frantzius, Alexander von. "El antiguo convento de la misión de Orosi en Cartago." In *Viajes por la República de Costa Rica*, edited by Elías Zeledón Cartín. 3 vols. San José: Academia de Geografía e Historia, 1997.

García Monge, Joaquín. *Abnegación*. San José: Imprenta de Padrón Pujol, 1902.

González, Luisa. *A ras del suelo*. 9th ed. San José: Editorial Costa Rica, 1989.

González Flores, Luis Felipe. *Paidofilaxis: Fundamentos sociales y científicos de la protección de la infancia*. San José: Imprenta Nacional, 1939.

Bibliography

La Gota de Leche: Memoria relativa a la actuación del año 1913–1914. San José: Tipografía Nacional, n.d.

Jiménez, Gerardo, and Enrique Jiménez. *Higiene de las habitaciones y del agua en Costa Rica.* San José: Tipografía Nacional, 1902.

Marr, Wilhelm. "Viajes a Centroamérica." In *Costa Rica en el siglo XIX: Antología de viajeros,* edited by Ricardo Fernández Guardia. 1929. Reprint, San José: Editorial Universitaria Centroamericana, 1985.

Meléndez Chaverri, Carlos, ed. *Mensajes presidenciales, 1896–1916.* San José: Academia de Geografía e Historia, 1983.

———. *Mensajes presidenciales, 1928–1940.* San José: Academia de Geografía e Historia, 1987.

Núñez, Solón. "La Ankylostomiasis." *Boletín de la Subsecretaría de Higiene y Salud Pública* 1, no. 1 (1923): 11–15.

———. *La tosferina.* San José: Imprenta Nacional, 1923.

———. *Mi catecismo higiénico.* San José: Imprenta Nacional, 1926.

Ortíz Cartín, Bienvenido. *Copilación de leyes, decretos y circulares referentes a medicina e higiene del año 1821 hasta 1920.* San José: Tipografía Nacional, 1924.

Peralta F., Genaro. *Guía-directorio de la ciudad de San José, 1905.* San José: Imprenta de Antonio Lehmann, 1905.

Pupo Pérez, Carlos. *Nuestras enfermedades evitables: Principios de higiene que nadie debe ignorar.* San José: Imprenta Alsina, 1913.

———. *Medios para desarrollar la medicina científica en Costa Rica.* San José: Imprenta Gutenberg, 1932.

———. *Nuestros males: Principios sanitarios que nadie debe ignorar.* 2d ed. San José: Tipografía Nacional, 1936.

Putnam, George Palmer. *The Southland of North America: Rambles and Observations in Central America during the Year 1912.* New York: G. P. Putnam and Sons, 1913.

Quesada, Gregorio. *La homeopatía en Costa Rica.* San José: Imprenta de Avelino Alsina, 1905.

Recuerdo del cincuagésimo aniversario de la Botica Francesca (1869–1918). San José: Imprenta Alsina, 1918.

Reglamento de la Escuela de Obstetricia de la Facultad de Medicina de la República de Costa Rica. San José: Imprenta María v. de Lines, 1907.

República de Costa Rica. *Censo general de la República de Costa Rica (27 de noviembre de 1864).* San José: Imprenta Nacional, 1868.

———. *Censo de la República de Costa Rica* [1883]. N.p., n.d.

———. *Censo general de la República de Costa Rica (1892).* San José: Tipografía Nacional, 1893.

———. *Memoria de Gobernación, Policía y Fomento, 1902–1903.* San José: Tipografía Nacional, 1903.

———. *Memoria de Gobernación y Policía correspondiente a los años de 1907 y 1908.* San José: Imprenta Nacional, 1909.

República de Costa Rica. *Memoria de Gobernación y Policía, 1919.* San José: Imprenta Nacional, 1920.

———. *Memoria de Gobernación y Policía, año 1920.* San José: Imprenta Nacional, 1921.

———. *Memoria de Gobernación y Policía, 1926.* San José: Imprenta Nacional, 1928.

———. *Memoria de Gobernación y Policía correspondiente al año 1923.* San José: Imprenta Nacional, 1924.

———. *Memoria de Gobernación, Policía, Trabajo y Previsión Social correspondiente al año 1932.* San José: Imprenta Nacional, 1934.

———. *Memoria de Salubridad Pública y Protección Social correspondiente al año 1927.* San José: Imprenta Nacional, 1928.

———. *Memoria de la Secretaría de Salubridad Pública y Protección Social correspondiente a los años de 1930–1931.* San José: Imprenta Nacional, 1932.

———. *Memoria de la Secretaria de Salubridad Pública y Protección Social, año 1936.* San José: Imprenta Nacional, 1937.

———. *Memoria de la Secretaria de Salubridad Pública y Protección Social del año administrativo 1937.* San José: Imprenta Nacional, 1938.

———. *Censo de la República de Costa Rica, 22 de mayo de 1950.* 2d ed. San José, 1975.

Rucavado, Francisco J. *Lecciones del Primero y del Segundo Curso: Escuela de Obstetricia de Costa Rica.* San José: Tipografía Nacional, 1903.

Sandino, Augusto. "Manifesto 'Luz y Verdad.' " In *El pensamiento vivo de Sandino,* edited by Sergio Ramírez. San José: Editorial Universitaria Centroamericana, 1974.

Schapiro, Louis. *Misión del maestro de escuela en el servicio de inspección sanitaria escolar.* San José: Tipografía Nacional, 1915.

Squier, Ephraim George. *Nicaragua; Its People, Scenery, Monuments, Resources, Condition, and Proposed Canal; with One Hundred Original Maps and Illustrations.* Rev. ed. New York: Harper and Brother Publishers, 1860.

Stephens, John Lloyd. *Incidents of Travel in Central America, Chiapas, and Yucatan.* 2 vols. New York: Harper and Brothers, 1841.

Valdizán, Hermilio, and Angel Maldonado. *La medicina popular peruana: Contribución al "folk-lore" médico del Perú.* 2 vols. Lima: Imprenta Torres Aguirre, 1922.

Valle, José Cecilio del. "Sabios, capitalistas y obreros (discurso pronunciado en el acto de la instalación de la Sociedad Económica, por su Director, el 29 de noviembre de 1829)." In *Pensamiento vivo de José Cecilio del Valle,* edited by Rafael Heliodoro Valle. 2d ed. San José: Editorial Universitaria Centroamericana, 1971.

Vasconcelos, José. *Indología: Una interpretación de la cultura ibero-americana.* Paris: Agencia Mundial de Librería, [1930].

———. *Memorias.* 2 vols. 2d ed. Mexico City: Fondo de Cultura Económica, 1983.

Zeledón Cartín, Elías, ed. *Viajes por la República de Costa Rica.* 3 vols. San José: Academia de Geografía e Historia, 1997.

Secondary Sources

Abel, Christopher. "External Philanthropy and Domestic Change in Colombian Health Care: The Role of the Rockefeller Foundation, ca. 1920–1950." *Hispanic American Historical Review* 75, no. 3 (1995): 339–76.

Ackerknecht, Erwin H. *A Short History of Medicine.* 2d ed. Baltimore, Md.: Johns Hopkins University Press, 1982.

Acuña de Chacón, Angela. *La mujer costarricense a través de cuatro siglos.* 2 vols. San José: Imprenta Nacional, 1969–1970.

Acuña Ortega, Victor Hugo. *Los orígenes de la clase obrera en Costa Rica: Las huelgas de 1920 por la jornada de ocho horas.* San José: Centro Nacional de Acción Pastoral, 1986.

Aguilar Bonilla, Manuel. "Centenario de la primera revista médica de Costa Rica." *Acta Médica Costarricense,* special issue (1982): 27–38.

Alexander, Robert J. *Juscelino Kubitschek and the Development of Brazil.* Ohio University, Monographs in International Studies, Latin America Series, no. 16.

Ameringer, Charles D. *A Political Biography of José Figueres of Costa Rica.* Albuquerque: University of New Mexico Press, 1978.

Anderson, Benedict. *Imagined Communities: Reflections on the Origin and Spread of Nationalism.* 2d ed. London: Verso Editions, 1991.

Anderson, John Lee. *Che Guevara: A Revolutionary Life.* New York: Grove Press, 1997.

Anderson, Warwick. "Where is the Postcolonial History of Medicine?" *Bulletin of the History of Medicine* 72, no. 3 (1998): 522–30.

Archila, Ricardo. *Historia de la medicina en Venezuela.* Mérida, Venezuela: Universidad de los Andes, 1966.

———. "Médicos alemanes en Venezuela: Siglos XVIII y XIX." *Humboldt* 21, no. 73 (1980): 74–79.

Arnold, David, ed. *Imperial Medicine and Indigenous Societies.* Manchester: Manchester University Press, 1988.

Armus, Diego. "Enfermedad, ambiente urbano e higiene social: Rosario entre fines del siglo XIX y comienzos del XX." In *Sectores populares y vida urbana,* edited by Diego Armus. Buenos Aires: Consejo Latinoamericana de Ciensias Sociales, 1984.

Arrom, Silvia Marina. *The Women of Mexico City, 1790–1857.* Stanford, Calif.: Stanford University Press, 1985.

Asturias, Francisco. *Historia de la medicina en Guatemala.* 2d ed. 1902. Reprint, Guatemala City: Editorial Universitaria, 1958.

Asua, Miguel J. C. de. "Influencia de la Facultad de Medicina de París sobre la de Buenos Aires." *Quipu* 3, no. 1 (1986): 79–89.

Austin Alchon, Suzanne. *Native Society and Disease in Colonial Ecuador.* Cambridge: Cambridge University Press, 1991.

Badilla, Gómez Patricia. "Ideología y derecho: El espíritu mesiánico de la reforma jurídica costarricense (1882–1888)." *Revista de Historia* (Costa Rica) no. 18 (Jan.–June, 1988): 187–202.

Barran, Pedro. *Historia de la sensibilidad en el Uruguay.* 2 vols. Montevideo: Ediciones de la Banda Oriental, 1990.

Barrow, Logie. "Socialism in Eternity: The Ideology of Plebeian Spiritualists, 1853–1913." *History Workshop* (spring 1980): 37–69.

Bartrip, P. W. J. *Mirror of Medicine: A History of the British Medical Journal.* Oxford: British Medical Journal, 1990.

Basadre, Jorge. *La multitud, la ciudad y el campo en la historia del Perú [1929].* 3d ed. Lima: Mosca Azul, 1980.

Bastien, Joseph W. *Healers of the Andes: Kallawaya Herbalists and Their Medicinal Plants.* Salt Lake City: University of Utah Press, 1987.

———. "Differences between Kallawaya-Andean and Greek-European Humoral Theory." *Social Science and Medicine* 28, no. 1 (1989): 45–51.

Benchimol, Jaime. "Domingo José Freire e os primórdios da bacteriologia no Brasil." *Manguinhos: História, Ciência, Saúde* 2, no. 1 (1995): 67–98.

———. *Dos micróbios aos mosquitos: Febre amarela e a revoluçao pasteuriana no Brasil.* Rio de Janeiro: Editorial Fiocruz, 1999.

———, ed. *Manguinos do sonho à vida.* Rio de Janeiro: Fiocruz, 1990.

Ben Plotkin, Mariano. "Freud, Politics, and the Porteños: The Reception of Psycho-analysis in Buenos Aires, 1910–1943." *Hispanic American Historical Review* 77, no. 1 (1997): 45–74.

Berman, Edward H. *The Influence of the Carnegie, Ford, and Rockefeller Foundations on American Foreign Policy: The Ideology of Philanthropy.* Albany: State University of New York Press, 1983.

Besse, Susan K. *Restructuring Patriarchy: The Modernization of Gender Inequality in Brazil, 1914–1940.* Chapel Hill: University of North Carolina Press, 1996.

Birn, Anne-Emanuelle. "A Revolution in Rural Health? The Struggle over Local Health Units in Mexico, 1928–1940." *Journal of the History of Medicine* 53, no. 1 (January 1998): 43–76.

Blécourt, Willem de, and Cornelie Usborne. "Preface: Situating 'Alternative Medicine' in the Modern Period." *Medical History* 43 (1999): 283–85.

Boileau, David A. *Cardinal Mercier: A Memoir.* No place of publication: Peeters, 1996.

Borges, Dain. *The Family in Bahia, Brazil, 1870–1945.* Stanford, Calif.: Stanford University Press, 1992.

Bowers, John Z., and Elizabeth F. Purcell, eds. *Aspects of the History of Medicine in Latin America.* New York: Josiah Macy Jr. Foundation, 1979.

Brandt, Allan M. *No Magic Bullet: A Social History of Venereal Disease in the United States since 1880.* New York: Oxford University Press, 1987.

Brannstrom, Christian. "Polluted Soil, Polluted Souls: The Rockefeller Hookworm Eradication Campaign in São Paulo, Brazil, 1917–1926." *Historical Geography* 25 (1997): 25–45.

Brenes Jiménez, María Cecilia. "Estudios sobre historia de la farmacia en Costa Rica, período 1917–1926." Licenciatura Thesis, University of Costa Rica, 1969.

Brown, E. Richard. "Public Health and Imperialism: Early Rockefeller Programs at Home and Abroad." *American Journal of Public Health* 66, no. 9 (September 1976): 897–905.

———. *Rockefeller Medicine Men: Medicine and Capitalism in America.* Berkeley: University of California Press, 1979.

Bullock, Mary Brown. *An American Transplant: The Rockefeller Foundation and Peking Union Medical College.* Berkeley: University of California Press, 1980.

Bulow, Tulio von. "Apuntes para la historia de la medicina en Costa Rica durante la colonia." *Revista de los Archivos Nacionales* (Costa Rica) 9, nos. 1–2 (1945): 43–63.

———. "Apuntes para la historia de la medicina en Costa Rica durante la colonia (4a parte)." *Revista de los Archivos Nacionales* (Costa Rica) 9, nos. 11–12 (1945): 89–111.

Burns, E. Bradford. *Patriarch and Folk: The Emergence of Nicaragua, 1798–1858*. Cambridge: Harvard University Press, 1991.

Buss, Fran Leeper, *La Partera: Story of a Midwife*. Ann Arbor: University of Michigan Press, 1980.

Bynum, W. F., and Roy Porter, eds. *Medical Fringe and Medical Orthodoxy, 1750–1850*. London: Croom Helm, 1987.

———. *Companion Encyclopedia of the History of Medicine*. 2 vols. London: Routledge, 1993.

Cabezas Solera, Edgar. *La medicina en Costa Rica hasta 1900*. San José: Editorial Nacional de Salud y Seguro Social, 1990.

Cabrera, Lydia. *La medicina popular de Cuba: Médicos de antaño, curanderos, santeros y paleros de hogaño*. Miami, 1984.

Cameron, H. C. *Mr. Guy's Hospital*. London: Longman, 1954.

Campos, Victor, and Alia Sarkis. *Curanderismo tradicional de Costa Rica*. San José: Editorial Costa Rica, 1978.

Campos Coelho, Edmundo. *As profissões imperiais: medicina, engenharia e advocacia no Rio de Janeiro (1822–1930)*. Rio de Janeiro: Record, 1999.

Campos Marín, Ricardo. "Vacunadores en Guerra: La lucha por el monopolio profesional de la vacunación antivariólica en España, 1870–1900." Paper presented at the Symposium on Practices of Healing in Latin America and Spain, New York University, April 2001.

Canal, Nestor Miranda, Emilio Quevedo Vélez, and Mario Hernández Alvarez. *Medicina (2): La institucionalización de la medicina en Colombia*, vol. 8 of *Historia social de la ciencia en Colombia*, ed. Emilio Quevedo Vélez (Bogotá: Instituto Colombiano para el Desarrollo de la Ciencia y la Tecnología Francisco José de Caldas, 1993), 243–44.

Canguilhem, Georges. *On the Normal and the Pathological*. London: D. Reidel Publishing Co., 1978.

Casas, Antonio, and Herman Vargas. "The Health System in Costa Rica: Toward a National Health Service." *Journal of Public Health Policy* 1, no. 3 (1980): 258–79.

Casey Gaspar, Jeffrey. "El ferrocarril al Atlántico en Costa Rica, 1871–1874." *Anuario de Estudios Centroamericanos* (Costa Rica) 2 (1976): 291–344.

Cerdas A., Ana Luisa. "El surgimiento del enclave bananero en el Pacífico Sur." *Revista de Historia* (Costa Rica) 28 (1993): 117–59.

Cerdas A., José Manuel. "La cuestión social y las condiciones de vida de los obreros de Costa Rica (1930–1960)." *ABRA* (Costa Rica) 21–22 (1995): 59–95.

Cerdas Cruz, Rodolfo. *Formación del Estado en Costa Rica (1821–1842)*. San José: Editorial de la Universidad de Costa Rica, 1985.

Chacón Trejos, Gonzalo. *Tradiciones costarricenses*. San José: Trejos Hermanos, 1956.

Bibliography

Chalhoub, Sidney. "The Politics of Disease Control: Yellow Fever and Race in Nineteenth-Century Rio de Janeiro." *Journal of Latin American Studies* 25, no. 3 (1993): 441–63.

———. *Cidade febril: Cortiços e epidemias na Corte imperial.* Rio de Janeiro: Companha das letras, 1996.

Chomsky, Aviva. *West Indian Workers and the United Fruit Company in Costa Rica, 1870–1940.* Baton Rouge: Louisiana State University Press, 1996.

Conniff, Michael L. *Urban Politics in Brazil: The Rise of Populism, 1925–1945.* Pittsburgh, Pa.: University of Pittsburgh Press, 1981.

Cooper, Donald B. "The New 'Black Death': Cholera in Brazil, 1855–1856." In *The African Exchange: Toward a Biological History of Black People,* edited by Kenneth F. Kiple. Durham, N.C.: Duke University Press, 1988.

Coto Montero, Fausto. *Homenaje a doña Amparo de Zeledón.* San José: Imprenta Nacional, 1951.

Crellin, John K., and Jane Philpott. *Herbal Medicine Past and Present.* 2 vols. Durham, N.C.: Duke University Press, 1990.

Cruz, Vladimir de la. *Las luchas sociales en Costa Rica, 1870–1930.* San José: Editorial Costa Rica, 1980.

Cruz, Yalena de la. *Los Forjadores de la Seguridad Social en Costa Rica.* San José: Caja Costarricense de Seguro Social, 1994.

———. *Guillermo Padilla Castro: Forjador de instituciones.* San José: ABC Ediciones, n.d.

Cruz-Coke, Ricardo. *Historia de la medicina chilena.* Santiago: Editorial Andres Bello, 1995.

Cueto, Marcos. "Nacionalismo y ciencias médicas: Los inicios de la investigación biomédica en el Perú, 1900–1950." *Quipu* 4, no. 3 (1987): 327–55.

———. *Excelencia científica en la periferia: Actividades científicas e investigación biomédica en el Perú, 1890–1950.* Lima: Tarea, 1989.

———. "Indigenismo and Rural Medicine in Peru: The Indian Sanitary Brigade and Manuel Núñez Butrón." *Bulletin of the History of Medicine* 65 (1991): 22–41.

———. "The Cycles of Eradication: The Rockefeller Foundation and Latin American Public Health." In *International Health Organizations and Movements, 1918–1939,* edited by Paul Weindling. Cambridge: Cambridge University Press, 1995.

———, ed. *Missionaries of Science: The Rockefeller Foundation in Latin America.* Bloomington: Indiana University Press, 1994.

———. *Salud, cultura y sociedad en América Latina.* Lima: Instituto de Estudios Peruanos, 1996.

Cunningham, Andrew. "Transforming Plague: The Laboratory and the Identity of Infectious Diseases." In *The Laboratory Revolution in Medicine,* edited by Andrew Cunningham and Perry Williams. Cambridge: Cambridge University Press, 1992.

Danielson, Ross. *Cuban Medicine.* New Brunswick, N.J.: Transaction Books, 1979.

Darnton, Robert. *Mesmerism and the End of the Enlightenment in France.* Cambridge: Harvard University Press, 1968.

———. *The Great Cat Massacre and Other Episodes in French Cultural History.* New York: Vintage Books, 1985.

Davies, Celia. "The Health Visitor as Mother's Friend: A Woman's Place in Public Health, 1900–1914." *Social History of Medicine* 1, no. 1 (April 1988): 39–59.

Dávila Cubero, Juan. *Viva Vargas! Historia del Partido Confraternidad Guanacasteca.* San José: Ediciones Guayacán, 1987.

Davis, Natalie Zemon. "The Reasons of Misrule: Youth Groups and Charivaris in Sixteenth-Century France." *Past and Present* 52 (1971): 41–75.

Delaporte, François. *The History of Yellow Fever: An Essay on the Birth of Tropical Medicine.* Cambridge, Mass.: MIT Press, 1991.

Diacon, Todd A. *Millenarian Vision, Capitalist Reality: Brazil's Contestado Rebellion, 1912–1916.* Durham, N.C.: Duke University Press, 1991.

Díaz, Fabián de Jesús. *Vida e historia de la medicina en la provincia.* Valencia, Venezuela: Secretaría de Educación y Cultura, 1966.

Dobles Segreda, Luis. *Medicina e higiene.* Vol. 9 of *Indice bibliográfico de Costa Rica.* San José: Imprenta Lehmann, 1927–1936.

Dow, James. *The Shaman's Touch: Otomi Indian Symbolic Healing.* Salt Lake City: University of Utah Press, 1986.

———. "Curandero/Curandeiro." In vol. 2 of *Encyclopedia of Latin American History and Culture,* edited by Barbara Tenenbaum. New York: Charles Scribner's and Sons, 1995.

Drake, Paul W. *Socialism and Populism in Chile, 1932–1952.* Urbana: University of Illinois Press, 1978.

Eakin, Marshall C. "The Origins of Modern Science in Costa Rica: The Instituto Físico-Geográfico Nacional, 1887–1904." *Latin American Research Review* 34, no. 1 (1999): 123–50.

Echavarría Campos, Trino. *Historia y geografía del Cantón de San Ramón.* San José: Imprenta Nacional, 1966.

Edelman, Marc. "A Central American Genocide: Rubber, Slavery, Nationalism, and the Destruction of the Guatusos-Malekus." *Comparative Studies in Society and History* 4, no. 2 (1998): 356–90.

Ellis, Jack D. *The Physician-Legislators of France: Medicine and Politics in the Early Third Republic, 1870–1914.* Cambridge: Cambridge University Press, 1990.

Enríquez, Francisco. "El Curandero de Moravia." *Actualidades del CIHAC* (Centro de Investigaciones Históricas de América Central, Universidad de Costa Rica) 1, no. 5 (1994): 1–2.

———. "Diversión pública y sociabilidad en las comunidades cafetaleras de San José: El caso de Moravia (1890–1930)." Master's thesis, University of Costa Rica, 1998.

Escudé, Carlos Andrés. "Health in Buenos Aires in the Second Half of the Nineteenth Century." In *Social Welfare, 1850–1950: Australia, Argentina, and Canada Compared,* edited by D. C. M. Platt. London: Macmillan Publishers Ltd., 1989.

Ettling, John. *The Germ of Laziness: Rockefeller Philanthropy and Public Health in the New South.* Cambridge: Harvard University Press, 1981.

Fallas Monge, Carlos Luis. *El movimiento obrero en Costa Rica, 1830–1902.* San José: Editorial Universidad Estatal a Distancia, 1983.

Farley, John. "Parasites and the Germ Theory of Disease." In *Framing Disease: Studies in Cultural History,* edited by Charles Rosenberg and Janet Golden. New Brunswick, N.J.: Rutgers University Press, 1992.

Finkler, Kaja. *Spiritualist Healers in Mexico: Success and Failure of Alternative Therapeutics.* New York: Praeger, 1985.

Fischel, Astrid. *Consenso y represión: Una interpretación socio-política de la educación costarricense.* San José: Editorial Costa Rica, 1987.

———. *El uso ingenioso de la ideología en Costa Rica.* San José: Editorial Universidad Estatal a Distancia, 1992.

Flores Mescal, Mario. "Historia de la Universidad en El Salvador." *Anuario de Estudios Centroamericanos* 1 (1976): 107–40.

Foster, George M. "On the Origin of Humoral Medicine in Latin America." *Medical Anthropology Quarterly* 1, no. 4 (December 1987): 355–93.

Frutos Verdesia, Juan Bautista. *Dr. Solón Núñez Frutos.* San José: Ministerio de Cultura, Juventud y Deportes, 1979.

Fumero Vargas, Patricia. "La ciudad en la aldea: Actividades y diversiones urbanas en San José a mediados del siglo XIX." In *Héroes al gusto y libros de moda: Sociedad y cambio cultural en Costa Rica (1750–1900),* edited by Iván Molina Jiménez and Steven Palmer. San José: Plumsock Mesoamerican Studies, 1992.

———, ed. *Centenario de la Facultad de Farmacia.* San José: Editorial de la Universidad de Costa Rica, 1997.

Gabb, William M. "On the Indian Tribes and Languages of Costa Rica." *Proceedings of the American Philosophical Society* 14 (1875): 483–601.

García, Juan César. *Pensamiento social en salud en América Latina.* Mexico City: Interamericana McGraw Hill, 1994.

Gevitz, Norman, ed. *Other Healers: Unorthodox Medicine in America.* Baltimore, Md.: Johns Hopkins University Press, 1988.

Gil Zúñiga, José Daniel. "La Virgen de los Angeles: Evolución de un mito." *Revista de Historia* (Costa Rica) 11 (1985): 47–129.

———. "Delito y control social en la provincia de Heredia, 1885–1941." Paper presented at the symposium Las sociedades centroamericanas siglos XIX y XX. San José, 1990.

Goldwater, Carmel. "Traditional Medicine in Latin America." In *Traditional Medicine and Health Care Coverage: A Reader for Health Care Administrators and Practitioners,* edited by Robert H. Bannerman et al. Geneva: World Health Organization, 1983.

Gómez A., Juan. "José C. Zeledón." In *Homenaje a don José C. Zeledón.* San José: Imprenta Trejos Hermanos, 1924.

González Flores, Luis Felipe. *Historia de la influencia extranjera en el desenvolvimiento educacional y científico de Costa Rica.* San José: Editorial Costa Rica, 1976.

González González, Gonzalo. "Algunos datos sobre historia de la farmacia y la medicina en Costa Rica." *Revista de la Universidad de Costa Rica* 1 (September 1945): 66–70.

González Leandri, Ricardo. *Curar, persuadir, gobernar: La construcción histórica de la profesión médica en Buenos Aires, 1852–1886.* Madrid: Consejo Superior de Investigaciones Científicas-Centro de Estudios Históricos, 1999.

González Pacheco, Carlos Eduardo. *Hospital San Juan de Dios: 150 años de historia.* San José: Editorial Nacional del Seguro Social, 1995.

González Villalobos, Paulino. *La Universidad de Santo Tomás.* San José: Editorial de la Universidad de Costa Rica, 1989.

Grandin, Greg. *The Blood of Guatemala: A History of Race and Nation.* Durham, N.C.: Duke University Press, 2000.

Gudmundson, Lowell. *Costa Rica before Coffee: Society and Economy on the Eve of the Export Boom.* Baton Rouge: Louisiana State University Press, 1986.

———. "De 'Negro' a 'Blanco' en la Hispanoamérica del siglo XIX: La asimilación afroamericana en Argentina y en Costa Rica." *Mesoamérica* 12, no. 7 (1986): 309–29.

Guerra, Francisco. "Drugs from the Indies and the Political Economy of the Sixteenth Century." In *Analecta Médico-Historica: I Materia Médica in the Sixteenth Century.* London: Pergamon Press, 1966.

———. *El médico político: Su influencia en la historia de Hispano-América y Filipinas.* Madrid: Afrodisio Aguado, 1975.

———. *Las medicinas marginales: Los sistemas de curar prohibidos a los médicos.* Madrid: Alianza Editorial, 1976.

Guy, Donna J. *Sex and Danger in Buenos Aires: Prostitution, Family, and Nation in Argentina.* Lincoln: University of Nebraska Press, 1990.

Hale, Charles A. "Political and Social Ideas in Latin America, 1870–1930." In vol. 4 of *The Cambridge History of Latin America,* edited by Leslie Bethell. Cambridge: Cambridge University Press, 1984–1995.

———. *The Transformation of Liberalism in Late-Nineteenth-Century Mexico.* Princeton, N.J.: Princeton University Press, 1989.

Hall, Carolyn. *El café y el desarrollo histórico-geográfico de Costa Rica.* 3d ed. San José: Editorial Costa Rica, 1982.

Hernández Rodríguez, Carlos. "Trabajadores, empresarios y Estado: La dinámica de clase y los límites institucionales del conflicto, 1900–1943." *Revista de Historia* (Costa Rica) 27 (1993): 51–86.

———. "Herbolarios, empíricos y farmacéuticos: Contribución a la historia de la farmacia en Costa Rica." In *Centenario de la Facultad de Farmacia, Universidad de Costa Rica, 1897–1997,* edited by Patricia Fumero. San José: Editorial de la Universidad de Costa Rica, 1998.

Hernández Sáenz, Luz María. "Learning to Heal: The Medical Profession in Colonial Mexico, 1767–1831." Ph.D. diss., University of Arizona, 1993.

———. *Learning to Heal: The Medical Profession in Colonial Mexico, 1767–1831.* New York: Peter Lang, 1997.

Hess, David J. *Spirits and Scientists: Ideology, Spiritism, and Brazilian Culture.* University Park, Pa.: Penn State University Press, 1991.

Hewa, Soma. "The Hookworm Epidemic on the Plantations in Colonial Sri Lanka." *Medical History* 38, no. 1 (1994): 167–83.

Historia general de la medicina argentina. 2 vols. Córdoba: Universidad nacional Autónoma de Córdoba, 1976–1980.

Hochman, Gilberto. *A era do saneamento: As bases da política de saúde pública no Brasil.* São Paulo: Editora Hucitec, 1998.

Incera Olivas, Eugenia. "El Hospital San Juan de Dios: Sus antecedentes y su evolución histórica, 1845–1900." Licenciatura Thesis, University of Costa Rica, 1978.

Jackson, Ralph. *Doctors and Diseases in the Roman Empire.* Norman: University of Oklahoma Press, 1989.

Jenkins, Gwynne L. "Changing Roles and Identities of Midwives in Rural Costa Rica." *Medical Anthropology* 20 (2001): 409–44.

Jones, Norman Howard. *The Pan-American Health Organization: Origins and Evolution.* Geneva: World Health Organization, 1981.

Joseph, Gilbert M., and Daniel Nugent, eds. *Everyday Forms of State Formation: Revolution and the Negotiation of Rule in Modern Mexico.* Durham, N.C.: Duke University Press, 1994.

Karasch, Mary C. *Slave Life in Rio de Janeiro, 1808–1850.* Princeton, N.J.: Princeton University Press, 1987.

Katz, Friedrich. *The Life and Times of Pancho Villa.* Stanford, Calif.: Stanford University Press, 1995.

Kiple, Kenneth F., ed. *The Cambridge World History of Human Disease.* Cambridge: Cambridge University Press, 1993.

Knight, Alan. "Populism and Neo-populism in Latin America, Especially Mexico." *Journal of Latin American Studies* 30 (1998): 223–48.

Koven, Seth, and Sonya Michel. "Womenly Duties: Maternalist Politics and the Origins of the Welfare State in France, Germany, Great Britain, and the United States." *American Historical Review* 95, no. 4 (1990): 1089–1108.

Koss, Joan D. "Religion and Science Divinely Related: A Case History of Spiritism in Puerto Rico." *Caribbean Studies* 16, no. 1 (April 1976): 23–43.

Láchner Sandoval, Vicente. "Apuntes de higiene pública: Organismos, institutos y profesiones en relación con este ramo." In *Revista de Costa Rica en el siglo XIX.* San José: Imprenta Nacional, 1902.

Lagarriga Attias, Isabel. *Medicina tradicional y espiritismo, Los espiritualistas trinitarios marianos de Jalapa, Veracruz.* Mexico City: Sociedad de Estudios Paranormales, 1975.

Lanning, John Tate. *Academic Culture in the Spanish Colonies.* Folcroft, Pa.: Folcroft Press, Inc., 1949.

———. *The Royal Protomedicato: The Regulation of the Professions in the Spanish Empire.* Edited by John Jay TePaske. Durham, N.C.: Duke University Press, 1985.

Lantaro Ferrer, Pedro. *Historia general de la medicina en Chile.* Talca, Chile: Imprenta Talca, 1904.

Láscaris, Constantino. *Desarrollo de las ideas en Costa Rica.* 2d ed. San José: Editorial Costa Rica, 1975.

Lastres, Juan B. *Historia de la medicina peruana.* 3 vols. Lima: Imprenta Santa María, 1951.

——. *La cultura peruana y la obra de los médicos en la emancipación.* Lima: Editorial San Marcos, 1954.

Leavitt, Judith Walzer. *The Healthiest City: Milwaukee and the Politics of Health Reform.* Princeton, N.J.: Princeton University Press, 1982.

——. *Brought to Bed: Childbearing in America, 1750–1950.* New York: Oxford University Press, 1986.

——. "Medicine in Context: A Review Essay of the History of Medicine." *American Historical Review* 95, no. 5 (December 1990): 1471–84.

Lehoucq, Fabrice, and Ivan Molina. *Stuffing the Ballot Box: Fraud, Electoral Reform, and Democracy in Comparative Perspective.* Cambridge: Cambridge University Press, 1992.

Levine, Robert M., and John J. Crocitti, eds. *The Brazil Reader: History, Culture, Politics.* Durham, N.C.: Duke University Press, 1999.

Lewis, Milton, and Roy Macleod, eds. *Disease, Medicine, and Empire: Perspectives on Western Medicine and the Experience of European Expansion.* New York: Routledge, 1988.

Loudon, Irvine. "The Nature of Provincial Medical Practice in Eighteenth-Century England." *Medical History* 29 (1985): 1–32.

Low, Setha M. "Dr. Moreno Cañas: A Symbolic Bridge to the De-medicalization of Healing." *Social Science and Medicine* 16, no. 5 (1982): 527–31.

——. "The Medicalization of Healing Cults in Latin America." *American Ethnologist* 15, no. 1 (1988): 136–55.

Luros, Pablo. "Nuestro problema médico-hospitalario." *Revista Médica* (Costa Rica) 9, no. 189 (1950): 11–28.

Malavassi, Paulina. "Entre la marginalidad social y los orígenes de la salud pública: Leprosos, curanderos y facultativos en el valle Central de Costa Rica, 1784–1845." Master's thesis, Universidad de Costa Rica, 1998.

Malloy, James M. *The Politics of Social Security in Brazil.* Pittsburgh, Pa.: University of Pittsburgh Press, 1979.

Marín Hernández, Juan José. "Prostitución y pecado en la bella y próspera ciudad de San José." In *El paso del cometa: Estado, política social y culturas populares en Costa Rica (1800–1950),* edited by Iván Molina Jiménez and Steven Palmer. San José: Plumsock Mesoamerican Studies, 1994.

——. "De curanderos a médicos: Una aproximación a la historia de la medicina en Costa Rica, 1800–1949." *Revista de Historia* (Costa Rica) 32 (1995): 65–108.

Marks, Shula. "What Is Colonial about Colonial Medicine? And What Has Happened to Imperialism and Health?" *Social History of Medicine* 10, no. 2 (1997): 205–19.

Marquez, Patricio V., and Daniel J. Joly, "A Historical Overview of the Ministries of Public Health and the Medical Programs of the Social Security Systems in Latin America." *Journal of Public Health Policy* 7, no. 3 (1986): 378–94.

Martínez Durán, Carlos. *Las ciencias médicas en Guatemala: Orígen y evolución.* 3d ed. Guatemala City: Editorial Universitaria, 1964.

McClellan, James E. *Colonialism and Science: Saint Domingue in the Old Regime.* Baltimore, Md.: Johns Hopkins University Press, 1992.

Meade, Teresa A. *"Civilizing" Rio: Reform and Resistance in a Brazilian City, 1889–1930.* University Park: Pennsylvania State University Press, 1997.

Meléndez Chaverri, Carlos. *Dr. José María Montealegre.* San José: Academia de Geografía e Historia, 1968.

Mercier, D. J. *Psicología: Vida orgánica y sensitiva; Vida intelectiva o racional.* Buenos Aires: Ediciones Anaconda, 1942.

Mesa-Lago, Carmelo. *Social Security in Latin America: Pressure Groups, Stratifications, and Inequality.* Pittsburgh, Pa.: University of Pittsburgh Press, 1978.

Molina Jiménez, Iván. *Costa Rica (1800–1850): El legado colonial y la génesis del capitalismo.* San José: Editorial de la Universidad de Costa Rica, 1991.

———. "Los catálogos de libros como fuentes históricas." *Revista de Filosofía de la Universidad de Costa Rica* 30, no. 71 (1992): 103–16.

———. "Vivienda y muebles: el marco material de la vida doméstica en el Valle Central de Costa Rica (1821–1824)." *Revista de Historia de América* no. 116 (July–December 1993): 60–91.

———. *"El que quiera divertirse": Libros y sociedad en Costa Rica, 1750–1914.* San José: Editorial de la Universidad de Costa Rica, 1995.

———. *La ciudad de los monos: Roberto Brenes Mesén, los católicos heredianos y el conflicto cultural de 1907 en Costa Rica.* San José: Editorial de la Universidad de Costa Rica, 2001.

Molina Jiménez, Iván, and Fabrice Lehoucq. *Urnas de lo inesperado: Fraude electoral y lucha política en Costa Rica (1901–1948).* San José: Editorial de la Universidad de Costa Rica, 1999.

Molina Jiménez, Iván, and Steven Palmer. *The History of Costa Rica: Brief, Up-to-Date and Illustrated.* San José: Editorial de la Universidad de Costa Rica, 1998.

Molina Jiménez, Iván, and Steven Palmer, eds. *Héroes al gusto y libros de moda: Sociedad y cambio cultural en Costa Rica (1750–1900).* San José: Plumsock Mesoamerican Studies, 1992.

———. *El paso del cometa: Estado, política social y culturas populares en Costa Rica (1800–1950).* San José: Plumsock Mesoamerican Studies, 1994.

———. *Educando a Costa Rica: Alfabetización popular, formación docente y género (1880–1950).* San José: Plumsock Mesoamerican Studies, 2000.

Moll, Aristides A. *Aesculapius in Latin America.* Philadelphia, Pa.: W. B. Saunders Company, 1944.

Monge Alfaro, Carlos. *Nuestra historia y los seguros.* San José: Editorial Costa Rica, 1974.

Mongeau, Beatrice Bell. "The 'Granny' Midwives: A Study of a Folk Institution in the Process of Social Integration." Ph.D. diss. University of North Carolina, 1973.

Morales, Gerardo. *Cultura oligárquica y nueva intelectualidad en Costa Rica, 1880–1914.* San José: Editorial de la Universidad Nacional Autónoma, 1993.

Morgan, Lynn Marie. *Community Participation in Health: The Politics of Primary Care in Costa Rica.* New York: Cambridge University Press, 1993.

Moya Gutiérrez, Arnaldo. "Cultura material y vida cotidiana. El entorno doméstico de los vecinos principales de Cartago (1750–1820)." In *Héroes al gusto y libros de moda: Sociedad y cambio cultural en Costa Rica (1750–1900)*, edited by Iván Molina Jiménez and Steven Palmer. San José: Plumsock Mesoamerican Studies, 1992.

Murdock, Carl J. "Physicians, the State, and Public Health in Chile, 1881–1891." *Journal of Latin American Studies* 27 (1995): 551–67.

Murillo Chaverri, Carmen. *Identidades de hierro y humo: La construcción del ferrocarril al Atlántico, 1870–1890*. San José: Editorial Porvenir, 1995.

Needell, Jeffrey. "The *Revolta Contra Vacina* of 1904: The Revolt against 'Modernization' in Belle-Epoque Rio de Janeiro." *Hispanic American Historical Review* 67, no. 2 (1987): 233–69.

Nye, Robert A. *Crime, Madness, and Politics in Modern France: The Medical Concept of National Decline*. Princeton, N.J.: Princeton University Press, 1984.

Oconitrillo, Eduardo. *Los Tinoco (1917–1919)*. San José: Editorial Costa Rica, 1982.

———. *El Bellavistazo*. San José: Editorial Costa Rica, 1983.

———. *Vida, muerte y mito del Dr. Moreno Cañas*. San José: Editorial Costa Rica, 1985.

———. *Julio Acosta: El hombre de la providencia*. San José: Editorial Costa Rica, 1994.

Orellana, Sandra L. *Indian Medicine in Highland Guatemala: The Pre-Hispanic and Colonial Periods*. Albuquerque: University of New Mexico Press, 1987.

Orlove, Benjamin, ed. *The Allure of the Foreign: Imported Goods in Postcolonial Latin America*. Ann Arbor: University of Michigan Press, 1997.

Ortíz de Montellano, Bernardo. *Aztec Medicine, Health, and Nutrition*. New Brunswick, N.J.: Rutgers University Press, 1990.

Ovares, Flora, and Margarita Rojas. *100 años de la literatura costarricense*. San José: Ediciones Farben, 1995.

Ovares, Flora, Margarita Rojas, Carlos Santander, and María Elena Carballo. *La casa paterna: Escritura y nación en Costa Rica*. San José: Editorial de la Universidad de Costa Rica, 1993.

Palmer, Steven. "A Liberal Discipline: Inventing Nations in Costa Rica and Guatemala, 1870–1900." Ph.D. diss., Columbia University, 1990.

———. "Getting to Know the Unknown Soldier: Official Nationalism in Liberal Costa Rica, 1880–1900." *Journal of Latin American Studies* 25 (1993): 45–72.

———. "Pánico en San José: El consumo de heroína, la cultura plebeya y la política social en 1929." In *El paso del cometa: Estado, política social y culturas populares en Costa Rica (1800–1950)*, edited by Iván Molina Jiménez and Steven Palmer. San José: Plumsock Mesoamerican Studies, 1994.

———. "Confinement, Policing, and the Emergence of Social Policy in Costa Rica, 1885–1935." In *The Birth of the Penitentiary in Latin America: Essays on Criminology, Prison Reform, and Social Control, 1830–1940*, edited by Carlos Aguirre and Ricardo Salvatore. Austin: University of Texas Press, 1996.

———. "Prolegómenos a toda futura historia de San José, Costa Rica." *Mesoamérica* 31 (1996): 181–213.

———. "Central American Encounters with Rockefeller Public Health, 1914–1921." In *Close Encounters of Empire: Writing the Cultural History of U.S.–Latin Amer-*

ican Relations, edited by Gilbert Joseph, Catherine Legrand, and Ricardo Salvatore. Durham, N.C.: Duke University Press, 1998.

———. "Adiós Laissez-faire: La política social en Costa Rica (1880–1940)." *Revista de Historia de América,* 124 (1999): 99–117.

Palmer, Steven, and Gladys Rojas. "Educating Señorita: Teacher Training, Social Mobility, and the Birth of Costa Rican Feminism, 1885–1925." *Hispanic American Historical Review* 78, no. 1 (1998): 45–82.

Peard, Julyan G. "Tropical Medicine in Nineteenth-Century Brazil: The Case of the 'Escola Tropicalista Bahiana,' 1860–1890." In *Warm Climates and Western Medicine: The Emergence of Tropical Medicine, 1500–1900,* edited by David Arnold. Amsterdam: Editions Rodopi, 1996.

———. "Tropical Disorders and the Forging of a Brazilian Medical Identity, 1860–1890." *Hispanic American Historical Review* 77, no. 1 (1997): 1–43.

———. *Race, Place, and Medicine: The Idea of the Tropics in Nineteenth-Century Brazilian Medicine.* Durham, N.C.: Duke University Press, 1999.

Perdiguero, Enrique. "The Popularization of Medicine during the Spanish Enlightenment." In *The Popularization of Medicine, 1650–1850,* edited by Roy Porter. New York: Routledge, 1992.

Pérez Brignoli, Héctor. "El crecimiento demográfico de América Latina en los siglos XIX y XX: Problemas, métodos y perspectivas." *Avances de Investigación* (Centro de Investigaciones Históricas, Universidad de Costa Rica) 48 (1989): 1–28.

Pérez Fontana, Velarde. *Historia de la medicina en el Uruguay con especial referencia a las comarcas del Río de la Plata.* 2 vols. Montevideo: Ministerio de Salud Pública, 1967.

Perone, Babette, H. Henrietta Stockel, and Victoria Krueger. *Medicine Women, Curanderas, and Women Doctors.* Norman: University of Oklahoma Press, 1989.

Picado Chacón, Manuel. *Dr. Clodomiro Picado: Vida y obra.* San José: Editorial de la Universidad de Costa Rica, 1980.

Pineo, Ronn F. "Misery and Death in the Pearl of the Pacific: Health Care in Guayaquil, Ecuador, 1870–1925." *Hispanic American Historical Review* 70, no. 4 (1990): 609–37.

———. *Social and Economic Reform in Ecuador: Life and Work in Guayaquil.* Gainesville: University Press of Florida, 1996.

Porter, Roy. "The Patient's View: Doing Medical History from Below." *Theory and Society* 14, no. 2 (1985): 175–98.

———. *Health for Sale: Quackery in England, 1650–1850.* Manchester: Manchester University Press, 1989.

———. *The Greatest Benefit to Mankind: A Medical History of Humanity from Antiquity to the Present.* London: Harper Collins, 1997.

Press, Irwin. "The Urban Curandero." *American Anthropologist* 73, no. 3 (1971): 741–56.

———. "Problems in the Definition and Classification of Medical Systems." *Social Science and Medicine* 14B (1980): 45–57.

Quesada Avendaño, Florencia. *En el Barrio Amón: Arquitectura, familia y sociabilidad del primer residencial de la elite urbana de San José, 1900–1935*. San José: Editorial de la Universidad de Costa Rica, 2001.

Quesada Soto, Alvaro. *La formación de la narrativa nacional costarricense (1890–1910): Enfoque histórico-social*. San José: Editorial Universidad de Costa Rica, 1986.

———. *La voz desgarrada: La crisis del discurso oligárquico y la narrativa costarricense, 1917–1919*. San José: Editorial de la Universidad de Costa Rica, 1988.

Quevedo, Emilio, and Amarillys Zaldúa. "Antecedentes de las reformas médicas del siglo XVIII y XIX en el Nuevo Reino de Granada: Una polémica entre médicos y cirujanos." *Quipu* 3, no. 3 (1986): 311–34.

Quirós, Claudia. *La era de la encomienda*. San José: Editorial Universidad de Costa Rica, 1990.

Ramírez, Victoria. *Jorge Volio y la revolución viviente*. San José: Editorial Guayacan, 1989.

Ramsey, Matthew. *Professional and Popular Medicine in France, 1770–1830: The Social World of Medical Practice*. Cambridge: Cambridge University Press, 1988.

———. "Alternative Medicine in Modern France." *Medical History* 43 (1999): 286–322.

Richardson, Miles, and Barbara Bode. "Popular Medicine in Puntarenas, Costa Rica: Urban and Societal Features." In *Community Culture and National Change*, edited by Richard N. Adams et al. New Orleans: Middle American Research Institute, 1972.

Risse, Guenter B. "Medicine in New Spain." In *Medicine in the New World*, edited by Ronald R. Numbers. Knoxville: University of Tennessee Press, 1987.

———. *Mending Bodies, Saving Souls: A History of Hospitals*. New York: Oxford University Press, 1999.

Risse, Guenter B., Ronald L. Numbers, and Judith Walzer Leavitt, eds. *Medicine without Doctors: Home Health Care in American History*. New York: Science History Publications, 1977.

Robles Soto, Arodys. "Patrones de población en Costa Rica, 1860–1930." *Avances de Investigación* (Centro de Investigaciones Históricas, Universidad de Costa Rica) 14 (1986): 1–39.

Rodríguez Sáenz, Eugenia. "'Tiyita, bea lo que me han echo': Estupro e incesto en Costa Rica (1800–1850)." In *El paso del cometa: Estado, política social y culturas populares en Costa Rica (1800–1950)*, edited by Iván Molina Jiménez and Steven Palmer. San José: Plumsock Mesoamerican Studies, 1994.

Roig de Leuchsenring, Emilio. *Médicos y medicina en Cuba: Historia, biografía y costumbrismo*. Havana: Museo Histórico de las Ciencias Médicas "Carlos J. Finlay," 1965.

Rojas Bolaños, Manuel. *Lucha social y guerra civil en Costa Rica*. San José: Editorial Porvenir, 1989.

Rojas Chaves, Gladys. *Café, ambiente y sociedad en la cuenca del río Virilla, Costa Rica (1840–1955)*. San José: Editorial de la Universidad de Costa Rica, 2000.

Ramón Trigo, Ana Cecilia. *Las finanzas públicas de Costa Rica: Metodología y fuentes (1870–1948)*. San José: Centro de Investigaciones de América Central, 1995.

Romero, José Luis. *Latinoamérica: Las ciudades y las ideas.* 3d ed. Mexico City: Siglo XXI, 1976.

Rosenberg, Charles E. *The Cholera Years: The United States in 1832, 1849, and 1866.* Chicago: University of Chicago Press, 1962.

———. "Medical Text and Social Context: Explaining William Buchan's Domestic Medicine." *Bulletin of the History of Medicine* 57 (1983): 22–42.

———. *The Care of Strangers: The Rise of America's Hospital System.* New York: Basic Books, 1987.

Rosenberg, Mark. *Las luchas por el seguro social en Costa Rica.* San José: Editorial Costa Rica, 1983.

———. "Social Reform in Costa Rica: Social Security and the Presidency of Rafael Angel Calderón Guardia." *Hispanic American Historical Review* 61, no. 2 (1981): 279–96.

Ruggiero, Kristin. "Honor, Maternity, and the Disciplining of Women: Infanticide in Late Nineteenth-Century Buenos Aires." *Hispanic American Historical Review* 72, no. 3 (1992): 353–73.

Ruiz Naufal, Victor M., and Arturo Gálvez Medrano. "La *Historia de la Medicina en México* dentro de la historiografía médica mexicana." In vol. 1 of *Historia de la Medicina en México desde la época de los indios hasta el presente,* edited by Francisco de Asis Flores y Troncoso. Mexico City: Instituto Mexicano de Seguro Social, 1982.

Russell-Wood, A. J. R. *Fidalgos and Philanthropists: The Santa Casa de Misericordia of Bahia, 1550–1755.* Berkeley: University of California Press, 1968.

———. *The Black Man in Slavery and Freedom in Colonial Brazil.* New York: St. Martin's Press, 1982.

Sabater Reyes, Miguel Angel. "Los primeros médicos chinos en Cuba," *Boletín del Archivo Nacional* (Cuba), no. 11 (1988): 23–29.

Salazar Mora, Jorge Mario. *Calderón Guardia.* San José: Ministerio de Cultura, Juventud y Deportes, 1980.

———. *Política y reforma en Costa Rica, 1914–1958.* San José: Editorial Porvenir, 1981.

———. *El significado de la legislación social de los cuarenta en Costa Rica.* San José: Ministerio de Educación Pública, 1993.

———. *Crisis liberal y Estado reformista, 1914–1949.* San José: Editorial Universidad de Costa Rica, 1995.

Salgado Pimenta, Tânia. "Barbeiros-sangradores e curandeiros no Brasil (1808–1828)." *Manguinhos: História, Ciencias, Saúde* 5, no. 2 (1998): 349–72.

Samper, Mario. "Generations of Settlers: A Study of Rural Households and Their Markets on the Costa Rican Frontier, 1850–1935." Ph.D. diss., University of California at Berkeley, 1987.

Samper, Mario, ed. *El censo de la población de 1927: Creación de una base nominal computarizada.* San José: Oficina de Publicaciones de la Universidad de Costa Rica, 1991.

Sanfilippo B., José. "Ocultismo y medicina." *Boletín mexicano de historia y filosofía de la medicina* 12, nos. 71–74 (1990): 47–53.

Santos Filho, Lycurgo de Castro. *História geral da medicina brasileira.* 2 vols. São Paulo: Editora de Universidade de São Paulo, 1977–1991.

———. "Medicine in Colonial Brazil: An Overview." In *Aspects of the History of Medicine in Latin America,* edited by John Z. Bowers and Elizabeth F. Purcell. New York: Josiah Macy Jr. Foundation, 1979.

Schendel, Gordon. *Medicine in Mexico: From Aztec Herbs to Betatrons.* Austin: University of Texas Press, 1968.

Sheridan, Richard B. *Doctors and Slaves: A Medical and Demographic History of Slavery in the British West Indies, 1680–1834.* Cambridge: Cambridge University Press, 1985.

Sherraden, Margaret S. "Social Policy in Latin America: Questions of Growth, Equality, and Political Freedom." *Latin American Research Review* 30, no. 1 (1995): 176–90.

Shortt, S. E. D. "Physicians and Psychics: The Anglo-American Medical Response to Spiritualism, 1870–1890." *Journal of the History of Medicine and Allied Sciences* 39, no. 3 (July 1984): 339–55.

Simmons, Ozzie G. "Popular and Modern Medicine in Mestizo Communities of Coastal Peru and Chile." *Journal of American Folklore* 68, no. 267 (1955): 57–71.

Siraisi, Nancy G. *Medieval and Early Renaissance Medicine: An Introduction to Knowledge and Practice.* Chicago: University of Chicago Press, 1990.

Skinner, Alanson. "Notes on the Bribri of Costa Rica," *Indian Notes and Monographs* 6, no. 3 (1920): 23–48.

Smith, Brian A. *A History of the Nursing Profession.* London: Heinemann, 1960.

Smith, Michael M. "The 'Real Expedición Marítima de la Vacuna' in New Spain and Guatemala." *Transactions of the American Philosophical Society* 64, no. 1 (1974): 1–65.

Sotela, José Enrique. *Reseña histórica de la anestesia en Costa Rica.* San José: Editorial Nacional de Salud y Seguro Social, 1997.

Sowell, David. "Miguel Perdomo Neira: Healing, Culture, and Power in the Nineteenth-Century Andes." *Anuario Colombiano de Historia Social y de la Cultura* 24 (1997): 167–88.

———. *The Tale of Healer Miguel Perdomo Neira: Medicine, Ideologies, and Power in the Nineteenth-Century Andes.* Wilmington, Del.: Scholarly Resources, 2001.

Stepan, Nancy Leys. "The Interplay between Socio-economic Factors and Medical Science: Yellow Fever Research, Cuba, and the United States." *Social Studies of Science* 8 (1978): 397–424.

———. *Beginnings of Brazilian Science: Oswaldo Cruz, Medical Research, and Policy, 1890–1920.* New York: Science History Publications, 1981.

———. *"The Hour of Eugenics": Race, Gender, and Nation in Latin America.* Ithaca, N.Y.: Cornell University Press, 1991.

———. "Tropical Medicine in Brazil, 1900–1930s: Foreign Models, Local Realities." Paper presented at the Commonwealth Fund Conference, Cultural Encounters and Resistance: The United States and Latin America, London, 2001.

Stern, Alexandra Minna. "Responsible Mothers and Normal Children: Eugenics, Nationalism, and Welfare in Post-revolutionary Mexico, 1920–1940," *Journal of Historical Sociology* 12, no. 4 (1999): 369–97.

Bibliography

Stone, Doris. *Los tribus talamanqueños de Costa Rica.* San José: Editorial Antonio Lehmann, 1961.

Stone, Samuel. *Dinastía de los conquistadores.* San José: Editorial Universiteria Centroamericana, 1983.

Taussig, Michael. *Shamanism, Colonialism, and the Wild Man: A Study in Terror and Healing.* Chicago: University of Chicago Press, 1987.

Tenorio-Trillo, Mauricio. *Mexico at the World's Fairs: Crafting a Modern Nation.* Berkeley: University of California Press, 1996.

Texera Arnal, Yolanda. "Médicos y cirujanos pardos 'en condición de por ahora' en la provincia de Venezuela, siglo XVIII." *Colonial Latin American History Review* 8, no. 3 (1999): 321–38.

Tjarks, German, et al., "La epidemia de cólera de 1856 en el Valle Central: Análisis y consecuencias demográficas." *Revista de Historia* (Costa Rica) 3 (1978): 81–127.

Trinidade Lima, Nísia, and Narra Britto. "Salud y nación: Propuesta para el saneamiento rural. Un estudio de la revista *Saúde* (1918–1919)." In *Salud, cultura y sociedad en América Latina,* edited by Marcos Cueto. Lima: Instituto de Estudios Peruanos, 1996.

Valladares, Manuel. "La causa del Dr. Esteban Cortí, alias Curti." *Revista de los Archivos Nacionales* (Costa Rica) 3, nos. 3–4 (1939): 132–69.

Vargas Arias, Claudio Antonio. *El liberalismo, La Iglesia y el Estado en Costa Rica.* San José: Guayacán, 1991.

Viales Hurtado, Ronny José. *Después del enclave: Un estudio de la region Atlántica costarricense, 1927–1950.* San José: Editorial de la Universidad de Costa Rica, 1998.

Vicuña Mackenna, Benjamín. *Médicos de antaño.* 1877. Reprint, Santiago: Editorial Francisco de Aguirre, 1974.

Viesca Treviño, Carlos. "Curanderismo in Mexico and Guatemala: Its Historical Evolution from the Sixteenth to the Nineteenth Century." In *Mesoamerican Healers,* edited by Brad R. Huber and Alan R. Sandstrom. Austin: University of Texas Press, 2001.

Voeks, Robert A. *Sacred Leaves of Condomblé: African Magic, Medicine, and Religion in Brazil.* Austin: University of Texas Press, 1997.

Walkowitz, Judith R. *City of Dreadful Delight: Narratives of Sexual Danger in Late-Victorian London.* Chicago: University of Chicago Press, 1992.

Warner, John Harley. "The Idea of Southern Medical Distinctiveness: Medical Knowledge and Practice in the Old South." In *Sickness and Health in America: Readings in the History of Medicine and Public Health,* edited by Judith Walzer Leavitt and Ronald R. Numbers. 2d ed. Madison: University of Wisconsin Press, 1985.

Wünderich, Volker. *Sandino: Una biografía política.* Managua: Editorial Nueva Nicaragua, 1995.

Zimmerman, Eduardo A. *Los liberales reformistas: La cuestión social en la Argentina, 1890–1916.* Buenos Aires: Editorial Sudamericana, 1995.

Zulawski, Ann. "Hygiene and the 'Indian Problem': Ethnicity and Medicine in Bolivia, 1910–1920." *Latin American Research Review* 35, no. 2 (2000): 107–28.

INDEX

Abel, Christopher, 159, 177
Acosta, Julio, 180–81, 191–92
Acuña, Irene, 200–202
African-based medicine, 2, 8,14, 19, 22, 31–33, 131–34, 144, 189, 198. *See also* Ethnicity; Obeah
Afro-Caribbeans: of Costa Rica, 11, 33, 146
Agricultural workers, 175–77, 223
Alajuela: epidemics in, 12–13, 76; hospital in, 108; licensed midwives in, 151; numbers of healers in, 62; physicians in, 93, 98, 99, 225; unlicensed empirics in, 26–30
Alberdi, Juan, 147
Allende Gossens, Salvador, 218–19
Alternative medicine: 15, 189, 214, 217, 231, 237. *See also* Carballo Romero, Carlos; Homeopaths; Spiritists; Unorthodox healers
Alvarado, Carlos, 161–62
Alvarado, Lucas, 40, 45, 52
Ancylostomiasis. *See* Hookworm disease
Anesthesia, 51, 73–74, 103, 115, 122, 142, 194
Antillón, Sotero, 183–84, 186, 200–203
Apothecaries, 53, 126–30, 136; use of term, 16
Aragón, Carlos, 109–13
Argentina, 8, 146, 147, 288 n.24; medi-

cal journals in, 78; medical reform in, 69–70, 82, 219–20
Arias, Arnulfo, 219
Arnold, David, 241–42 n.12

Bacteriology, 4–7, 25, 117, 158, 181, 211; and increased stature of physicians, 124; revolution in, and medical and hospital reform, 68–69, 74, 83–93, 159, 222, 233
Bahia, 19, 51, 95. *See also* Tropicalista School (Bahia)
Bananas, 11, 13, 93, 146, 159, 161. *See also* Afro-Caribbeans; Limón; United Fruit Company
Barber-surgeons, 26–29, 47, 59, 125, 132, 137; licensing of, by Protomedicato, 53–56; predominance of blacks and mulattoes among, 33. *See also* Brenes, Nicolás; Empirics; Ethnicity; Tooth pullers
Barboza Meléndez, Ramona, 129, 134
Barreda, Gabino, 68
Bastos, Francisco, 58–59
Benchimol, Jaime, 117
Billings, John S., 73–74.
Biomedicine, 3, 4, 8, 23, 25, 117, 155–56, 190, 231–32, 235–36; as arm of neocolonialism, 6, 9, 234; popular responses to, 8, 184; and positivism, 25,

Biomedicine (*cont.*)
67, 218. *See also* Bacteriology; Imperial medicine; Medical systems

Borges, Dain, 83, 95, 96

Bourbon reforms: of hygiene, medicine and surgery, 53, 57; and midwife education, 141–42; and proliferation of Protomedicatos, 53

Brandt, Allan, 146–47

Brazil, 219; domestic medicine in, 21; empirics in, 26, 135; homeopathy and spiritism in, 123; hookworm research in, 157; medical education in, 83; medical identity of, 51; medical reform in, 69–70, 78; surgeons in, 28. *See also* African-based medicine; Ethnicity; Tropicalista School (Bahia)

Brealey, Richard, 41–45

Brenes, Nicolás, 28

British Medical Journal, 78, 264 n.33

Buchan, William: popularity of *Domestic Medicine*, 21–22

Buenos Aires, 14, 43, 99; practitioners in, 17, 67, 83; urbanization and hygiene reform in, 70

Calderón Guardia, Rafael Angel, 205–09, 217–18, 226–29, 236; and introduction of Social Security, 1, 192. *See also* Catholicism; Social Security

Calderón Muñoz, Rafael, 80, 104, 117, 217, 227

Calnek, Tomás, 87, 106

Cansancio. See Hookworm disease

Carballo Romero, Carlos, 183–91, 200–206, 209–16. *See also* Calderón Guardia, Rafael Angel; Empirics; Homeopaths; Magic; Policing; Spiritists

Carbell, Carlos (professor). *See* Carballo Romero, Carlos

Cardona, José María, 58

Carit, Adolphe, 21, 64–65

Carranza, Bruno, 46, 51, 52, 59, 63–65, 73

Cartago, 39, 149; epidemics in, 12–13; first generation of native physicians from, 39–43, 52, 65–66, 72; foreign practitioners resident in, 41, 43, 59; hookworm campaign in, 170; hospital in, 108; physicians in, 93, 99, 225; suppression of curanderos in, 60; unlicensed empirics in, 28–30

Carter, Henry, 164–65, 168–69

Catholicism, 19, 25, 74, 135; among physicians, 25, 117; and medical reform, 208, 217–18, 236. *See also* Calderón Guardia, Rafael Angel; Ethnomedicine, Religion; Religious healers

Céspedes, Benjamín de, 100, 113, 115, 138, 147

Chalhoub, Sidney, 8

Charity: of physicians, 40, 45, 98, 112; of state, 57, 105

Charlatans. *See* Quackery

Childbirth, 104, 112, 138, 145–48, 152. *See also* Infant mortality; Midwives; Physicians; School of Obstetrics

Chile, 33, 99, 135, 182, 219, 228

Chinese medicine, 2, 131, 198

Cholera, 12, 13, 24, 41–42, 49, 50, 54; Costa Rican epidemic of 1856, 29, 46, 48, 53, 61–64, 124; and humoral medicine, 23, 50

Chomsky, Aviva, 133

Civil War of 1948, 228–29

Clinical medicine, 50, 51, 57, 83

Coffee, 3, 11, 13, 21, 26, 70, 110; epidemics as threat to export of, 49, 108; physicians and cultivation of, 40, 44–45; and political economy of public health, 159, 223; processing facilities and miasmas, 24, 112

Colegio de Santo Tomás. *See* University of Santo Tomás

College of Pharmacists, 121–22, 196

Comadronas. See Midwives

Comte, Auguste, 68–69, 214

Corredor, Juan (father), 29–30, 63, 134

Cortés, León, 217, 220

County Health Units, 222–23

Courtí, Esteban, 34, 36

Cruz, Oswaldo, 70, 84

Cuba, 19, 55, 182, 220; immigrant practitioners from, 94–95, 100–101, 113, 137, 146; medical education in, 44, 83. *See also* Carballo Romero, Carlos; Town doctors

Cueto, Marcos, 10, 83, 87, 117, 159

Curanderas. *See* Women healers

Curanderos, 1–5, 110, 112, 117, 119, 184, 195, 231; definition of, 6–9, 15–16, 190, 243–44 n.18; numbers of, 26

Danielson, Ross, 44, 55, 137

Dentists, 48, 62, 92–93, 119; numbers of, 122, 197. *See also* Empirics

Department of Ancylostomiasis, 167, 177, 220, 227. *See also* Hookworm disease; Rockefeller Foundation

Diphtheria: 14, 91–92, 102, 223

Disease eradication. *See* Hookworm disease

District physicians. *See* Town doctors

Domestic medicine, 2, 18–22, 26, 35

Dorila (wisewoman), 143–44

Dow, James, 190, 243–44 n.18

Durán, Carlos, 72–74; 77, 95–97, 126, 144, 157, 191, 194; and discovery of hookworm disease, 87–89, 146, 159–62; and hospital reforms, 78–79, 106–08; private practice of, 91–92, 102. *See also* Faculty of Medicine (Costa Rica); Hospital San Juan de Dios (Costa Rica); Medical professionalism

Echavarría, María, 30

Echeverría, Emilio, 91, 115–16, 191, 194

Echeverría, Juan, 47–48

Ecuador: medical education and reform in 82–84, 141

Elmendorf, John, 155–56

Empirics: 1, 3, 9, 10, 92, 122, 149, 186, 190, 195; definition of, 15–16; and hookworm campaign, 177–78; licensing of, 18, 37, 56–61, 93, 95, 119, 134–38, 150, 157, 198, 232, 233, 252 n.1; likened to surgeon-apothecaries, 28; persecution of, 125–30, 133, 183–85; and rivalry with physicians, 48, 200–203; state mobilization and training of, 38, 58, 60–61, 235. *See also* Curanderos; Policing

England: immigrant practitioners from, 41–42; as place of study of Costa Rican physicians, 70–71

Epidemics: in Costa Rica, 12–14, 38, 49, 76, 161; and state mobilization of empirics, 60

Ernesto, Pedro, 219

Espinach, José Ventura, 43, 45, 106

Ethnicity: and popular medicine, 7, 14, 130–34; of practitioners, 2, 31–33, 144, 251 n.67, 256–57 n.56, 357–58 n.70, 258–59 n.83. *See also* African-based medicine; Ethno-medicine; Race

Ethno-medicine, 14, 19, 22, 30, 31, 35, 133, 231, 237, 276 n.21

Ettling, John, 88, 165

Eugenics, 140, 145–48, 159

Faculty of Medicine (Costa Rica), 77–81, 98, 100, 115, 133, 150–51, 155, 159, 161, 189, 197, 206, 217, 221, 227; decline in influence of, 180, 191–92; and homeopathy, 124–25, 149; licensing by, 80–81; and promotion of scientific activity, 86, 138, 147; and prosecution of illegal practice, 81, 183–84; and Social Security, 228. *See also* Medical professionalism; Pharmacists; Physicians

Faculty of Medicine, Surgery and Pharmacy. *See* Faculty of Medicine (Costa Rica)

Fermín Meza, José, 61
Fernández, Mauro, 72, 113, 115, 160–63
Figueres, José, 229
Figueres, Mariano, 163, 195, 229
Finlay, Carlos, 70, 99
Flores, Juan, 100–104, 145
Foreign healers, 26–27, 33–36, 62, 72, 127–30, 183, 231. *See also* Carballo Romero, Carlos; Courtí, Esteban; Empirics; Salisch, Adolfo (Count)
Franco, Roberto, 157
Franklin, Spencer, 116–17
Frantzius, Alexander von, 39, 43, 45, 50, 52, 62, 106
Freire, Domingo José, 70

Gaceta Médica de Costa Rica, 86, 97, 104, 191; and clinical case studies, 91–92, 101; and medical publishing, 86, 193. *See also* Faculty of Medicine (Costa Rica); Medical professionalism; Medical science
García, Juan César, 6, 158–59
García Granados, Carlos, 129–30
Gender, 2, 85, 153,184, 187, 200–203, 211, 234–35; and hookworm sufferers, 172–73; and hospital admissions, 107. *See also* Midwives; Physicians; Women healers
Germany: immigrant practitioners from, 39–42, 49–50, 104–05; as place of study of Costa Ricans, 194, 200
Germ theory, 4, 6, 73, 158, 163. *See also* Bacteriology; Hookworm disease; Medical systems
González, Luisa, 139, 143, 152
González Flores, Luis Felipe, 178, 227, 279–80 n.60
González Leandri, Ricardo, 8, 117, 274 n.56
González Víquez, Cleto, 147, 148, 160, 162, 210
Grecia, 108–11, 223

Guanacaste, 112, 225; empirics in, 59, 140–41
Guatemala, 157. *See also* Immigrants; Protomedicato; University of San Carlos (Guatemala)
Guevara de la Serna, Ernesto, 220
Guy, Donna, 146
Guy's Hospital, 72–74, 97, 106
Gynecology, 100, 103–04

Hahnemann, Samuel, 123–24
Hale, Charles, 68
Hegemony: and counterhegemonic cultures, 14; medical, 10
Herbal medicine, 1, 6, 14, 18–20, 35; and empirics, 26–31, 60, 118, 128–30, 132, 143. *See also* Curanderos; Midwives
Herbal medicines, 50, 189; international trade in, 20, 35
Heredia: epidemics in, 12–13, 61; hospital in, 108; practitioners in, 24, 61, 80, 93, 99–100, 103, 128, 145, 225
Hernández, José Gregorio, 217
Hernández Sáenz, Luz María, 44, 140
Higienistas, 69–70, 76, 112, 117, 146, 153, 167, 227
Historiography: Costa Rican revisionist, 13
History of medicine: in Latin America, 6–10, 156, 243 n.16; new social history of, 2, 17
Hochman, Gilberto, 279–80, n.7
Hoffman, Karl, 42, 43, 49–52
Home care. *See* Domestic medicine
Home guides, 20–21, 197. *See also* Buchan, William; Domestic medicine
Homeopaths, 120, 122–25, 185, 190, 199, 203, 237. *See also* Hahnemann, Samuel; Unorthodox healers
Hookworm disease, 4, 7, 74, 236; in Brazil, 280–81 n.7; Costa Rican campaigns against, 90, 161–65, 229; Costa Rican discovery of, 86–90, 146,

Limón (*cont.*)
  physicians in, 80, 93, 100, 115, 225.
  See also Afro-Caribbeans; Bananas;
  Obeah; United Fruit Company
Lister, Joseph, 73, 78
Listerism, 264 n.33; at Guy's Hospital,
  73. *See also* Durán, Carlos; Germ the-
  ory
López Calleja de Zeledón, Amparo: as
  pharmacist and popular healer, 121–
  22, 279–80 n.60
Louvain: and medical studies, 84, 207,
  217–18
Luján, Mario, 192, 227, 279–80 n.60

Magic, 183, 210; in medicine, 6, 9, 18,
  26, 132, 184–85, 190; in midwifery,
  142; and shamanism, 31. *See also* Carballo Romero, Carlos
Malaria, 12, 13, 35, 88, 107, 109, 180,
  195, 223
Mariana (midwife), 139, 143–44
Marín, Isaura, 149, 151
Medical Association (Costa Rica), 41,
  49, 77, 120–21
Medical eclecticism, 5, 19, 117, 184
Medical education, 16, 48; in Costa Rica,
  41, 43, 48, 75, 81–82, 193, 224; of
  Costa Ricans abroad, 39–40, 66, 68,
  70–75, 83–85, 96–97, 193–94, 220,
  224, 232; of empirics, 57; in Latin
  America, 14, 43–44, 56, 82–85; of
  Latin Americans abroad, 84; of mid-
  wives, 141–42, 147–52, 235. *See also*
  School of Obstetrics; School of Phar-
  macy; University of San Carlos
  (Guatemala); University of Santo
  Tomás
Medical ethics, 80–81, 199
Medicalization: of childbirth, 140–41,
  151–54; of everyday life, 4, 157; of
  healing cults, 217, 294 n.32. *See also*
  Hookworm disease; Midwives; School
  of Obstetrics; Women healers

Medical marketplace, 2, 5, 48, 112, 120,
  185, 187, 195, 197, 207, 233; in
  Bahia, 95; in Costa Rica, 35, 61–63;
  and drugs, 20–21, 43; participation of
  empirics in, 6, 31, 32, 131, 191, 200;
  in San José, 95. *See also* Physicians;
  Specialization
Medical monopoly, 4, 10, 137, 157, 231,
  237; in Argentina, 274 n.56; attack
  on, by empirics, 135, 209, 211, 214–
  16; attack on, by homeopaths, 123;
  and gender, 202–03, 232; and professionalization, 67, 90, 119, 184–85;
  and Protomedicato licensing, 55. *See
  also* Faculty of Medicine (Costa Rica);
  Medical marketplace; Medical professionalism; Physicians
Medical pluralism, 190, 232, 236–37
Medical populism, 206–09, 218–19,
  226–29, 234. *See also* Calderón
  Guardia, Rafael Angel; Carballo
  Romero, Carlos
Medical professionalism, 2–9, 232; in
  Costa Rica, 25, 49, 55, 67, 77–81, 90;
  of midwives, 151; and political power,
  119–20, 191–94; and popular medicine, 184–85; and stratification of
  practitioners, 92–93, 121. *See also* Faculty of Medicine (Costa Rica); Physicians
Medical science, 9; in Costa Rica, 48, 51,
  68, 74, 79–80, 83, 86–90, 156, 159,
  221; in Latin America, 37, 87, 158–
  59; politics of, 2; and professional
  identities, 48, 88–89, 98, 140, 150–
  51, 235; and professional journals,
  78, 89; romance narrative of, 92. *See
  also* Durán, Carlos; Tropicalista School
  (Bahia)
Medical systems, 6, 20, 22–25; marriage
  of, 117. *See also* Biomedicine; Ethno-
  medicine; Homeopaths; Humoral
  medicine; Town doctors
Mercier, D. J. Desiré Joseph (Cardinal),

Pharmacies, 21, 30; and association with empirics, 129; immigrant proprietors of, 45, 63–64; numbers in San José, 43; operated by physicians, 44–45, 63–65, 105, 190; and Protomedicato, 53. *See also* College of Pharmacists; Pharmacists

Pharmacists, 1, 3, 33, 4, 47, 62, 185; licensing of, by Protomedicato, 53; in Medical Association, 49; in Mexico, 20–1; numbers of, 17–18, 62–64, 197; rivalry with physicians, 48, 55, 92–93, 119–22; use of term, 16. *See also* College of Pharmacists; Medical Association (Costa Rica); Medical monopoly

Phlebotomists. *See* Barber-surgeons

Physicians: biomedical stereotype of, 6, 9; earnings of, 45–47, 52, 55, 99, 112–13, 115–17, 162, 208, 254 n.26; and gender, 85, 153, 192, 279 n.59; geographical distribution of, 42–43, 80, 93–96; licensing of, 37; nationalization of, 67, 70–72, 90, 114; numbers of, 17–18, 62–63, 93–96, 184–85, 191–93, 208, 224–26, 252 n.1, 288 n.24; place of study of, 68, 70–72, 83–85; and political power, 4, 6, 41, 69–72, 98, 159, 207, 215–216, 228; professional hierarchy of, 96–101; professional and public appointments available to, 48, 53, 96, 98; and rivalry with empirics, 48, 59, 104, 112, 117, 126–30, 183–85; and rivalry with homeopaths, 124–25; and rivalry with pharmacists, 48, 63–64, 119–22, 196–97; scientific identity of, 67, 86–90; and social class, 4, 6, 72, 85, 89, 96–102. *See also* Medical marketplace; Medical monopoly; Medical professionalism; Social stature

Picado, Clodomiro, 192, 221

Picado, Jadwisia de, 85, 153

Policing: of medicine, 9–10; and prosecution of unlicensed healers, 120, 125–30, 133, 138, 183–84, 199, 206, 215, 233. *See also* Empirics; Medical ethics; Ministry of Public Health and Social Protection; Protomedicato

Political economy: of public health, 158–59

Popularization: of germ theory, 4, 163, 171; of hygiene, 162; of learned medicine, 21, 182. *See also* Buchan, William; Hookworm disease

Popular medicine: as counterhegemonic, 8; of mestizos, 22; suppression of, 9–10. *See also* Empirics; Ethno-medicine; Herbal medicine; Humoral medicine; Indigenous healers; Medical systems

Porter, Roy, 185

Positivism, 8, 214, 233, 237; in Costa Rica, 13, 147; and medical profession, 67–69, 74, 93, 126, 203, 237. *See also* Bacteriology; Liberal state; Physicians

Practice, 45, 91; in ports, 115–16; private, 40, 190, 218, 228; in rural areas, 93, 103, 109–15; in urban areas, 95–96, 101–105. *See also* Physicians

Press, Irwin, 5, 9, 243–44 n.18

Priests: as healers, 24, 29, 32, 62, 105, 189; and hookworm campaign, 176; in vaccination campaign, 60. *See also* Catholicism; Empirics; Religious healers

Professionalization. *See* Medical professionalism

Prostitution, 100. *See also* Higienistas; Venereal disease

Protomedicato, 30, 32, 38, 43, 58, 60, 257–58 n.70; in the colonial period, 37, 53; retention of, in republican Latin America, 53–55. *See also* Empirics; Midwives; Protomedicato of the Republic of Costa Rica

Protomedicato of the Republic of Costa Rica, 34–41, 49, 52–56, 61, 73, 76,

127, 232, 254 n.26; dissolution of, 79; and licensing of empirics, 56–61, 119, 137; and licensing of titled practitioners, 45, 122. *See also* Empirics; Medical Association (Costa Rica); Midwives

Prowe, Herbert, 88, 157

Psychiatry, 104, 202

Public health, 4–7, 67, 84, 119, 147, 206, 225, 233–34, 236; and campaign against hookworm disease, 56, 90, 158; centralization of, 181–82, 207, 221–22; and latrine construction, 164, 170, 172, 175; organizations in the Americas, 76, 162; popular responses to, 8; and town doctors, 77, 223; and vaccination, 111–12. *See also* Hookworm disease; Immigration; Ministry of Public Health and Social Protection; Rockefeller Foundation

Puerto Rico: hookworm campaign in, 163, 169; practitioners in, 17

Puntarenas, 215; domestic medicine in, 18; empirics in, 126–27; epidemics in, 12–13; hookworm campaign in, 155; licensed empirics in, 63, 136; pharmacies in, 21; physicians in, 80, 225; town doctors in, 47, 108, 115–17; yellow fever in, 49, 50

Pupo Pérez, Carlos, 103, 113, 115, 161–65, 179, 196

Quackery, 3, 131, 134, 173, 199–200

Quacks, 15, 26, 27, 120, 127, 137. *See also* Empirics; Foreign healers

Querétaro (Mexico): practitioners in, 17, 62

Quesada, Gregorio, 124–25

Race, 85, 146–47, 160

Racism. *See* Eugenics

Ramsey, Matthew, 9, 26

Recetarios. *See* Domestic medicine

Religion: in medicine, 6, 9, 19, 217, 236, 246 n.6.

Religious healers, 128, 135, 139, 199, 272 n.19

Reynantes, Tiburcia ("María la Gachupina"), 30–31

Rio de Janeiro: 14; Medical School, 85; practitioners in, 17, 29, 219; urbanization and hygiene reform in, 70, 117

Risse, Guenter, 106

Rockefeller Foundation, 6, 7, 105, 117, 155–58, 162–82, 192–94, 222, 224. *See also* Hookworm disease; Imperial medicine: and public health

Rosenberg, Charles, 21, 50

Rosenberg, Mark, 208, 226–27

Roux, Pierre Paul Emile: and diphtheria antitoxin, 92

Salguero, Dorotea, 30, 60

Salisch, Adolfo (Count), 27, 34

Salmon, Charles, 41–42

Sanitary Code, 100, 191, 196

San José: as center of coffee economy, 39, 70; as center of medical profession, 93, 226; epidemics in, 12–13; contracting licensed practitioners for, 27, 39; and first generation of native physicians, 40; licensed midwives in, 151–52; medical marketplace in, 62–64; as new capital, 39; as origin of second generation of native practitioners, 70–71; settlement of immigrant practitioners in, 41, 43, 65–66

San Ramón, 108, 127

Santos Filho, Lycurgo de, 26, 28

Schapiro, Louis, 157, 165–72. *See also* Hookworm disease; Rockefeller Foundation

School Health Department, 165, 176–81, 222–23, 227. *See also* Hookworm disease; Rockefeller Foundation

School of Obstetrics, 81–82, 86, 98,

Typhoid, 155; in Costa Rica, 12, 13, 223

Ulloa Giralt, Juan, 74–81, 89, 95, 96, 106, 144, 155–159, 191
United Fruit Company, 6, 11, 90, 115, 161, 226; hospital in Limón, 108–109; medical department of, 116, 194
United States of America, 7, 156; as place of study of Costa Rican physicians, 70–71, 194; specialization in, 48. *See also* Imperial medicine: and public health; Rockefeller Foundation
University of León (Nicaragua): 17, 43, 82
University of San Carlos (Guatemala): 17, 41, 66; and Guatemalan medical Enlightenment, 39; and influence on system of medical regulation, 52; medical education of Costa Ricans at, 39–40, 70–72, 99
University of San Marcos (Lima), 44, 82–83, 85
University of Santo Tomás: closure of, 82; medical instruction of Costa Ricans at, 41, 46, 48, 57
Unorthodox healers, 120, 190, 231. *See also* Homeopaths; Spiritists

Vaccination: in Costa Rica, 12–13, 32, 38, 50, 53, 124, 180, 223; 1805 campaign, 58, 60; popular reactions against, in Latin America, 8, 111; and town doctors, 39, 47, 58, 109–12. *See also* African-based medicine; Empirics; Indigenous healers; Medicalization; Town doctors
Vargas, Petronila, 128–29, 134
Vargas Vargas, Francisco, 217
Venereal disease, 13, 29–32, 46, 98, 111, 147, 186, 190, 195, 289 n.35; Law on Venereal Prophylaxis, 76, 146
Villalobos, América, 152
Virgen of Los Angeles, 19
Volio, Jorge (general), 210, 213, 292 n.7

Walker, William. *See* War of 1856–57
War of 1856–57, 49, 53, 58, 59. *See also* Cholera; Surgeons
Whooping cough: in Costa Rica, 12, 14
Witchcraft, 34, 187, 276 n.21
Women healers, 234, 250 n.55; as dentists, 122; as physicians, 85, 153, 192, 279 n.59; as sorceresses, 26, 276 n.21; unlicensed, 27, 30–31, 61, 128–30, 134, 138, 139; as wisewomen, 141–44, 189. *See also* Empirics; Midwives
Wucherer, Otto, 88–89, 157

Yellow fever, 8, 70, 160; in Costa Rica, 12, 13, 51, 76; and medical science, 49, 78, 102

Steven Palmer is Assistant Professor in the Department
of History at the University of Windsor, Canada.

Library of Congress Cataloging-in-Publication Data
Palmer, Steven Paul.
From popular medicine to medical populism : doctors,
healers, and public power in Costa Rica, 1800–1940 / Steven Palmer.
p. : cm.   Includes bibliographical references and index.
ISBN 0-8223-3012-1 (cloth : alk. paper)
ISBN 0-8223-3047-4 (pbk : alk. paper)
1. Medicine — Costa Rica — History. 2. Traditional
medicine — Costa Rica — History. 3. Social medicine — Costa
Rica — History. [DNLM: 1. History of Medicine, 19th Cent. —
Costa Rica. 2. History of Medicine, 20th Cent. — Costa Rica.
3. Faith Healing — history — Costa Rica. 4. Health Services —
history — Costa Rica. 5. Physicians — history — Costa
Rica. WZ 70 DC8 P176f 2003] I. Title.
R471.C8 P35 2003   610′.97286 — dc21
2002010078